MIDWIFE PUBLICATIONS

Nell Tharpe

Clinical Practice Guidelines for Midwifery & Women's Health

Clinical Practice Guidelines for Midwifery & Women's Health 2004-2005

This edition is dedicated with boundless love and appreciation to my children, who set me on the Path, and to my husband, who continues to walk beside me.
Also, to those who have met me on the Path and sustained me on my Journey.

Deep thanks go to all of the families who have honored me by allowing my presence at their births; the midwives I have had the pleasure to know and work with; the educators who have guided my growth; and my colleagues from all walks of life who have mentored me.

Especial thanks go to my dearest friends, who provided me with their love, their unqualified support, and unparalleled inspiration. I cherish you and will hold you each in my heart forever.

Carolyn Farina, RN

Patricia Kirby, RN

Meg Lutes, RN

Cover illustration by isa maria

MIDWIFE PUBLICATIONS, INC.

Producing professional education programs and publications for midwives.

Midwife Publications, Inc
P.O. Box 348
East Boothbay, ME 04544
Phone or Fax 207-633-3749
e-mail: midwifepub@gwi.net
www.midwifepublications.com

Library of Congress Cataloguing-in-Publication Data

Tharpe, Nell L. 1956-

Clinical Practice Guidelines for Midwifery & Women's Health 2004-2005/Nell L. Tharpe

Included bibliographical references and index

Midwifery, Women's Health, Maternity, Newborn, Birth

ISBN 0-9701417-3-4

Forward

The *Clinical Practice Guidelines for Midwifery and Women's Health* have grown out of a desire to have a concise reference guide that reflects current practice, and provides support and guidance in the day to day practice of midwifery and women's health with diverse populations.

The American College of Nurse-Midwives (ACNM) and the Midwives Alliance of North America (MANA) both recommend that midwives utilize written policies and/or practice guidelines. The *Clinical Practice Guidelines for Midwifery & Women's Health* are updated and published every two years. Comments and suggestions are always appreciated, with references and resources whenever possible. Regional differences in practice styles occur, therefore the guidelines are broad-based, and designed to reflect current practice and literature as much as possible.

The *Clinical Practice Guidelines for Midwifery & Women's Health* are designed to be kept where you practice; a copy in your exam room(s), one copy for your birth setting, another by the phone at home. Customize the guidelines further with your written additions, deletions, highlighter etc. This is a working practice tool, one that was created to be *used*.

Midwives are blessed with a love for their work. It is the same patience and perseverance that a laboring mother so appreciates that has helped midwifery to grow. It is my hope that this book will make your professional practice simpler and more rewarding.

This book is written for all of the midwives, wherever they practice, and the women, children and families that they care for.

Nell L. Tharpe, MS, CNM, CRNFA

Table of Contents

Women First!

Midwifery and women's health is first and foremost about caring for women.

Every woman deserves to receive care that is safe, satisfying, and fosters her ability to care for herself. Such care, to be effective, must address women's own cultural and developmental needs. As we care for women in our diverse communities the ability to listen, and to integrate women's concerns into the care we provide, is essential.

As midwives we practice within a healthcare continuum that is increasingly complex, both for ourselves as professionals, and for the clients we guide through the system. Many women do not have a frame of reference that allows them to formulate the questions that concern them. They look to their care provider to provide direction that is consistent with their perceived needs and internal beliefs.

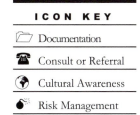

ICON KEY	
🗀	Documentation
☎	Consult or Referral
🌐	Cultural Awareness
🌢	Risk Management

Throughout this book symbols will be used to indicate key areas for particular attention. The purpose of the symbols is to heighten awareness, and stimulate critical thinking in areas that hold potential pitfalls. Safe midwifery practice includes not only providing quality care to the women we serve, but also practicing in a manner that protects the midwife from undue risk whether it be from infectious disease, fear of persecution, or professional liability.

🗀 Documentation of care is an essential element to quality midwifery and women's health practice. Documentation skills allow the midwife to review her or his own records at a later date and have a clear view of the women's presentation, the midwifery evaluation process, midwifery care plan development, implementation and results. Documentation also allows others to follow the care provided, and the client response. This is an essential communication tool for the midwife in a group practice. For those midwives or students who seek to improve documentation skills, recommendations for documentation are addressed later in Chapter 2.

☎ Collaborative practice is what connects midwives to those who can provide on-going or specialty care that is not within the midwife's scope of practice. Midwives function within the current health care system. Women's health care forms a continuum that extends from home birth and alternative care, through general medical and community-based medicine and midwifery, to high-tech tertiary care and specialty services. Not all services are appropriate for all women.

The midwife has a responsibility to provide access to services as indicated by the woman's health, preferences, and the midwife's scope of practice. Throughout this book the driving philosophy will be that of the International Confederation of Midwives:

> *A midwife is a person who, having been regularly admitted to a midwifery educational programme, duly recognized in the country in which it is located, has successfully completed the prescribed course of studies in midwifery and has acquired the requisite qualifications to be registered and/or legally licensed to practice midwifery.*
>
> *She must be able to give the necessary supervision, care and advice to women during pregnancy, labour and the postpartum period, to conduct deliveries on her own responsibility and to care for the newborn and the infant. This care included preventive measures, the detection of abnormal conditions in mother and child, the procurement of medical assistance and the execution of emergency measures in the absence of medical help.*
>
> *She has an important task in health counseling and education, not only for the women, but within the family and the community. The work should involve antenatal education and preparation for parenthood and extends to certain areas of gynecology, family planning and childcare. She may practice in hospitals, clinics, health units, domiciliary conditions or in any other service.(1)*

⊕ Cultural awareness is essential for quality care of women in our multicultural world. We need to consider each woman as an individual, who exists, not in our practice settings, but in her own corner of the world. Cultural influences may affect birth choices, birth control methods, sexual orientation, etc. Cultural awareness includes consideration of the client's race, religion, ethnic heritage, age, generation, geographic location (i.e., rural versus urban.), and cultural mores.

☙ Risk management includes the thoughtful consideration of factors that increase risk to the mother or baby, the well woman, or the midwife providing care. Identification of risk factors is the first step in reducing their potential impact on midwifery practice.

Essential components of risk management include a thorough knowledge-base of basic midwifery; the pathophysiology of commonly encountered conditions; and current recommendations for care. Careful documentation of care provided, active listening to each woman as an individual, and clearly stated expectations regarding your role as a midwife and the woman's role when receiving care are integral components of risk management as applied to midwifery practice.

A word about evidence-based midwifery practice.

"Evidence-based" practice is the catchword of the day. Goode (2000) offers a multidisciplinary practice model that addresses nine key factors to consider when evaluating current research for clinical application. These include:

- Pathophysiology

- Retrospective or Concurrent Record Review

- Risk Management Data

- Local, National & International Standards

- Infection Control Data

- Patient or Client Preferences

- Clinical Expertise

- Benchmarking Data

- Cost Effectiveness Analysis

By integrating all of these factors into evaluation of current research the midwife can validate her or his clinical decision-making using an evidence-based practice model that also fits the midwifery model of care. Clinical expertise comes with time and attention to practice. The new practitioner or novice must maintain a heightened awareness of her or his limitations, and boundaries of practice.

The Purpose of Clinical Practice Guidelines

Clinical practice guidelines are used to direct and define parameters for midwifery care. This may be influenced by the recommended parameters of the midwife's professional organization(s) such as the American College of Nurse Midwives (ACNM), the Midwives Alliance of North America (MANA), or the International Confederation of Midwives (ICM). State laws, both statute and regulations, may affect the scope of midwifery practice, as may hospital by-laws, birth center rules and regulations, health insurance contracts, and liability insurance policies.

Each individual midwife must define her or his scope of practice based on philosophy of midwifery practice, educational preparation, experience, skill level, and the individual practice setting. A midwife's scope of practice may vary from one practice location to another, and may change throughout her career.

Each client who comes to a midwife for care has the right to information regarding the midwife's scope of practice, usual practice location(s), and provisions for access to medical or obstetrical care should this become necessary. Development of working relationships with area health care providers can be a valuable asset in fostering continuity of care.

Developing a Collaborative Practice Network

Midwives do not practice in isolation. Every midwife, regardless of practice location needs a network of contacts to help provide ongoing care and services. Collaborative practice models allow for a wide variety of contact categories that range from informal relationships to highly structured arrangements. Collaborative practice means that the relationship format is developed jointly between the attending midwife and the physician or health care provider in question.

Consultation, or Referral?

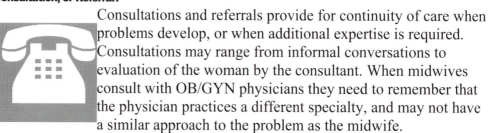

Consultations and referrals provide for continuity of care when problems develop, or when additional expertise is required. Consultations may range from informal conversations to evaluation of the woman by the consultant. When midwives consult with OB/GYN physicians they need to remember that the physician practices a different specialty, and may not have a similar approach to the problem as the midwife.

Development of professional relationships with physicians in your area begins with you. Make arrangements to meet and introduce yourself. Show consideration of the doctor's busy schedule, make a breakfast date, or offer to bring lunch to the office. Make good eye contact, shake hands firmly and present yourself as a professional and a colleague.

Your goal is to make a positive impression, so that when you have a woman who needs service, you have already smoothed the way. It is not required that you agree on philosophy of care or management styles, but it is important that you establish a good working relationship. It helps to introduce yourself to the office staff, for those times you will need to interrupt the doctor during office hours.

Determining in advance what type of call is indicated will impact what information is needed. Couch your conversation in terms that directs the care you are looking for. If you do not provide this direction, the physician will manage the patient as she or he would her or his usual patients

Forms of consultations may include:

Informational: "Just letting you know that Mrs. B is here in labor. She is a G3, P2002 at term and is at 5 cms after one hour of labor. I expect an uneventful birth shortly." In this instance you already have a professional relationship established, and have defined your collaborative relationship to include notification of specified information.

Heads Up: " Miss R. has meconium-stained fluid. I've called the Pediatric Service. Baby looks fine, the fetal heart rate baseline is in the 140s with good accelerations. Mom was 7 cms at last exam and labor is progressing nicely. I'll let you know if anything changes." In this instance you are aware that you may need additional support or expertise, and provide information in advance in case an emergency call is required later.

Request for Information or Opinion: "Ms. K. has Atypical Glandular Cells on her most recent pap smear. I've never seen this before. What do you recommend for her follow-up?" In this example, you are looking for information to guide your client's care when you have reached the limits of your scope of practice, or when you work in a collaborative practice where you tailor the care you provide to both the client and the practice setting.

Request for Evaluation: "I'm sending Mrs. S. to you for evaluation of her enlarged uterus. She is a 43 year-old G2 P2002, who has had severe menorrhagia for the past 5 months. Her pelvic ultrasound is consistent with large uterine fibroids. We have discussed the potential for hysterectomy and she does/does not prefer hysterectomy for definitive treatment of this problem. I am referring her to you for evaluation & treatment."

In this example, your client has a problem that requires evaluation, and potentially treatment, not within your scope of practice. Clearly stating previous discussions, client preferences, and your expectations can influence the physician's approach to the client.

Transfer of Care: "Mary R has cervical cancer. I am transferring her to you for continued care of this problem. I will continue to be available to provide ongoing support."

Emergency: "Keisha P. has a post partum hemorrhage. I think she may have retained placental parts. Her EBL is currently at 1000ml. I need you to see her immediately."

For those midwives who practice in the out of hospital setting, calling the OB/GYN on-call may be preferable to simply calling 911 or the emergency room. If you have an established working relationship a direct admission to the maternity unit may be possible.

Other collaborative practice relationships are important to establish. Primary care providers will commonly care for midwifery clients in the event of a general medical problem such as hypertension, diabetes, or heart disease. While some midwives have expanded their practice to include primary care services this is often limited to treatment of acute conditions such as back pain, upper respiratory infections and the like.

Every practitioner caring for women, regardless of their scope of practice, should develop a network of care providers that may include physicians, chiropractors, naturopaths, acupuncturists, dieticians, mental health professionals, social service personnel, clergy, support & self-help groups, local emergency services, homeless shelters, addiction centers, etc. This network provides the mechanism by which midwives may address the varied needs of the women who come to us for care.

Key to providing woman-oriented care is to connect women with the services they require and may not know how to access. This may include a combination of mainstream medical care, alternative or complementary modalities, and non-medical services. The role of the midwife is to listen to women, clarify their needs, and facilitate meeting those needs in a caring and non-judgmental manner. Individual philosophy of midwifery care should direct, but not drive, the care you provide.

Clear discussion of the parameters of midwifery practice, the practice location(s), practice limitations or boundaries required by collaborative relationships, practice agreements, and clinical options of midwifery care (including privileges) goes a long way toward evaluating if a particular midwifery practice is appropriate for the individual client.

Women may come from settings where there is very limited access or availability of health care, and accept whatever care is provided. Other women may have a strong need to direct their health care, and mandate their active participation in all health related decisions. Most women fall somewhere in the middle of these two examples.

Healthcare as a Continuum

Healthcare can be thought of as a continuum that runs from alternative or self-care to general medical care to specialty and technologically sophisticated care. One example of this concept is the continuum of birth locations which may range from the client's home through a freestanding or hospital based-birth center, small community hospitals to larger community hospitals, and finally to regional perinatal referral centers.

In an ideal world our clients would be able to move back and forth along this continuum as best met their needs. They would have access to the full range of services and providers necessary for their care, from within a supportive health care system and environment, where there was true collaborative practice based on meeting the needs of the client. Few of us practice in such an ideal setting. However, it remains imperative that we understand the continuum of services that are available, no matter where we stand ourselves on the continuum.

The women who come to us for care, our clients, do not live in the health care world, and their awareness of what services are available may be influenced by issues of access, impact of advertising, social and cultural beliefs, the experiences of their friends or relatives, and the ever present television and movie world. Unless we have an idea of the options out there, we will be less able to listen and hear what women are saying to us, and less able to address their concerns in language that they can understand.

Clients who are oriented toward alternative care may be influenced toward medical care when necessary in a trusting relationship with their midwife or health care provider. Clients who are comfortable and familiar with highly interventive care may be influenced toward self-care and non-interventionist care when it is recommended in an environment of trust and ready access to medical care if necessary.

Midwifery care is traditionally based on providing care that begins from non-interventionist care and includes interventions only as necessary or indicated. Deciding what interventions are 'necessary' and when they are 'indicated' defines our individual practice as midwives.

Cultural Diversity

The world is fast becoming an international society. No matter where we practice, it is likely that each of us will provide care to women who come from different countries or cultures from ourselves or from the location where we obtained our basic midwifery education & training.

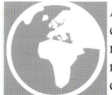

Awareness and sensitivity to cultural practices and beliefs can enhance client satisfaction and build a trusting professional relationship. Cultural diversity encompasses a wide range of reference points, which may include social and emotional development, age, race, religion, sexual orientation, ethnic heritage, country of origin, geographic location, and cultural beliefs and mores. Becoming culturally competent involves a certain level of interest, inquiry and awareness of cultural differences.

Cultural differences may be considered as cross cultural, meaning the midwife and the client come from different ethnic or racial backgrounds, or they may be intercultural, where the midwife and the client come from similar ethnic or social backgrounds but have developed disparate views and beliefs, especially in regard to healthcare. An example of this is the homebirth midwife whose client reveals that she wants access pharmacological pain relief for labor, or a hospital-based midwife whose client calls following a surreptitiously planned homebirth.

Cultural competence requires that the midwife remain open-minded, an active listener, and evaluate each woman's needs in light of the practice setting. Access to culturally competent interpreters to translate language, social customs and mores related to women's health care can be extremely helpful. A minimum standard requires that language interpreters be available. Literal translation, however, may not always provide correct or accurate information about women's needs.

Developmental Considerations

Attention to developmental changes throughout a woman's life is essential in order to address the concerns that are most pressing to her. The needs of adolescent women are vary different from those of the woman of childbearing age, and those of the woman who is past menopause, even when they each present for the same type of visit.

Individualizing care involves taking into account the woman's chronological age, developmental stage, emotional development, sexual orientation and preferences, and social factors. Midwives who frequently care for the under-served, should remember that the effects of poverty and marginal nutrition may impact the aging process.

Ageism can occur at any point in the age spectrum.

- **Adolescents** may present at various developmental stages based on age, emotional development, ethnicity, and other social and cultural factors. Compliance is frequently an issue as authority is challenged, and the young woman seeks to explore the boundaries and limits put upon her.

- **The mentally challenged** may require coordination of specialized services in order to be provided appropriate reproductive health care. Intimate exams may require sedation or anesthesia in order to avoid emotional trauma, especially in the woman with a history of sexual violence.

- **The physically challenged** may or may not have developmental delays depending on the cause of the physical challenge. Women with brain injuries may be unpredictable and volatile, while those with spinal cord injuries may not have noticeable developmental issues.

- **Older women** often have a change of focus from reproductive health care to concerns surrounding general health and the fear of illness, disability, and death. Women may regress into dependence as they age, or they may continue to be independent, or dependent as they were previously.

- **Immigrant and refugee women** may have culturally mediated variations in development, which may make interpretation of developmental stages more challenging. Accessing resources to learn about cultural variations may aid in appropriate client assessment.

- **Socioeconomic challenges** may impact the rate and progression of a woman's physical, emotional and social development. Remaining non-judgmental offers the optimum opportunity to determine how best to identify each individuals unique needs, and provide or direct women to the services that might best meet those needs.

Risk Management

Risk management means identifying and managing the potential risk to each woman we care for, the unborn and newly born infants of those women, ourselves as midwives and each of the other health professionals that become involved in the care of the women and families we serve.

The term "**risk management**" has acquired a bad name in recent years, as many liability insurance companies use this term to identify 'risk factors' that may indicate an increased likelihood for a less than optimal outcome, or chance of litigation. As midwives, we need to recognize that life entails risk, for ourselves as professionals, and for those who come to us for care.

We need to each determine what level of risk we are willing to accept in our lives, knowing that ultimately, we are not in control of the multiple factors that put ourselves & those we care for and about "at risk". For some midwives this may mean practicing in an environment where there is a physician present 24/7 "just in case", and for others it may mean caring for women often thought of as "high risk" in the home environment. For most midwives, this choice is somewhere in the middle.

Risk to the Client

Identification of risk to our clients is nearly impossible. Even with the surge in the number of double-blind case controlled studies in women's health, we are not able to successfully identify which women are in fact at risk for which problems. New data is continually being compiled about risks associated with race, ethnicity, genetics, lifestyle, behaviors, and the list goes on.

Keeping abreast of new data, and incorporating it into our knowledgebase is one way of managing risk. In this way we can provide information to our clients to help them identify health care decisions and choices that are appropriate for them. Frank discussions about the relative risk of options for care should include the potential for unexpected outcomes, the unpredictability of individual response, and the impact and importance of self-determination.

Risk to the Unborn and Newborn

If calculating risk to the client who we can see and test and talk with is difficult, quantifying risk to the unborn, and by extension to the newly born, is virtually impossible. However, pregnant women look to their midwives as skilled professionals with the ability to identify potential problems and take corrective action to safeguard their babes in the womb.

How information is presented during pregnancy may influence the mother's attitude about the safety of birth, the ability of the health care system to meet her and her baby's needs, and her ability to parent. Risk should be addressed in a realistic fashion that is supportive of birth, in every location, and does not undermine either alternative or medical providers. We can foster the concept that birth works, while still addressing the fact that there are no guarantees of a perfect outcome, and that access to medical services is an option we are fortunate to have.

Risk to the Midwife

Each midwife needs to determine what is included in her own individual scope of practice. Most often the midwife's scope of practice is consistent with the guidelines recommended by her or his professional midwifery organizations. Not every midwife will provide every service. A midwife's scope of practice is a dynamic entity, one that changes with experience, practice location, fatigue, staffing, or distance to specialty care, etc. Each midwife must manage individual professional risk by constantly assessing the scope of her or his midwifery practice, and whether it meets the midwife's needs as well as those of the community served.

Identification of women with risk factors may impact midwifery management of risk in a number of ways, it may result in a transfer of care, a consultation, or continued independent management of the women's care. It all depends on the midwife's expertise and self-determined scope of practice, state laws regarding midwifery practice, and the midwife's comfort level with the level of risk involved in caring for the particular risk factor in this individual, health care setting, community, and legal climate.

Examples of midwife risk *may* include one or a combination of the following:

- Not defining your scope of practice
- Providing care outside your scope of practice
- Providing solo practice with 24/7 call & no relief coverage
- Homebirth or birth center practice
- Attending VBAC births
- Not pursuing continuing education
- Expanding services without obtaining education &/or training

- Providing care outside of what is legally authorized by state or other jurisdiction

- Not seeking consultation or referral when a problem presents

- Seeking consultation or referral when a problem presents

- Practicing in a hostile medical community, regardless of legal status of midwifery

- Providing services that were previously seen as medical care

Midwives vary tremendously in the amount of risk, and therefore stress, they are willing live with on a day-to-day basis. Some may prefer to work in settings where there is a physician available for 'back-up' at all times, while others may practice in isolated settings where the nearest physician is miles away. Increased midwife autonomy may be associated with increased midwife risk. Development of mechanisms to reduce midwife risk can offer the opportunity for the midwife to rest better at night, and continue a career for decades.

Think about what services you include in your scope of practice. If someone were to ask you for a summary of what is included in your scope of practice as you practice in your current setting would you have such a document available? Would you defer to ACNM or MANA, or perhaps the International Confederation of Midwives? Have you read those documents recently? Do you know what they hold you accountable for?

Think about the benefits and risks associated with defining your scope of practice, no matter what your credentials or practice setting. You are held accountable to national, state, and local standards, are you active in helping to define & set those standards?

References

1. Jointly developed by the International Confederation of Midwives and the International Federation of Gynaecology and Obstetrics. Adopted by the World Health Organization.

2. Goode, Colleen (2000). What constitutes the "evidence" in evidence-based practice? Applied Nursing Research 13:222-225.

3. International Confederation of Midwives (2002)

Chapter
2

Exemplary Midwifery Practice

Exemplary midwifery practice is care that is woman-oriented and focuses on excellence in the processes of providing care, improving maternal and child health, and professionalism as a means of promoting the midwifery model of care.

Exemplary midwifery practice, according to Kennedy,[1] encompasses several key concepts. These concepts include the philosophy of midwifery and its expression through the individual midwife's choice and use of therapeutic measures; the quality of caring for and about women; and support for midwifery as demonstrated through practice and professional involvement in midwifery.

Midwives who provide exemplary midwifery care were found by Kennedy to create balance between their professional lives as midwives and their personal lives. They were able to both support the normal process of birth, while at the same time remaining vigilant for the unexpected, and attuned to the small details that might signify a change.

Exemplary midwives were described as having the qualities of integrity, honesty, compassion, understanding, the ability to communicate effectively, flexibility, and were seen as non-judgmental. These qualities were coupled with excellent clinical skills including attentive and thorough assessment, exceptional screening, preventive health counseling, and the ability to be patient with the process of labor and birth. Interventions and technology were used only when necessary.

---

[1] Kennedy, HP (2000). A model of exemplary midwifery practice: Results of a Delphi study. Journal of Midwifery & Women's Health. 45; 4-19.

Finally, exemplary midwives were found to personalize care. In every setting they endeavored to create a setting that engendered respect and was focused primarily on meeting the needs of the mother and family.

As a goal, we should each strive toward exemplary midwifery practice. It is a goal that requires development of excellent clinical skills, and coupling them with sound clinical judgment. We each need the ability to make critical decisions, and act upon them, in a manner that is appropriate for the setting in which we practice and honors the uniqueness of the woman and family under our care.

As a profession we need to work toward the goal of educating our clients and colleagues about how midwifery is different from medicine and nursing, and to ensure that difference is reflected in the midwifery education programs and clinical experiences of those learning midwifery. Midwifery encompasses an attitude of belief that birth is essentially normal, that women have the right to be listened to and heard, and that birth and well woman care are important events in the lives of women.

As a profession can be remarkably different from obstetrics, yet seemingly demonstrates many of the same behaviors, we need to show how the care we provide is different. One way of doing that is through the documentation of midwifery care.

Documentation as Risk Management

Midwives hear the words 'risk management' and invariably they groan. Risk management is a dynamic process that affects how we provide care on a day-to-day basis. This section will attempt to identify ways in which you can maintain your practice while providing quality care in this litiginous society.

Exemplary midwifery practice includes understanding, and implementing, essential components of a risk management program to enhance midwifery care and outcomes.

Documenting Culturally Competent Care

Midwives and other health professionals have a legal and moral obligation to provide culturally competent care. An excellent resource for women's health providers is Hill's *Caring for Women Cross Culturally*. Cultural competence means that professionally you are able to step outside of your own culture, and obtain the vision & skills necessary to provide care in a context that is appropriate for the women who come to you for care.

The attitudes and behaviors needed to do this include a sincere interest in other cultures, the ability to communicate, and a sense of honor for the customs of others. On a more practical level the ability to access interpreter services is a key behavior that is both essential and legally mandated. Each midwife is expected to obtain or have access to information on specific health care problems that are racially or ethnically more prevalent, and familiarity with historical events and cultural practices that may effect health in the populations served.

Each of these components should be addressed in the medical record when they are applicable. It can be a simple check box, such as:

☐ Interpreter service offered

Documentation of cultural competence may also entail detailed description such as the informed consent process when provided through an interpreter prior to surgery or a procedure. It may be culturally appropriate to exclude the father from the birth room, or to ensure a family member is present as a chaperone during intimate exams. Documentation of the cultural indications for changes or differences in care serves to protect the midwife and to reinforce the need for respect and awareness of cultural differences.

The essential characteristic of the culturally competent midwife is an ability to embrace diversity while retaining one's sense of personal cultural identity. In order to do this it may be necessary to relinquish control in client encounters. Contemplation of any sense of failure, fear, frustration, anger or embarrassment can serve to help the midwife become more culturally sensitive and foster personal growth.

Documentation Skills and Techniques

Clear, concise documentation is the key to validating quality care, and is an integral part of any risk management program.

Thorough documentation allows midwives and other health care professionals to have a clear view of each woman's individual presentation, concerns, and preferences for care, as well as a means of following the health care professional's thought processes regarding working diagnosis and on-going plans for care.

Each note should provide essential information that could potentially guide another care professional in the event of a transfer of care, such as might occur following referral for evaluation of an abnormal pap smear, transfer to physician care for a high risk condition, or simple cross-coverage arrangements between midwives.

In the event of legal action, the client's medical record should ideally provide a clear picture of the client presentation, concerns, and response to care or treatment, as well as identifying the midwife's evaluation process, working diagnoses, anticipatory thinking, planning for diagnosis and treatment, follow-up care and evaluation, and initiation of collaborative practice as indicated.

Both ACNM and MANA offer *minimum data sets* (MDS) that can be used as a tool to evaluate the adequacy of documentation. These minimum data sets have been developed to provide a tool for collecting data about the care midwives provide. Midwives seeking to improve their documentation skills may also use the MDS as a self-evaluation instrument by performing retrospective chart or medical record audits to determine documentation weaknesses and areas for improvement

Documentation Basics

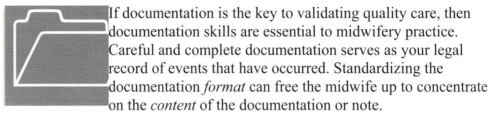If documentation is the key to validating quality care, then documentation skills are essential to midwifery practice. Careful and complete documentation serves as your legal record of events that have occurred. Standardizing the documentation *format* can free the midwife up to concentrate on the *content* of the documentation or note.

Thorough and complete documentation can be relatively brief and to the point. It is rarely necessary to provide lengthy notes. Notes can be handwritten, typed, entered into a computer data collection system, or dictated and transcribed. They may be written on a form that provides a general guide, such as a *labor flow sheet*, or written on a blank sheet of paper such as a *progress note*. Notes should reflect your findings, and your thinking as you care for this woman. All notes should have, at a minimum, the following information:

- Client Identification: i.e., name, date of birth, medical record number where applicable

- Date of Service: date & time are necessary for time-sensitive situations such as labor care, or during newborn resuscitation.

- Reason for Encounter: this is often described in the client's own words, i.e., 'The client states "It burns when I pee,"' or as a simple statement, such as "Onset of labor".

- Client History: this includes an expansion of reason for the encounter and includes the relevant history and subjective information provided by the client or family, including the review of systems (ROS).

- Objective Findings: this may include the results of the physical exam, mental status evaluation, labs, ultrasounds or other testing as indicated by the history and physical.

- Clinical Impression: this is also known as the assessment or working diagnosis, and may include several differential diagnoses under consideration pending lab or testing results. This is generally documented as primary symptoms, or conditions, with differential diagnoses listed to validate testing and communicate anticipatory thinking.

- Midwifery Plan of Care: the plan of care may be subdivided into several categories, but essentially, it should outline the diagnostic and therapeutic measures initiated at the visit, along with anticipated results and further actions that are anticipated based on potential results.

Client History
Components of the History to Consider

The history can be divided into several history types: the comprehensive health history, the interval history, and the problem-oriented or event-specific history.

Within these categories the history can be further subdivided into the personal medical and surgical history, personal social history, and family medical history. These sub-types of the history can be again subdivided to allow for focus on specific areas of concern such as the menstrual history, obstetrical history, or genetic history.

The *review of systems* (ROS) is a brief review of the major body systems with the client to determine the presence or absence of signs and symptoms of disease. The review of systems generally includes the following categories: Head, eyes, ears nose & throat (HEENT), skin, chest or thorax, and respiratory, cardiac, gastrointestinal, genitourinary, musculo-skeletal, endocrine, and neurologic systems.

Identifying which components of the history to pursue is a skill that can assist the midwife in efficiently identifying problems or concerns and developing a working list of differential diagnoses. Components of the history that are included in the client interview should be documented, including the client's response. The skilled diagnostician is an active listener, who can discern which client responses are pertinent, and use directed inquiry to elicit further information.

Physical Examination
Components of the Physical Exam to Consider

Every body system has both general and specific elements that may be evaluated during the physical examination. Thorough evaluation of the area(s) of concern is an integral part of client or patient evaluation.

While many midwives typically deal primarily with conditions related to childbearing, comprehensive well-woman health care may also include evaluation and treatment of many other general gynecologic or medical problems and conditions.

Documentation of the physical exam is most frequently organized in a head-to-toe manner. Following a consistent format allows for easier client evaluation, documentation of results, and review of information. Terms used should be standard medical terms that describe the presence or absence of findings in an objective manner that is consistent with the anatomic area under evaluation. "Normal" is not an objective finding, as the range of normal varies widely from client to client.

Standard terminology should be used whenever possible to identify areas of note i.e., right lower quadrant (RLQ), periumbilical, sub-sternal. Left (L) and right (R) should be clearly identified whenever applicable. Instruments and tests used during the physical exam should be identified when necessary to describe the technique used for evaluation, for example: "A speculum was inserted in the vagina to expose the cervix" or alternatively, "Speculum exam demonstrated…."

The language should be clear, descriptive, and indicate any unusual client response to the exam, or unusual findings. Notes should reflect your critical thinking during the exam i.e., "the left breast was noted to have an irregular fixed mass in the upper outer quadrant, into the axillary tail. The mass was approximately 3x6 cms, with bluish discoloration over the area, which may represent increased vascularity. The mass was firm but not hard, however, it was accompanied by palpable axillary lymph nodes. The clinical picture is highly suspicious for breast cancer in spite of a negative mammogram last week."

Clinical Impression
Differential Diagnoses to Consider

The clinical impression may be more familiar as the *assessment*, or the *diagnostic impression*. This should be a brief summary of the working diagnoses or description of presenting symptoms. These may be presented in a numbered running list from most to least important.

The clinical impression is also used for coding purposes, and 'rule-out' is not acceptable for coding purposes, although it may be documented as a way of listing the differential diagnoses under consideration.

The clinical impression should identify what you believe is going on with the client, based on the client history, physical examination, and any testing performed on-site. The clinical impression and differential diagnosis will then direct further evaluation and testing, the follow-up plan, and need for consultation or referral. Examples of differential diagnoses includes:

1. Preventive health visit, no other symptoms (NOS)

2. Urinary burning, urgency, and frequency; R/O cystitis

3. Pregnancy, 10 weeks gestation by LMP

4. Breast mass, L

5. Pregnancy, at 12 weeks with RLQ pain. Rule out

    a. Appendicitis

    b. Ectopic pregnancy

    c. Ovarian cyst

Diagnostic Testing
Diagnostic Tests and Procedures to Consider

Diagnostic testing includes any tests or procedures that are done to elicit additional information to accurately diagnose a problem, or evaluate an on-going treatment plan.

Testing should be documented in a brief, straightforward manner with additional explanations necessary only in unusual situations. Testing is often documented as a numbered running list, but should be clear enough that tests ordered can be clearly identified by other health care professionals. One area where this can be confusing is when 'panels' are ordered, which are often not consistent from facility to facility. "PIH labs" may include different arrays of tests at different locations. This becomes especially important when a transfer of care is necessary, and test results are pending.

Test results should be clearly documented in an easy to find location, especially when they pertain to on-going care of a problem. Test results come under the heading of *Objective Findings* when you are writing or dictating a note.

Providing Treatment
Therapeutic Measures to Consider

Therapeutic measures include the administration, ordering, or prescription of medications or treatments. Documentation of medications should include the medication name, dosage, timing, and route of administration. If off-label medication use is prescribed this should be documented, including discussion with client and documentation of the informed consent process.

Other treatments, such as physical therapy, or respiratory therapy treatments should be documented as ordered, including the indication for the treatment. An example might include: "Incentive spirometry TID post-op to prevent pulmonary atelectasis".

Providing Treatment
Alternative Measures to Consider

Alternative treatment measures include complementary and alternative therapies such as acupuncture, acupressure, homeopathy, herbal remedies, massage, etc. When possible, document resources for suggested measures. Include client instructions and discussion regarding alternative, traditional and empiric treatments.

Lack of randomized controlled trials may limit use of alternative measures in some practices, while in other practices these time-honored methods of caring for pregnant women may be used on a regular & frequent basis. Ethical practice requires discussion of known risks and benefits of all therapeutic measures, and thorough documentation of the same.

"Client inquired about use of castor oil to stimulate labor at term. The FHR was reactive today, cervix is soft and 1 cm. We discussed her options: expectant care, herbal or homeopathic remedies to stimulate cervical change, and the parameters for use of cervical ripening medications, or induction of labor. She was advised she may use 2-4 oz of Castor oil po. (see JNM Vol XX, pp xx). She was instructed to call with the onset of labor or…"

Providing Support
Education and Support Measures to Consider

Client education is an integral part of most midwifery practices, and as such should be clearly documented. Use of standardized client education materials can make documentation simpler and less time consuming. A simple reference to a brochure will suffice in this instance, i.e., "Client was given the Bleeding in Early Pregnancy handout, with instructions to call if bleeding should persist or worsen".

A master file should be kept of regularly used client education materials, so the midwife may refer back as needed to see what materials were used during a specific time period. Documentation should indicate whether education and support measures were provided verbally or in writing. Written instructions or recommendations allow the client to refer back to them after the visit, and refresh her memory about what happened at the visit. Many practices provide non-carbon forms to document client education with a copy of the form retained in the medical record.

Follow-up Care
Follow-up Measures to Consider

The instructions of when a client should return for care or when follow-up care is anticipated are key in the clear documentation of the midwifery plan of care. Clients must know what is expected of them in order to comply with care. Follow-up may include returning for a scheduled visit, such as a prenatal visit, or it may be that the midwife is going to contact the client following test results, such as after a mammogram performed on a client with a suspicious breast mass.

When there is any deviation from normal or expected findings, a clear plan for follow-up should be documented. In the example above of a woman with a breast mass, the documentation might include the date that results were received, discussion with the client about options for care, plan for referral to a breast specialist, the date and time of the specialist appointment, documentation of the consult including records transferred to the specialist, and a mechanism to follow-up to verify client compliance.

For midwives who provide comprehensive women's health care, a follow-up file may be necessary in order to track clients and their problems. In this instance, documentation in the client record that the follow-up file has been utilized can help with tracking. A follow-up file may be a simple index card file or a software program that automatically generates reminders, identifies no-shows, and provides a comprehensive record of problems and follow-up contacts.

Collaborative Practice
Consider Consultation or Referral

Any consultations or referrals should be clearly documented. Referrals include such things as counseling, smoking cessation, nutritional evaluation, substance abuse treatment, alternative therapies, and evaluation for reproductive, medical or surgical problems.

Documentation should include the name and specialty of the provider, how the contact was made, i.e., phone or letter, or directly by the client, as well as the indication for the consult or referral and the expected type of care. Formal consultation requests are often in letter format and should include a brief history of the problem, essential information about the client, the type of service the client is being referred for, and your expectations regarding care.

Sample referral letter

Dear Dr. B.,

I am referring Emma Shol to you for evaluation of her abnormal pap smear.

Emma is a 25 year old G0, P0 who has had regular pap smears since she was 19. Her pap of July 02 was returned with LGSIL. At that time I performed colposcopy, and CIN I was confirmed on biopsy. The exam was satisfactory and her ECC was negative. Her initial 2 follow-up paps were normal, until this last one, which was returned with HGSIL. I have enclosed copies of those reports for you.

> OB/GYN Hx: Neg STI screen, HPV testing + for high risk types, monogamous relationship x 2 years. Hormonal contraception.
>
> PMH: Allergies: PCN, Medications: Lunelle. No other medical problems
>
> PSH: T&A as child
>
> Family Hx: Mother with breast cancer, Father with hypertension

I am referring her to you for evaluation & treatment of this problem. Emma & I have discussed the need for repeat colposcopy and I have advise her that you will likely perform a LEEP excision of the area for definitive diagnosis and treatment. I have scheduled this with your office, and instructed Emma to take 2 ibuprofen prior to her visit.

Thank you for seeing Emma. I look forward to hearing back from you. Please let me know your preference for follow-up after Emma's evaluation so we can coordinate our care. If you have questions or need further information I can be reached at XXX-XXXX.

Sincerely Yours,

Midwife R., CNM, CPM

Recommendations for Basic Documentation

Demographic Info:

    Name: Age/DOB: Date of Visit:

    Address

    Marital Status

    Next of Kin/Person to Contact in Emergency

    Primary Care Provider

Reason/indication for visit:

    History of Chief Complaint or Current Concern:

History/Subjective Data

    Past Medical History (PMH)

    Past Surgical History (PSH)

    OB/GYN or Reproductive Health History

    Social Hx

    Review of Systems (ROS)

Objective Data

    Physical Exam (PE)

    Laboratory or other diagnostic testing results

Assessment

    Primary Signs or Symptoms

    Clinical Impression

    Diagnosis

Midwifery Plan of Care, (based on midwife scope of practice, client/patient needs & preferences, and practice setting)

    Diagnostic Testing/Anticipated Results

    Therapeutic Measures/Recommendations for Care

    Client Education/Support/Informed Consent

    Follow-Up/Anticipated Plan for Continued Care

    Referrals/Indications for Consultation or Referral

**A Note About
Informed Consent**

Informed consent is a specific process designed to ensure that the client or patient is provided with adequate information with which to make an informed decision or choice about their care. Documentation of informed consent should include information about the procedure, medication, or treatment recommended that covers:

- Indications for the proposed procedure, medication, or treatment

- The accepted or experimental use of the proposed procedure, medication, or treatment

- The potential benefits, actions, or effects of the proposed course of action

- The potential risks and adverse effects of the proposed course of action

- The alternatives to the proposed course of action, including potential effectiveness, risk, and benefit, and including no action, expectant care, or 'watchful waiting'

- Client understanding of discussion, best demonstrated by the client paraphrasing information received, and documented by direct quote i.e., "You're going to try to turn my baby so she isn't butt first."

- Midwife and client signatures witnessed by third party

Informed consent can be revoked by the client at anytime, potentially placing the midwife at a disadvantage in a challenging situation. Be sure to document your take on client understanding and willingness to participate in the recommended care, especially if there is any hesitation expressed.

For example:

Informed consent discussion was held regarding options for care at 42 weeks gestation. Client was provided with written and verbal information about the risks, benefits and alternatives to:

Fetal testing; Continued 'watchful waiting'; Cervical ripening using: Herbal remedies (evening primrose oil, blue cohosh), Mechanical devices (foley catheter, laminaria), Prostins (cervidil, misoprostol, prepidil), Induction of labor using misoprostol, oxytocin, castor oil, etc.

We discussed the indications for cervical ripening and induction of labor in this setting. The following discussion the client expressed her preference as X. However, she appeared somewhat uncomfortable and uncertain about X *(induction or waiting for example)*. At this point we will do

> *X (perhaps cervical ripening or watchful waiting)*, and re-evaluate in *X (will be dictated by cervical status, fetal well-being, etc.)* hours/days/or for specific practice, fetal, or maternal parameters.

A preprinted form for the most common indications using informed consent may be helpful. Including current references may be helpful as well.

References

1. Caroll, R. (Ed). (2001). Risk management handbook for healthcare organizations. American Society for Healthcare Risk Management. Josey-Bass: San Fransisco.

2. Kennedy, HP (2000). A model of exemplary midwifery practice: Results of a Delphi study. Journal of Midwifery & Women's Health. 45; 4-19.

Care of the Woman During Pregnancy

Prenatal means 'before birth. Prenatal care is an opportunity to teach the woman how to care for her baby before she or he is born.

There are basic components of prenatal care that are included in the core competencies of midwifery practice. For further information, the midwife is encouraged to compare the standards for basic midwifery practice that have been developed by ACNM, MANA and the ICM.

By comparing these three important standards (all available on-line by accessing the respective organizations web sites) one can gain an understanding of the expected standards for midwifery practice in the United States.

Each midwife must provide locally appropriate care. One of the limitations of a book like this is that care varies from location to location, and from provider to provider. Attempts to standardize care must, by nature, ignore the needs of individual. The purpose of prenatal care is to identify that small, but significant, number of women whose pregnancy will deviate from the wide range of normal in a manner that may jeopardize maternal or fetal well-being.

Every woman has unique needs during pregnancy. It is a time of many changes and adjustments. Caring for women during this time of transition can foster individual autonomy and enhance self-care practices. This may improve her ability to care for her child, and to recognize her strengths as a woman and a mother.

Many of the women we see are unfamiliar with the expectations of the health care system and will need some guidance in order to navigate the system, or negotiate for care that is appropriate to their needs. Building a strong professional relationship allows for trust to develop. Should the woman encounter challenges during her pregnancy, she will be more likely to heed the recommendations of the midwife.

The provision of prenatal care varies widely from practice to practice; based on the type of women's health care professional(s) in the practice, the practice setting, and the anticipated location for labor and birth. Regional variations are also common. Be sure to familiarize yourself with local or regional resources and standards. These are not meant to dictate practice, but to provide guidelines for care that is appropriate for the majority of women.

Providing women care during pregnancy includes respecting each woman's individual desires in relation to the preferred type of health care provider; the amount of active participation in her care that she desires, her planned and preferred location of labor and birth, and methods to access medical services should they be needed. Each midwife is responsible for outlining to the pregnant client the scope of her practice, and usual parameters for care.

The amount and types of testing performed during pregnancy should be determined by indications for testing or evaluation, current recommendations for practice, as well as discussion with the client regarding the risks, benefits and alternatives to testing or evaluation processes.

Maternal participation in prenatal care encourages self-determination, and may foster her resolve to surrender to the forces of labor and birth. The process of participation also builds trust. Discussion with the client demonstrates the multitude of potential options that are available, and encourages flexibility on the part of both the mother-to-be and the midwife.

Diagnosis of Pregnancy

Key Clinical Information

Nature is highly motivated to maintain the species, and pregnancy can occur in spite of valiant attempts to prevent it. The diagnosis of pregnancy may be a welcome event, or devastating news. Most women have mixed feelings about the changes that pregnancy will bring to their lives.

Client History:

Components of the History to Consider

- Reproductive history
  - G, P
  - Last menstrual period
  - Method of birth control
  - Symptoms of pregnancy
  - Previous STDs
- Signs or symptoms of complications, i.e.
  - Pain or cramping
  - Bleeding
  - Social history
  - Client feelings about possible pregnancy
  - Drugs or medications taken since LMP
  - Support systems
- Relevant medical/surgical history
  - Allergies
  - Medications
  - Medical conditions
  - Surgeries
- Social history
- Review of Systems

Physical Examination:

Components of the Physical Exam to Consider

- Vital signs

- Thyroid
- Pelvic evaluation
  - Uterine sizing
  - Consistency of uterus
  - Color of cervix
  - Cervical motion tenderness
  - Vaginal or cervical discharge
  - Adnexal tenderness
- Abdominal exam
  - Fetal heart tones
  - Fundal height
  - Abdominal tenderness

Clinical Impression:

Differential Diagnoses to Consider

- Pregnancy, no other symptoms (NOS)
- Pregnancy complicated by
  - Ectopic pregnancy
  - Unplanned pregnancy
  - Molar pregnancy
  - Blighted ovum
- Secondary amenorrhea, secondary to
  - Thyroid dysfunction
  - Ovarian dysfunction
  - History of contraceptive hormone use
  - Oral contraceptives
  - Depo Provera

Diagnostic Testing:

Diagnostic Tests and Procedures to Consider

- Urine or serum HCG
- Quantitative B-HCG
- TSH
- Pelvic or vaginal ultrasound

Providing Treatment:

Therapeutic Measures to Consider

- Prenatal or other vitamin supplement with folic acid
- Iron replacement therapy
- Treatment of any underlying infection or condition as indicated

Providing Treatment:

Alternative Measures to Consider

- Natural prenatal vitamin supplement
- Whole foods diet
- High folate foods
- Red raspberry leaf tea
- For herbal remedies to prevent or avoid pregnancy see A Difficult Decision: A Compassionate Book About Abortion by Joy Gardner

Providing Support:

Education and Support Measures to Consider

- Pregnancy options counseling as indicated
- Diet and nutrition counseling
- Prenatal care
  - o Usual care
  - o Prenatal testing
  - o Family involvement
- Practice
  - o Providers
  - o Medical affiliations
  - o Billing arrangements
- Birth options
  - o Location(s)
  - o Providers
  - o Philosophy of care
- Parent rights and responsibilities

Follow-up Care:

Follow-up Measures to Consider

- Document
  - o Anticipated EDC
  - o Relevant history
  - o Clinical findings
  - o Clinical impression
  - o Discussion & client preferences
  - o Midwifery plan of care
- Return for continued care
  - o 6-12 weeks gestation for initial prenatal visit
  - o ASAP if >12 weeks gestation
  - o Prenatal testing as indicated & desired

Collaborative Practice:

Criteria to Consider for Consultation or Referral

- As requested, and indicated, following discussion for
  - o Genetic counseling
  - o Amniocentesis
  - o Adoption services
  - o Abortion services
  - o Specialty care
- Social services
- Addiction resources

Initial Evaluation of the Pregnant Woman

Key Clinical Information

The initial evaluation provides the basis for ongoing pregnancy care. Careful attention to client history, and client response to the intimate questions asked during the initial interview, and to the physical exam can alert the midwife to unspoken issues. Gentle touch, coupled with an organized, systematic, yet unhurried manner is ideal during the first visit.

Careful documentation of all information is essential to allow for clear communication with other health care providers, and to serve as a comprehensive background of information for the busy midwife.

Client History:

Components of the History to Consider

- Client demographic information
- OB/GYN history
  - o Present pregnancy history
    - ▪ LMP
  - o G, P, pregnancy information and complications
  - o GYN disorders or problems
  - o Sexual history
  - o Contraceptive history
- Health risk evaluation
- Past medical/surgical history
- Family history
- Social history
- Review of systems

Physical Examination:

Components of the Physical Exam to Consider

- Vital Signs
- Observation of general status

- HEENT
- Skin
  - o Striae
  - o Scars or bruises
- Cardiorespiratory system
- Breasts
- Abdomen
  - o Fundal Height
  - o FHT
  - o Fetal lie
- GI system
- Genitourinary system
  - o Speculum exam
    - ▪ Vagina
    - ▪ Cervix
    - ▪ Collection of lab specimens
  - o Bimanual exam
  - o Uterine size, contour
  - o Tenderness
  - o Pelvimetry
- Rectal exam prn
- Musculoskeletal system

Clinical Impression:

Differential Diagnoses to Consider

- Pregnancy
  - o Viable
  - o Non-viable
  - o Ectopic
- Other diagnosis related to
  - o History
  - o Physical exam
  - o Diagnostic testing

Diagnostic Testing:

Diagnostic Tests and Procedures to Consider

- Pregnancy testing
  - o Urine or serum HCG
  - o Quantitative β-HCG
- STI testing
  - o Chlamydia and gonorrhea testing
  - o VDRL or RPR
  - o HIV testing
  - o Hepatitis B surface antigen
- Pap Smear
- Wet prep for BV
- Hematology & titers
  - o Hemoglobin and hematocrit or CBC
  - o Blood type, Rh factor and antibody screen
  - o Sickle cell prep
  - o Rubella titer
  - o Varicella antibody screen
  - o TSH
- Fetal & genetic testing
  - o Alfa fetal protein testing
  - o Cystic fibrosis testing
  - o Amniocentesis
- Ultrasound, vaginal or pelvic

- Tuberculosis testing
  - o PPD
  - o History of + PPD or BCG vaccine consider chest x-ray
- Urinalysis, with culture as indicated by history
- Group B strep culture

Providing Treatment:

Therapeutic Measures to Consider

- Prenatal vitamins with folic acid
- Iron supplementation
- Treatment of existing conditions as indicated

Providing Treatment:

Alternative Measures to Consider

- Whole foods diet
- Dietary sources of
  - o Folate
  - o Iron
  - o Calcium
  - o Fiber

Providing Support:

Education and Support Measures to Consider

- Discussion regarding
- Diet and activity recommendations
- Danger signs and when to call
- How to access care providers
- Usual return visit schedule
- Recommended prenatal visits
- Recommended Prenatal testing
  - o Usual tests
  - o HIV counseling
  - o Amnio counseling, as indicated
  - o Collaborative medical providers
  - o Birth
    - ▪ Location of birth
    - ▪ Waterbirth
    - ▪ VBAC counseling prn

Follow-up Care:

Follow-up Measures to Consider

- Schedule return prenatal visits
  - o Q 4-6 weeks through 32 weeks
  - o Q 2-3 weeks 32-36 weeks
  - o Weekly 36 weeks-onset of labor
  - o More frequent visits for women with risk factors
- Document risk factors & plan for care
- VBAC
  - o Obtain and review operative notes
  - o Surgical consultation
- Document informed consents

Collaborative Practice:

Criteria to Consider for Consultation or Referral

- Genetic or other counseling, as indicated
- Prenatal amniocentesis or CVS, as indicated
- VBAC or planned repeat Cesarean
- History or presence of serious risk factors

Evaluation of Health Risks in the Pregnant Woman

Key Clinical Information

Prenatal care is primarily concerned with the identification of health risks to the mother, fetus, or infant that may be modified or diminished by prompt diagnosis and treatment. Health risks have the potential to affect the health of the mother, her unborn baby, or newborn infant. Health risks may be related to behavior, but are often related to genetic heritage, cultural or ethnic background. Prenatal identification of health risks may offer the opportunity to diagnose or treat actual or potential conditions, or provide parents with information and support to help cope with unexpected outcomes.

Client History:

Components of the History to Consider

- Maternal demographic information
- Age
- Partner status
- Education
- Review of personal medical history
- Diseases or health disorders
- Medication use, OTC or Rx
- Alternative therapies
  - Herbs
  - Homeopathy
  - Acupuncture
- OB/GYN history
  - Prior pregnancy losses
  - Prior pregnancy conditions or complications
  - Birth defects
  - Infertility
  - STIs
  - GYN procedures
    - LEEP
    - Myomectomy
    - Hystosalpingogram
- Review of family medical history
  - Ethnic heritage
  - Hereditary or genetic health conditions
  - Cultural health habits or conditions
- Pregnancy related problems
  - Review of health habits
  - Smoking, alcohol, and/or drug use
  - Nutritional status/caffeine use
  - Pica
  - Physical activity
- Review of social situation and support
  - Presence of caring partner
  - Number & relationship of people in the home
  - Economic situation
  - Risk factors for abuse

Physical Examination:

Components of the Physical Exam to Consider

- Compete physical exam, including
  - Vital signs
  - Weight

-      Weight/height ratio (BMI)
- Evidence of
  - Malnutrition
  - Exhaustion
  - Abuse
- Skin exam for signs of
  - Needle tracks
  - Bruising
  - Burns
  - Petechia
  - Lesions
- Smell for signs of
  - Tobacco or alcohol use
  - Ketosis
  - General hygiene

Clinical Impression:

Differential Diagnoses to Consider

- Pregnancy at risk for adverse pregnancy outcome secondary to
- Health habits
- Genetic disorders
- Maternal age
- Health conditions
- Prior uterine or cervical surgery
- GYN disorder or infection
- Abuse
  - Physical
  - Sexual
  - Emotional
- Substance abuse
- Poor social support
- Non-compliance secondary to
  - Communication
  - Transportation
  - Maternal age
- Other diagnoses as indicated

Diagnostic Testing:

Diagnostic Tests and Procedures to Consider

- Drug screening
- Cotenine testing for smokers
- HIV testing
- Hepatitis testing

- Sickle cell prep
- Hemoglobin A1c
- Alfa fetal protein, triple or quadruple screen
- Group B Strep testing
- SDI testing
- Level I or Level II ultrasound
- Amniocentesis
- Chorionic villus sampling

Providing Treatment:

Therapeutic Measures to Consider

- Prenatal or multivitamin with folic acid
- Smoking cessation medications
- Other medications or treatments based on diagnosis

Providing Treatment:

Alternative Measures to Consider

- Nutritional support
- Hypnosis to change health habits
- Other treatments based on diagnosis

Providing Support:

Education and Support Measures to Consider

- Allow private time to encourage disclosure
- Provide information about risks and benefits of
  - o Current health behaviors
  - o Prenatal tests
  - o Testing options
  - o Treatment options
- Genetic counseling

- Social support services
- Cultural support services
- Diagnosis related support groups

Follow-up Care:

Follow-up Measures to Consider

- Document
  - o Presence of risk factor(s)
  - o Physical findings
  - o Discussions
  - o Clinical impression
  - o Midwifery plan for care
  - o Indications for consultation
- Return visits
  - o Frequency determined by client condition
  - o Evaluation of mother and fetus
  - o Time to develop cooperative relationship
  - o Observation for as risk behaviors
  - o Serial drug, cotenine, or STI testing

Collaborative Practice:

Criteria to Consider for Consultation or Referral

- For conditions not within the scope of the midwife's practice
- Genetic screening
- As indicated by lifestyle & social indicators
  - o Detox
  - o Counseling or therapy
  - o Women's shelter
- As requested for termination of abnormal pregnancy
- As indicated by evaluation for medical or specialty care

Ongoing Care of the Pregnant Woman

Key Clinical Information

The routine prenatal visit is any but routine for the pregnant woman. It is her brief opportunity to have her needs met and her concerns addressed, while at the same time having her pregnancy evaluated for the well-being of herself and her child. The midwife is alert to subtle signs or symptoms that may indicate a deviation from normal for this individual woman. Group prenatal care provides a unique opportunity to bring together women from diverse backgrounds, who can meet on the common ground of childbearing.

Client History:

Components of the History to Consider

- Interval history since last visit
  - o Maternal well-being
  - o Fetal motion
  - o Contractions
  - o Vaginal bleeding or discharge
  - o Dysuria
  - o Constipation
  - o Edema
  - o Exposure to any infectious diseases
- Client and/or family
  - o Concerns
  - o Questions
  - o Nutrition

  - o Activity patterns
  - o Plans related to pregnancy, labor & birth

Physical Examination:

Components of the Physical Exam to Consider

- Vital signs, including BP and weight
- General well-being
- Abdominal exam
  - o Fundal height
  - o Fetal heart tones
  - o Estimated fetal weight
  - o Fetal lie, presentation, position and variety
- CVA tenderness
- Examination of extremities for
  - o Edema
  - o Varicosities, phlebitis

- o Reflexes

Clinical Impression:

Differential Diagnoses to Consider

- Pregnancy
  - o Low risk
  - o Complicated by risk factors
- Other diagnoses based on
  - o History
  - o Physical exam
  - o Diagnostic testing

Diagnostic Testing:

Diagnostic Tests and Procedures to Consider

- Dip urinalysis, culture prn
- Urine culture for
  - o History of asymptomatic bacteriuria
  - o History of pylonephritis
  - o Urinary symptoms
- Glucose challenge
  - o First trimester
    - Previous gestational diabetic
    - High risk for gestational diabetes
  - o 25-28 weeks gestation
    - Routine screen
    - Repeat testing in high risk groups
- Blood type & antibody screen
  - o Initial prenatal labs
  - o 25-58 weeks for Rh negative mothers
- Hematocrit and hemoglobin
  - o Initial prenatal labs
  - o 25-28 weeks
  - o Q 4-6 weeks to evaluate iron replacement therapy
- Repeat STI testing as indicated
- Repeat wet mount as indicated
- Group B strep testing at 34-37 weeks gestation
- Ultrasound evaluation
  - o Pregnancy dating
  - o Genetic evaluation/amniocentesis
  - o Fetal growth and development
  - o Placental location
  - o Biophysical profile
  - o Amniotic fluid index
- Additional testing as indicated
  - o Sickle cell
  - o TIBC, indices
  - o Thyroid

Providing Treatment:

Therapeutic Measures to Consider:

- Prenatal vitamins with folic acid
- Iron supplementation as indicated
  - o Ferro-sequels 1-2 PO daily
  - o Niferex 150 1-2 PO daily
  - o Ferrous gluconate 1-2 PO daily
- Calcium supplements as indicated
  - o Citracal – 200-400 mg bid
  - o Tums – 500 mg 1-2 tabs daily
  - o Os-cal – 1 tab 2-3 x daily
- Influenza vaccine in the fall for those patients who:
  - o Currently have a chronic respiratory disorder (i.e. asthma, chronic bronchitis)
  - o Will be in the third trimester of pregnancy in December - April
  - o Will be early postpartum in December – April
- Immunization update if at significant risk

Providing Treatment:

Alternative Measures to Consider

- Dietary sources of
- Iron
  - o Organ meats & meats
  - o Eggs
  - o Blackstrap molasses
  - o Dried fruits (raisins, apricots, prunes)
  - o Deep green leafy vegetables
  - o Sea vegetables
- Folate
  - o Deep green leafy vegetables
  - o Root vegetables
  - o Whole grains
  - o Organ meats
  - o Nutritional yeast
- Calcium
  - o Dairy products
  - o Deep green leafy vegetables
  - o Shellfish, fish with bones (i.e. sardines)
  - o Deep green leafy vegetables
  - o Sea vegetables
- Third trimester/labor herbal support
- Red raspberry leaf
- Blue Cohosh

Providing Support:

Education and Support Measures to Consider

- Pregnancy discussion:
  - o Planned schedule of prenatal visits
  - o Expectations related to care
  - o Client/family expectations
  - o Midwife/practice expectations
  - o Any anticipated testing
- Social services available
- Fee & payment information
- Importance of fetal movement
- Nutrition and exercise
- Bowel & bladder function
- Feelings about pregnancy, birth, family and relationship changes
- Sexual relations
- Labor discussion:
  - o Planned location of birth
  - o Preparation for labor
  - o Signs and symptoms of labor
  - o Midwife call system
  - o When and how to call
  - o Anticipated labor care & birth options
  - o Pain relief
    - Labor support
    - Hydrotherapy
    - Massage
    - Positioning
    - Accupressure
    - Medication options
  - o Perineal support
  - o Episiotomy indicators
  - o Transport indicators
  - o Emergency physician coverage
- Anticipated infant care
  - o Vitamin K & route if given
  - o Erythromycin ophthalmic ointment
  - o Planned method of infant feeding
  - o Transport indicators
  - o Circumcision options
  - o Newborn evaluation at home
- Anticipated postpartum care

- o   Homebirth
- o   Birth center
- o   Hospital
- o   Vaginal birth
- o   Cesarean birth
- o   Planned help at home, resources
- o   Post partum method of birth control
- o   Anticipated visits for follow-up care
- o   Home visits
- o   Mother post-partum visits
- o   Infant evaluation

Follow-up Care:

Follow-up Measures to Consider

- Document
  - o   Findings
  - o   Client education
  - o   Plan for continued care
  - o   Pregnancy risk factors
  - o   Discussions with client/family
    - ▪   Informed consents
    - ▪   Preferences for labor & birth
    - ▪   Alternate providers/location for birth
    - ▪   Newborn care provider
- Midwifery plan of care

- o   Return visits
  - ▪   Q 4-6 weeks until 32 weeks gestation
  - ▪   Q 2-3 weeks from 32-36 weeks gestation
  - ▪   Weekly from 36 weeks until birth occurs
  - ▪   More frequent visits as indicated
- o   Informed consent or consultation, as indicated, for
  - ▪   Home birth
  - ▪   Birth center birth
  - ▪   VBAC
  - ▪   Tubal ligation

Collaborative Practice:

Criteria to Consider for Consultation or Referral

- For problems not within the scope of the midwife's practice
- For Rx not within the scope of the midwife's practice
- As indicated for
  - o   Surgical and/or anesthesia consultation
  - o   VBAC, or planned repeat Cesarean birth
  - o   Tubal ligation
  - o   Epidural or spinal anesthesia for labor & birth
- For pregnancy and/or childbirth education classes
- Diabetes education for the gestational diabetic
- Social service support prn

Care of the Pregnant Woman with Backache

Key Clinical Information

Backache during pregnancy is a common occurrence. Client posture, body mechanics and muscle tone may impact the strain on the back from the growing belly. Other causes of backache during pregnancy should not be dismissed without consideration, as this general symptom may be the only indication of a more serious condition.

Client History:

Components of the History to Consider

- LMP, EDC, gestational age
- Duration, severity and location of back ache
  - o   Precipitating event, if any
  - o   Timing of symptoms
  - o   Activities that aggravate backache
  - o   Medications or self-help measures used, and relief obtained
  - o   Presence of other associated symptoms
    - ▪   Presence or absence of contractions
    - ▪   Urinary symptoms
    - ▪   Presence of neurologic signs or symptoms
- Past medical history
  - o   Back injury, or disease
  - o   Kidney stones
- Social factors
  - o   Lifting at work
  - o   Physical abuse

Physical Examination:

Components of the Physical Exam to Consider

- VS, including weight
- General evaluation
  - o   Posture; presence of lordosis
  - o   Abdominal muscle tone
- Uterine size

- CVA tenderness
- Presence of muscle spasm
- Pelvic evaluation
  - o   When backache accompanied by contractions
  - o   History suggestive of pre-term labor
  - o   Cervical status
- Evaluation of neurologic status
  - o   Muscle tone
  - o   Strength
  - o   Coordination
  - o   Reflexes
- Signs of physical abuse
  - o   Bruising
  - o   Burns
  - o   Partner presence for entire visit

Clinical Impression:

Differential Diagnoses to Consider

- Backache of pregnancy
- Muscle strain or spasm, secondary to
  - o   Pregnancy
  - o   Injury
  - o   Pylonephritis
  - o   Renal calculi
  - o   Herniated disc

Diagnostic Testing:

Diagnostic Tests and Procedures to Consider

- Urinalysis
- Urine culture in the patient with a history of UTIs
- Fetal/uterine monitoring
- Ultrasound if renal calculi are suspected

Providing Treatment:

Therapeutic Measures to Consider:

- Pain Relief
- Acetaminophen
- Naproxen/Naproxen sodium
  - o   200-375 mg q 8-12 hs
  - o   Pregnancy Cat. B
- Ketoprofen (Orudis)
  - o   75 mg tid
  - o   Pregnancy Cat. B
  - o   Avoid in late pregnancy
- Muscle spasm
  - o   Flexeril
  - o   10 mg tid
  - o   Pregnancy Cat. B
- Osteopathic manipulation
- Chiropractic manipulation
- Physical therapy
  - o   For posture & lifting evaluation
  - o   For symptom management
  - o   For exercise training
- As appropriate for other confirmed diagnosis

Providing Treatment:

Alternative Measures to Consider

- Hot packs (moist heat, castor oil, vinegar)
- Massage
- Liniments
- Chiropractic or osteopathic adjustment
- Adequate calcium & magnesium intake
- Calcium
  - o   Sea vegetables
  - o   Broccoli, kale, sesame seeds
  - o   Raspberry leaf, oatstraw, borage
- Magnesium
  - o   Beets, dried beans, broccoli
  - o   Cornmeal, tofu, sweet potato
  - o   Dandelion greens, cashews, summer squash
- St. John's wort
  - o   Tincture 15-25 gtts 3-4 x daily
  - o   Infused oil for massage

Providing Support:

Education and Support Measures to Consider

- Back exercises
  - o   Yoga
  - o   Pelvic tilt
  - o   Stretching
  - o   Swimming
- Use of good body mechanics
  - o   Low heeled shoes
  - o   Posture to minimize lordosis
  - o   Avoid lifting with back
  - o   Bend knees to lift using leg muscles
  - o   Avoid bending or turning from waist
- Supportive sleep environment
  - o   Firm mattress
  - o   Pillows between knees
- Mechanical support measures
  - o   Well fitting, supportive bra
  - o   Prenatal abdominal cradle
  - o   Lumbar support in chair/car
  - o   Footstool to raise

Follow-up Care:

Follow-up Measures to Consider

- Document
  - o   Primary complaint & symptoms
  - o   Clinical findings
  - o   Client education/recommendations
  - o   Treatments
  - o   Plan for continued care
- Notify adult protective as needed for evidence of abuse
- Return for care
  - o   As scheduled for gestation
  - o   With worsening symptoms
    - ▪ Pain
    - ▪ Urinary symptoms
    - ▪ Numbness or tingling
    - ▪ Signs of preterm labor

Collaborative Practice:

Criteria to Consider for Consultation or Referral

- Persistent backache with contractions
- Development of fever and chills
- Positive testing for kidney involvement
  - o   Hematuria
  - o   Bactiuria
  - o   Calculi
- Sciatica or presence of other neurologic symptoms
  - o   Weakness
  - o   Numbness or tingling of extremities

Care of the Pregnant Woman with Constipation

Key Clinical Information

Constipation frequently occurs due to decreased motility of the intestine, as well as pressure from the growing uterus. Prevention of constipation requires attention to intake of both fluid and fiber, and adequate physical activity to stimulate the bowels. Determining acceptable fiber sources for your client is central to the prevention effort.

Client History:
Components of the History to Consider
- LMP, EDG, gestational age
- Nature of abdominal discomfort
  o Onset of problem
  o Location, severity
  o Other associated symptoms
- Bowel habits
  o Frequency and consistency of bowel movements
    ▪ Straining
    ▪ Hard stools
    ▪ Abdominal cramping w/ BM
  o Passage of flatus
  o Presence of blood in the stool
- Remedies tried
- Contributing factors
  o Iron therapy
  o Inactivity
  o Inadequate fluid intake
  o Inadequate fiber intake
  o Narcotic use

Physical Examination:
Components of the Physical Exam to Consider
- Vital signs, including temp
- Auscultate bowel sounds
- Palpate presence of hard stool in rectum
- Cervical evaluation if cramping present
- Palpate for presence of abdominal pain
  o Location
  o Rebound
  o Guarding

Clinical Impression:
Differential Diagnoses to Consider
- Constipation
- Irritable bowel syndrome
- Fecal impaction
- Ectopic pregnancy
- Appendicitis
- Intestinal obstruction

Diagnostic Testing:
Diagnostic Tests and Procedures to Consider
- Urine for specific gravity
- Stool for
  o Blood
  o Culture
  o Ova and parasites
- Quantitative β-HCG

- CBC, with differential
- Pelvic ultrasound

Providing Treatment:
Therapeutic Measures to Consider:
- NOTE: Acute abdomen must be ruled out before recommending therapies for constipation 🔖
- Fiber therapy
  o Citrucel - 1 TBS in 8 oz fluid 1-3 x daily
  o Metamucil - 1 tsp. in 8 oz fluid 1-3 x daily
  o Fibercon - 1 tab with 8 oz fluids 1-4 x daily
- Stool softeners
  o Docusate sodium 50-100 mg 1 PO QD or BID
  o Docusate calcium 240 mg 1 PO QD
- Laxatives
  o Senokot – 1 tab at hs
  o Milk of magnesia
- Glycerin suppositories
- Fleet enema if stool impacted

Providing Treatment:
Alternative Measures to Consider
- Increase fiber in diet
  o Dried fruit, prune juice
  o Whole grains, bran cereals, muffins
  o Uncooked vegetables
  o Psyllium seed 1 tsp. tid
- Increase fluid intake
  o Hot liquid in morning
  o Herb tea
  o Decaffeinated coffee
  o Hot prune juice
- Increase physical activity
- Bowel training
  o Allow regular time for toileting
  o Follow natural urges

Providing Support:
Education and Support Measures to Consider
- Prevention is key
- Walking helps stimulate natural peristalsis
- Fiber
  o Maintain adequate fiber intake
  o Helps to keep stool soft
  o Must be used with adequate fluid intake
- Stool softeners
  o Bring fluid to the stool to soften
  o Coat stool with surfactant to help move
- Laxatives
  o Stimulate peristalsis

o Should be used with caution during pregnancy
o May cause cramping
- Suppositories
  o Stimulate evacuation of lower bowel
  o May cause cramping
- Enemas
  o Flush the lower bowel
  o May cause cramping
- Lifestyle recommendations
  o Need for increased fiber and fluid
  o Need for activity to stimulate bowels
  o Hot drink in AM may stimulate bowels
  o Need for time for toileting
- Warning signs of
  o Pre-term labor
  o Acute abdomen

Follow-up Care:

Follow-up Measures to Consider

- Document
  o Presenting symptoms
  o Clinical findings

o Client education
o Treatments & recommendations
o Plan for continued care
- Return for care
  o As scheduled for gestation
  o Return sooner if symptoms worsen
- For emergency care
  o Symptoms of acute abdomen
  o Obstipation
  o Symptoms of preterm labor

Collaborative Practice:

Criteria to Consider for Consultation or Referral

- Threatened pre-term labor
- Positive occult blood on stool
- Abdominal pain that is:
  o Severe or persistent
  o Accompanied by fever
  o Abdominal rigidity or guarding
  o Accompanied by obstipation

Care of the Pregnant Woman with Dyspnea

Key Clinical Information

Shortness of breath becomes common in the later stages of pregnancy as the uterus pushes against the diaphragm. Anemia may also contribute to dyspnea. Evaluation of shortness of breath during pregnancy is necessary to determine whether is it physiologic or pathologic.

Client History:

Components of the History to Consider

- LMP, EDC, gestational age
- Timing of onset, duration and severity of symptoms
  o With activity vs at rest
  o Supine vs upright
  o Syncope
  o Other associated symptoms, i.e. fever, chills, cough
- Cardiopulmonary history
  o History of asthma
  o History of smoking
  o Environmental exposure to allergens, smoke, fumes
  o History of cardiac disorders and/or symptoms
- Anxiety or panic symptoms
- Self-help measures or medications used
- Review of systems

Physical Examination:

Components of the Physical Exam to Consider

- Vital signs, including temperature
- Color
- Auscultation and percussion of the chest
  o Presence of abnormal breath sounds
  o Respiratory rate, depth & volume
  o Respiratory effort
  o Presence of cough
- Observation for signs of respiratory distress

Clinical Impression:

Differential Diagnoses to Consider

- Physiologic SOB of pregnancy
- Upper respiratory infection
- Anemia
- Respiratory or cardiac disease process
  o Asthma
  o Valvular heart disease
  o Coronary artery disease
- Anxiety or panic attacks

Diagnostic Testing:

Diagnostic Tests and Procedures to Consider

- CBC with differential
- Sputum cultures
- TB testing
- Chest x-ray

Providing Treatment:

Therapeutic Measures to Consider:

- As indicated by diagnosis (See *Respiratory Disorders*)

Providing Treatment:

Alternative Measures to Consider

- Stretch periodically
- Maintain good posture
- Maintain daily physical activity
- Walking
- Yoga

- Swimming
- Use pillows as needed for comfort while at rest

Providing Support:

Education and Support Measures to Consider

- Reassurance
- Physiologic basis of shortness of breath
- Deliberate intercostal breathing
- Warning signs
  o Flu-like symptoms
  o Productive cough
  o Chest pain, SOB diaphoresis
  o Anxiety

Follow-up Care:

Follow-up Measures to Consider

- Document
  o Presenting complaint & symptoms
  o Clinical findings
  o Treatments
  o Client education & recommendations
- Plan for continued care
  o Return for care
  o As scheduled for gestation
  o Sooner for
    ▪ Presence of warning signs
    ▪ Persistence or worsening of symptoms
    ▪ As needed for support

Collaborative Practice:

Criteria to Consider for Consultation or Referral

- Diagnosis not within the scope of the midwife's practice
- Rx of medications not within the scope of the midwife's practice
- History or symptoms of asthma
- Evidence of significant respiratory infection
- Evidence of cardiac decompensation
- Anxiety or panic attacks

Care of the Pregnant Woman with Edema

Key Clinical Information

Physiologic edema of pregnancy occurs secondary to fluid retention as the body works to maintain adequate circulating fluid volume. Pressure of the pregnant uterus may cause venous stasis, and leakage of fluid into the soft tissue. Physiologic edema and the edema associated with pregnancy induced hypertension may be indistinguishable. Careful evaluation of additional signs and symptoms of PIH is necessary.

Client History:

Components of the History to Consider

- LMP, EDC, gestational age
- Prior history of
  o PIH
  o Edema with pregnancy
  o Varicose veins
- Onset, location, duration and severity of edema
- Usual sodium intake or restriction
- Symptoms of PIH
  o Headaches
  o Visual disturbances
  o Epigastric pain
- Other associated symptoms
- Self-help measures used and their effects
- Review of systems

Physical Examination:

Components of the Physical Exam to Consider

- Vital signs
- Compare BP & WT to baseline
- Presence or absence of facial edema
- Examination of extremities
- Deep tendon reflexes
- Presence of pitting edema
- Measurement of leg circumference
- Varicosities
- Signs of phlebitis

Clinical Impression:

Differential Diagnoses to Consider

- Physiologic edema of pregnancy
- Edema related to
  o Excessive sodium intake
  o Pregnancy induced hypertension
  o Thrombophlebitis

Diagnostic Testing:

Diagnostic Tests and Procedures to Consider

- Urinalysis, for proteinuria
- PIH labs (See Pregnancy Induced Hypertension)

Providing Treatment:

Therapeutic Measures to Consider:

- Prescription support hose

Providing Treatment:

Alternative Measures to Consider

- Diuretic foods
  o Asparagus
- Herbal support
  o Oatstraw
  o Red raspberry
  o Dandelion
  o Stinging nettle

Providing Support:

Education and Support Measures to Consider

- Discussion regarding
  o Physiologic basis of edema in pregnancy

o   Warning signs of PIH
- Self-help measures
  o   Rest, elevate extremities, pillow under right hip
  o   Increase fluids
  o   Add salt to diet to taste if low salt intake
  o   Decrease salt intake if high salt diet
  o   Avoid constrictive clothing
  o   Regular daily physical activity

Follow-up Care:

Follow-up Measures to Consider
- Document
  o   Symptoms
  o   Clinical findings

o   Treatments or recommendations
o   Client education
o   Plan for continued care
- Return for care
  o   As scheduled for gestation
  o   For increasing edema
  o   Symptoms of PIH

Collaborative Practice:

Criteria to Consider for Consultation or Referral
- Symptoms of PIH
- Severe varicosities
- Symptoms of phlebitis or thrombophlebitis

Care of the Pregnant Woman with Epistaxis

Key Clinical Information

Nosebleeds may occur with regularity in some pregnant women. While they are rarely of a serious nature, most women are anxious about the blood loss, and may require treatment if the bleeding does not stop promptly.

Client History:

Components of the History to Consider
- Frequency, duration and severity of bleeding
- Self-help measures used
- Use of inhaled drugs (i.e. cocaine, glue)
- Signs and symptoms of anemia

Physical Examination:

Components of the Physical Exam to Consider
- Vital signs, compare BP & P to baseline
- Examination of nares for
  o   Polyps
  o   Trauma
  o   Erosion
  o   Inflammation

Clinical Impression:

Differential Diagnoses to Consider
- Simple epistaxis
- Nasal polyps
- Inhalation drug use

Diagnostic Testing:

Diagnostic Tests and Procedures to Consider
- Hematocrit if persistent, recurrent copious flow
- Drug screen

Providing Treatment:

Therapeutic Measures to Consider:
- Normal saline nasal spray

- Nasal packing

Providing Treatment:

Alternative Measures to Consider
- Increase dietary intake of
  o   Vitamin C
  o   Calcium

Providing Support:

Education and Support Measures to Consider
- Discussion regarding
  o   Physiologic basis for epistaxis
  o   Avoid vigorous blowing or picking of nose
- Self-help measures
  o   Ice to bridge of nose to stop bleeding
  o   Pinch bridge of nose
  o   Use of humidifier or vaporizer

Follow-up Care:

Follow-up Measures to Consider
- Document
  o   Findings
  o   Education
  o   Plan for continued care
- Return for care
  o   As scheduled for gestation
  o   For severe bleeding unresponsive to above measures

Collaborative Practice:

Criteria to Consider for Consultation or Referral
- Severe cases for electrocautery of bleeding vessel

Care of the Pregnant Woman with Heartburn

Key Clinical Information

The pregnancy hormone relaxin may increase the incidence of heartburn or reflux in pregnant women. Women with a history of gastro esophageal reflux disease may require treatment during pregnancy. Small meals and bland diet may help with this problem.

Client History:

Components of the History to Consider

- LMP, EDC, gestational age
- Frequency, timing, duration and severity of symptoms
- Presence of symptoms prior to pregnancy
- Usual diet
- Self-help measures used & results

Physical Examination:

Components of the Physical Exam to Consider

- Vital signs including weight
- Fundal height

Clinical Impression:

Differential Diagnoses to Consider

- Physiologic heartburn of pregnancy
- Gastro-esophageal reflux disease
- Hiatal hernia

Diagnostic Testing:

Diagnostic Tests and Procedures to Consider

- H. Pylori testing if symptoms preceded pregnancy

Providing Treatment:

Therapeutic Measures to Consider:

- Antacid preparations
  - o Tums
  - o Maalox, not recommended
  - o Gelusil
  - o Amphojel
  - o Milk of magnesia, not recommended
- H2 Blockers (Preg. Cat B)
  - o Axid 150 mg PO BID
  - o Pepcid 20 mg PO BID
  - o Tagamet 300 mg PO QID
  - o Zantac 150 mg PO BID

Providing Treatment:

Alternative Measures to Consider

- Herbal remedies

  - o Lemon juice or cider vinegar in water
  - o Chamomile tea
  - o Oatstraw tea
  - o Red raspberry leaf tea
  - o Papaya chewable tablets
  - o *Avoid* licorice in pregnancy

Providing Support:

Education and Support Measures to Consider

- Physiologic basis of heartburn
- Comfort measures not cure
- Self-help measures
  - o Small frequent meals
  - o Maintain good posture
  - o Decrease intake of fatty or spicy foods
  - o Take food and fluids separately
  - o Elevate head of bed 10-30°
- Indications for referral

Follow-up Care:

Follow-up Measures to Consider

- Document
  - o Findings
  - o Education
  - o Plan for continued care
- Return for care
  - o As scheduled for gestation
  - o If persistent reflux or vomiting occurs

Collaborative Practice:

Criteria to Consider for Consultation or Referral

- If symptoms become severe
- For suspected or documented
  - H. pylori infection
  - Hiatal hernia
  - GERD
  - Gastric ulcer

Care of the Pregnant Woman with Hemorrhoids

Key Clinical Information

Hemorrhoids are varicosities of the anal region. They may be within the rectum, or outside the anal sphincter. The pressure of the pregnant uterus, and constipation may aggravate hemorrhoids causing bleeding, itching & burning. Thrombosed hemorrhoids are extremely painful, and are frequently treated with incision & drainage.

Client History:

Components of the History to Consider

- LMP, EDC, gestational age

- Prior history of hemorrhoids
- Duration, severity of symptoms
- Presence of bleeding, pain, itching

- Toileting habits
- Constipation or diarrhea
- Usual diet
- Medication use (i.e. iron supplements, stool softeners, enemas)

Physical Examination:

Components of the Physical Exam to Consider

- Examination for presence of
  o Hemorrhoids
  o External
  o Internal
  o Strangulated
  o Thrombosed
  o Anal lesions consistent with
    ▪ STD
    ▪ Trauma
- Anal fissure
- Anal fistula

Clinical Impression:

Differential Diagnoses to Consider

- Hemorrhoids
- Anal fissures
- Anal trauma
- Anal herpes
- Anal fistula
- Rectal polyp
- Rectal malignancy

Diagnostic Testing:

Diagnostic Tests and Procedures to Consider

- Stool for occult blood
- Herpes culture
- STD screen
- Anoscopy

Providing Treatment:

Therapeutic Measures to Consider:

- Anusol HC
- Lidocaine gel

- Manual reduction of hemorrhoids

Providing Treatment:

Alternative Measures to Consider

- Herbal remedies
  o Bilberry tablets or capsules tid
  o Witch hazel compresses
  o Comfrey compresses
  o Nettle tea
- Herbal or warm water sitz baths
- Knee chest position
- Epsom salt compresses
- Homeopathic remedies
  o Hamamelis 30x
  o Arnica 30x

Providing Support:

Education and Support Measures to Consider

- High fiber diet
- Avoid constipation
- Avoid straining at stool
- Options for treatment
- Topical medication use

Follow-up Care:

Follow-up Measures to Consider

- Document
  o Findings
  o Education
  o Plan for continued care
- Return for care
  o As scheduled for gestation
  o ASAP for thrombosed hemorrhoids

Collaborative Practice:

Criteria to Consider for Consultation or Referral

- For incision and drainage of thrombosed hemorrhoids
- Evaluation of severe, strangulated, or bleeding hemorrhoids
- Blood in stool with no evidence of hemorrhoids or rectal fissure
- Pathologic process causing symptoms

Care of the Pregnant Woman with Insomnia

Key Clinical Information

Insomnia affects many pregnant women as they approach term. It may help to think of it as nature's way of preparing for 2 am feedings. However, for the woman with significant sleep deprivation the ability to function on a daily basis may be significantly impaired. Starting labor with severe sleep deprivation is less likely to result in a smooth progression of labor.

Client History:

Components of the History to Consider

- LMP, EDC, gestational age
- Sleep/wake patterns
  o Difficulty falling asleep
  o Wakefulness
  o Fitful sleep
  o Interruptions

  o Bedtime
  o Naps
  o Total hours sleep/24 hrs
- Nocturia
- Emotional response to sleep deprivation
- Social issues
- Nutritional evaluation
- Caffeine intake and timing

- Meal patterns & content

Physical Examination:

Components of the Physical Exam to Consider
- Routine prenatal evaluation
- Evaluation for:
  o Adequate nutrition and hydration
  o Evidence of sleep deprivation
  o Evidence of other causes of sleep deprivation

Clinical Impression:

Differential Diagnoses to Consider
- Insomnia
- Anxiety
- Depression
- Obsessive-compulsive disorder
- Substance abuse
- Social concerns related to pregnancy

Diagnostic Testing:

Diagnostic Tests and Procedures to Consider
- Insomnia: None
- Other diagnosis: As indicated by diagnosis

Providing Treatment:

Therapeutic Measures to Consider:
- For sleep
  o Ambien
    ▪ 5-10 mg hs
    ▪ Pregnancy category B
  o Benadryl
    ▪ 25-50 mg hs
    ▪ Pregnancy category B
- For therapeutic sleep
  o Morphine Sulfate
    ▪ 10-15 mg IM
    ▪ Pregnancy category C
    ▪ May combine with Vistaril
  o Ambien

Providing Treatment:

Alternative Measures to Consider
- Increase vitamin B intake
- Herbal remedies
  o Chamomile tea
  o Hops tea or tincture (after 20 weeks gestation)

- Lemon balm tea
  o Skullcap tincture
  o Passion flower tea, tincture or fluid extract tid
- Hypnotherapy
- Aromatherapy
- Massage

Providing Support:

Education and Support Measures to Consider
- Physiologic basis of insomnia
- Other factors that may interfere with sleep
  o Work hours
  o Caretaking requirements
    ▪ Small children
    ▪ Elderly or ill parents/family
  o Sleeping arrangements
  o Nighttime hunger
- Encourage a positive approach to this difficult problem
  o Self-help measures
  o Nap during day to maintain rest
  o Warm bath
  o Warm milk
  o Massage
  o Extra pillows for support
  o Regular daily physical activity
  o Adequate dietary intake

Follow-up Care:

Follow-up Measures to Consider
- Document
  o Primary complaint & symptoms
  o Findings
  o Education
  o Plan for continued care
- Return for care
  o As scheduled for gestation
  o Increased visits for
    ▪ Evaluation and monitoring of medication use
    ▪ Emotional support

Collaborative Practice:

Criteria to Consider for Consultation or Referral
- For Rx not within the midwife's scope of practice
- For exhaustion
- For mental health issues
- As indicated for social issues

Care of the Pregnant Woman with Leg Cramps

Key Clinical Information

Leg cramps are a common occurrence during pregnancy, and may interfere with a woman's ability to sleep. They are more common during the nighttime hours. Cramping may be related to an imbalance of calcium in the muscle cells, causing muscle spasms.

Client History:

Components of the History to Consider
- LMP, EDC, gestational age
- Frequency, duration and severity of cramps
- Treatments or self-help measures used
- Calcium and sodium intake
- Physical activity level

Physical Examination:

Components of the Physical Exam to Consider
- Vital signs
- Evaluate for clonus
- Evaluate for muscle spasm

Clinical Impression:

Differential Diagnoses to Consider

- Physiologic leg cramps
- Leg cramps
- Varicose veins
- Restless leg syndrome
- Phlebitis
- Thrombophlebitis
- Deep vein thrombosis

Diagnostic Testing:

Diagnostic Tests and Procedures to Consider

- Serial calf measurments
- Venous ultrasound
- Clotting studies

Providing Treatment:

Therapeutic Measures to Consider:

- Calcium supplement
- Magnesium supplement

Providing Treatment:

Alternative Measures to Consider

- Dietary sources of calcium & magnesium
  - o Sea vegetables
  - o Tofu
  - o Sesame seeds (unhulled)
- Homeopathic remedies
  - o Calcarea Phos. 30x tid or with acute symptoms
  - o Calcarea Carb. 30x tid or with acute symptoms
- Herbal remedies

  - o Raspberry leaf
  - o Nettle
  - o Dandelion

Providing Support:

Education and Support Measures to Consider

- Physiologic nature of leg cramps
- Warning signs:
  - o Increasing muscle spasms
  - o Swelling or pain in leg
- Self-help measures
  - o Massage, stretching
  - o Increase calcium and sodium intake
  - o Regular daily activity, i.e. walking or swimming

Follow-up Care:

Follow-up Measures to Consider

- Document
  - o Findings
  - o Education
  - o Plan for continued care
- Return for care
  - o As scheduled for gestation
  - o For persistent leg pain

Collaborative Practice:

Criteria to Consider for Consultation or Referral

- For non-pregnancy related cause
- Phlebitis
- Thrombophlebitis
- Deep vein thrombosis

Care of the Pregnant Woman with Nausea and Vomiting

Key Clinical Information

While nausea and vomiting are considered a classic early pregnancy occurrence, they may cause significant dehydration and contribute to poor nutrition. In a few women the nausea and vomiting of pregnancy continue throughout the pregnancy. Hyperemesis of pregnancy most often occurs in the presence of a large amount of circulating pregnancy hormones. Prompt treatment is required to restore fluid and electrolyte balance.

Client History:

Components of the History to Consider

- LMP, EDC, gestational age
- History of thyroid disorders
- Duration and severity of symptoms
- Presence and frequency of vomiting
- Symptoms of dehydration
- Self-help measures used & results
- Nutritional intake
- Activity level
- Bowel & bladder pattern

Physical Examination:

Components of the Physical Exam to Consider

- Vital signs, including WT & BP
- General prenatal evaluation, including examination for
  - o Weight loss

  - o Skin turgor
  - o Fundal height for gestational age
  - o Bowel sounds
  - o General well-being

Clinical Impression:

Differential Diagnoses to Consider

- Morning sickness
- Hyperemesis gravidarum
- Molar pregnancy
- Bulimia
- Anxiety
- Depression
- Obsessive compulsive disorder

Diagnostic Testing:

Diagnostic Tests and Procedures to Consider

- For suspected hyperemesis:
  - o BUN and electrolytes

- o   Urine dip for ketones and glucose
- o   Serum albumin
- o   TSH
- Ultrasound

Providing Treatment:

Therapeutic Measures to Consider:

- Vitamin B6 (pyridoxine)
  - o   10-30 mg/day –
  - o   Pregnancy category A
- Meclizine
  - o   12.5. mg bid –
  - o   Pregnancy category B
- Prochlorperazine
  - o   5-25 mg q 4-6 h –
  - o   Pregnancy category C
- Chlorpromazine
  - o   10-25 mg q 4-6 h –
  - o   Pregnancy category C
- Zofran (
  - o   4-16 mg P.O. q 8 hrs, prn
  - o   Pregnancy category B
- IV hydration when indicated

Providing Treatment:

Alternative Measures to Consider

- Ginger tea
- Accupressure wristbands (Seabands®)

Providing Support:

Education and Support Measures to Consider

- Small bland meals, primarily carbohydrate
- Keep something in stomach i.e., saltines

- Electrolyte replacement
  - o   Pediolyte
  - o   Gatorade
  - o   Fluids with
    - ▪   Sugar
    - ▪   Salt
    - ▪   Salt substitute (adds potassium)
  - o   Take as sips only
- Restrict fats
- Advise family of need for support
- Review when to call for persistent symptoms

Follow-up Care:

Follow-up Measures to Consider

- Document
  - o   Primary complaint & symptoms
  - o   Clinical findings
  - o   Treatments & recommendations
  - o   Client education
  - o   Plan for continued care
  - o   Indications for prompt follow-up
- Return for care
  - o   As scheduled for gestation
  - o   If symptoms worsen
- Consider hospital care for dehydration

Collaborative Practice:

Criteria to Consider for Consultation or Referral

- For conditions not within the midwife's scope of practice
- Hyperemesis
- Dehydration
- Molar pregnancy

Care of the Pregnant Woman with Pica

Key Clinical Information

Pica is frequently a sign of iron deficiency anemia. The non-food items craved or eaten may be culturally directed. Here in Maine, women may crave not just earth, but salt-marsh clay from the edges of the tidal estuaries that feed the ocean. The most common substances craved are ice, clay, and laundry starch.

Client History:

Components of the History to Consider

- LMP, EDC, gestational age
- Previous H&H
- Prior history of anemia
- Identify non-food substance patient is eating or craving
- Common cultural or ethnic expressions of pica
- Evaluate patient's diet and nutritional resources
- Social issues

Physical Examination:

Components of the Physical Exam to Consider

- VS, including pulse
- Evaluate for symptoms of anemia
  - o   Color
  - o   Capillary refill
  - o   Orthostatic hypotension
  - o   Elevated heart rate

Clinical Impression:

Differential Diagnoses to Consider

- Pica, secondary to
  - o   Anemia
  - o   Nutrient deficiency
  - o   Social issues

Diagnostic Testing:

Diagnostic Tests and Procedures to Consider

- H&H
- Lead screening

Providing Treatment:

Therapeutic Measures to Consider:

- Iron replacement therapy if anemia present (See Anemia)

Providing Treatment:

Alternative Measures to Consider

- Iron rich foods

- Sea vegetables (high in iron and trace minerals)
- Red raspberry leaf tea

Providing Support:

Education and Support Measures to Consider

- Reassure if pica is not interfering with good nutrition
- Nutritional education
- Caution patient to avoid non-food items
- Try offering substitute items
  - Laundry starch, ice > frozen fruit pops
  - Clay > food grade seaweed

Follow-up Care:

Follow-up Measures to Consider

- Document
  - Findings
    - Education
    - Plan for continued care
- Return for care
- As scheduled for gestation
- As necessary to follow anemia

Collaborative Practice:

Criteria to Consider for Consultation or Referral

- Referral to social services as indicated
  - WIC
  - Food stamps
  - Food bank
- For severe pica accompanied by anemia
- For elevated lead levels

Care of the Pregnant Woman with Round Ligament Pain

Key Clinical Information

Round ligament pain can be a frequent occurrence at about 16-20 weeks gestation. It may mimic, or less frequently mask, more serious conditions such as appendicitis or ovarian torsion. It may cause significant distress, especially in the athletic woman who continues to jog, or those who have highly physical jobs such as waitresses or nurse's aides. An objective pain scale is recommended to measure and document client pain.

Client History:

Components of the History to Consider

- LMP, EDC, Gestational age
- Evaluation of the pain
  - Onset
  - Location
  - Severity
  - Duration
  - Characteristics
- Associated symptoms
  - Cramping
  - Backache
  - Nausea & vomiting
  - Change in bowel habits

Physical Examination:

Components of the Physical Exam to Consider

- Vital signs, including temp
- Verify location of pain
- Abdominal exam
  - Fundal height
  - FHR
  - Presence of contractions
  - Consistency of uterus
  - Palpate for tenderness
    - Fundus
    - Adnexa
    - Right upper quadrant
    - Right lower quadrant
- Pelvic exam
  - Cervical or vaginal discharge
  - Dilation and/or effacement

Clinical Impression:

Differential Diagnoses to Consider

- Round ligament pain
- PID
- Ectopic pregnancy
- Preterm labor
- Placental abruption
- Appendicitis
- Gallbladder disease
- Acute abdomen

Diagnostic Testing:

Diagnostic Tests and Procedures to Consider

- Urinalysis
- If pathology suspected
  - Chlamydia & gonorrhea testing
  - CBC, with diff
  - Ultrasound evaluation
    - Gallbladder
    - Appendix
    - Abdomen
    - Pelvis

Providing Treatment:

Therapeutic Measures to Consider:

- Maternity abdominal support or girdle
- Osteopathic manipulation

Providing Treatment:

Alternative Measures to Consider

- Yoga
- Acupuncture
- Herbal remedies
  - Red raspberry leaf tea

o   St. John's wort tincture

Providing Support:

Education and Support Measures to Consider

- Physiologic cause of round-ligament pain
- *Warning signs*
    o   Onset of contractions
    o   Persistent abdominal pain
    o   Fever
    o   Onset of nausea and vomiting
    o   Vaginal bleeding or discharge
    o   Pain with intercourse or BM
- Provide reassurance
- Self-help measures
    o   Pelvic tilt
    o   Warm baths
    o   Applying heat to area
    o   Positioning
    o   Knees to abdomen

o   Bending toward pain to ease ligament
o   Side-lying with pillow under abdomen

Follow-up Care:

Follow-up Measures to Consider

- Document
    o   Findings
    o   Education
    o   Plan for continued care
- Return for care
    o   As scheduled for gestation
    o   As indicated by test results
    o   With onset of *Warning signs*

Collaborative Practice:

Criteria to Consider for Consultation or Referral

- For abdominal pain inconsistent with round ligament pain
- For abnormal test results

Care of the Pregnant Woman with Varicose Veins

Key Clinical Information

Round ligament pain can be a frequent occurrence at about 16-20 weeks gestation. It may mimic, or less frequently mask, more serious conditions such as appendicitis or ovarian torsion. It may cause significant distress, especially in the athletic woman who continues to jog, or those who have highly physical jobs such as waitresses or nurse's aides. An objective pain scale is recommended to measure and document client pain.

Client History:

Components of the History to Consider

- LMP, EDC, gestational age
- Onset and location of varicose veins
- Use of medications
    o   Aspirin (ASA)
    o   NSAIDS
- Use of herbs that may affect clotting
- Changes with pregnancy
- Associated symptoms
    o   Pain
    o   Edema
    o   Redness
- History of superficial phlebitis or thrombophlebitis
- Current relief measures and their effects

Physical Examination:

Components of the Physical Exam to Consider

- Serial calf measurements
- Examination of varicosities
    o   Number
    o   Location(s)
    o   Size
    o   Severity
- Evaluate for symptoms of
    o   Superficial phlebitis
        ▪   Heat
        ▪   Redness
        ▪   Tenderness
    o   Deep vein thrombosis
        ▪   Pain

▪   + Homan's sign
▪   Leg edema

Clinical Impression:

Differential Diagnoses to Consider

- Varicose veins
- Superficial phlebitis
- Deep vein thrombosis

Diagnostic Testing:

Diagnostic Tests and Procedures to Consider

- Ultrasound prn to R/O deep vein thrombosis (DVT)

Providing Treatment:

Therapeutic Measures to Consider:

- Support hose, applied after elevating legs 10 minutes
- Foam pad to support vulvar varicosities
- Maternity abdominal support or girdle to relieve pressure on pelvic veins
- Low dose aspirin 80 mg
    o   1 PO daily x 7 days
    o   For symptoms of early superficial phlebitis

Providing Treatment:

Alternative Measures to Consider

- Herbal remedies
    o   Bilberry tablets or capsules tid
    o   Nettle tea or tincture daily
- Positioning
    o   Leg elevation
    o   Leg inversion (right angle position)

o   Inverted yoga postures (shoulder stand against support)

Providing Support:

Education and Support Measures to Consider

- Use & application of support hose
- Avoiding constrictive clothing
- Avoiding long periods of standing
- Rest with legs elevated
- Regular exercise, especially walking or swimming
- Medication instructions
- Patient *warning signs*
  - o   Persistent pain
  - o   Swelling
  - o   Redness
  - o   Fever

Follow-up Care:

Follow-up Measures to Consider

- Document
  - o   Findings
  - o   Education
  - o   Plan for continued care
- Return for care
  - o   As scheduled for gestation
  - o   4-7 days for suspected early superficial phlebitis
  - o   With any warning signs
- Evaluate closely in early post-partum period

Collaborative Practice:

Criteria to Consider for Consultation or Referral

- Suspected phlebitis or thrombophlebitis
- Severe vulvar varicosities

References

1. Barger, M. K. Ed. (1988). <u>Protocols for Gynecologic and Obstetric Health Care.</u> Philadelphia, PA: W. B. Saunders.

1. Briggs, G.G., Freeman, R. K., Yaffe, S. J. (1994) <u>Drugs in Pregnancy and Lactation</u> (4th Ed.). Philadelphia, PA: Williams & Wilkins.

2. Enkin, M., Keirce M., Renfrew, M., Neilson, J. (1995). <u>A Guide to Effective Care in Pregnancy and Childbirth</u> (2nd Ed.). New York, NY: Oxford University Press.

3. Foster, S. (1996). <u>Herbs for Your Health.</u> Loveland, CO: Interweave Press.

4. Frye, Anne. (1998). <u>Holistic Midwifery</u>. Portland, OR. Labrys Press

5. Frye, Anne. (1997). <u>Understanding Diagnostic Tests in the Childbearing Year.</u> (6th Ed.) Portland, OR. Labrys Press

6. Gordon, J. D., Rydfors, J. T., et al. (1995) <u>Obstetrics, Gynecology & Infertility</u> (4th Ed.) Glen Cove, N.Y., Scrub Hill Press.

7. Murphy, J. L., Ed. (2002). <u>Nurse Practitioner's Prescribing Reference.</u> New York, NY. Prescribing Reference, Inc.

8. Myles, M.F., (1985). <u>Textbook for Midwives</u> (10th ed.). Edinburg: Churchill Livingstone.

9. Scoggin, J., Morgan, G., (1997). <u>Practice Guidelines for Obstetrics and Gynecology.</u> Philadelphia, PA, Lippincott.

10. Scott, J. R., Diasaia, P.J., et al. (1996). <u>Danforth's Handbook of Obstetrics and Gynecology</u>. Philadelphia, PA, Lippincott - Raven.

11. Soule, D. (1996). <u>The Roots of Healing.</u> Secaucus, NJ: Citadel Press.

12. Varney, H., (1997). <u>Varney's Midwifery</u> (3rd ed.). Boston, MA: Jones and Bartlett.

13. Weed, S. (1985). <u>Wise Woman Herbal for the Childbearing Year.</u> Woodstock, NY: Ashtree Publishing.

Chapter
4

Care of the Pregnant Woman
with Prenatal Variations

Not every pregnancy remains uneventful. Prompt identification and
treatment of prenatal variations that may result in harm to mother or baby
ensures the best possible outcome.

The ability to pick up problems in pregnancy is an essential component of skilled midwifery practice. Midwives must simultaneously retain their belief that pregnancy is a normal physiologic condition while retaining a healthy respect for the problems and complications that may develop. Evaluation of potential problems requires the participation of the mother, and involving her in decision-making regarding options for care.

One of the hallmarks of midwifery practice is fostering client autonomy and participation in self-care. While the mother may have no control over the development of select problems, and may feel threatened by their development, the midwife can offer a sense of control by presenting options in the areas where client choice is possible. Respect for women's needs is especially important when an unexpected problems develops during what was 'supposed' to be a normal, uneventful pregnancy.

Care of the Pregnant Woman with Anemia, Iron Deficiency

Key Clinical Information

Anemia is a common diagnosis in women of childbearing age that may become worse during pregnancy Anemia may affect the oxygenation of both mother & fetus, and result in diminished fetal growth, maternal exhaustion, and other complications. The diagnosis and treatment of anemia, with attention to the overall nutritional status of the mother is urgently important for fetal well-being

Client History:
Components of the History to Consider
- LMP, EDC, gestational age
- Tobacco use

- History of closely spaced pregnancies
- History of anemia
- Presence of associated symptoms:
  o Fatigue
  o Dizziness

o   Headache
o   Pica (eating non-food items such as starch or clay)
o   Dyspnea
o   Palpitations
- Usual dietary patterns
  o   General nutrition
  o   Dietary iron sources
  o   Prenatal vitamin use
  o   Iron supplement use

Physical Examination:

Components of the Physical Exam to Consider

- Vital signs, including pulse & BP
- Pallor of skin and mucous membranes
- Examination for potential causes of anemia:

Clinical Impression:

Differential Diagnoses to Consider

- Physiologic anemia of pregnancy
- Iron deficiency anemia related to medical cause

Diagnostic Testing:

Diagnostic Tests and Procedures to Consider

- CBC with indices
- Indices in simple iron deficiency anemia:
  o   Normocytic
  o   Normochromic
- Serum ferritin
- Stool for occult blood, ova & parasites
- CDC range for lower limits of normal for Hematocrit & Hemoglobin during pregnancy

WEEK OF GESTATION	HGB (G/DL)	HCT (%)
12	11.0	33.0
16	10.6	32.0
20-24	10.5	32.0
28	10.7	32.0
32	11.0	33.0
36	11.4	34.0
40	11.9	36.0

Providing Treatment:

Therapeutic Measures to Consider

- Iron replacement therapy
  o   60-120 mg elemental iron daily
  o   Iron salts
  o   Ferrous sulfate 300mg
  o   Ferrous gluconate 300 mg
  o   Ferrous fumarate 300 mg

Providing Treatment:

Alternative Measures to Consider

- High iron food sources:
  o   Sea vegetables

o   Dried fruit (i.e. apricots or prunes)
    - High in iron
    - Add fiber to prevent constipation
o   Heme iron best absorbed
    - Meat
    - Poultry
    - Fish
o   Non-heme iron
    - Egg yolk
    - Grains
    - Vegetables
- Herbal sources of iron for pregnancy
  o   Alfalfa
  o   Nettle leaves
  o   Yellow dock root
  o   Parsley
  o   Dandelion
- Cast iron cookware
  o   Non-enamel surface
  o   Adds elemental iron

Providing Support:

Education and Support Measures to Consider

- Physiologic nature of anemia in pregnancy
- Pica decreases iron absorption
- Iron supplementation
  o   Avoid taking iron products with
      - Dairy
      - Food
      - Other supplements (i.e. prenatal vitamins)
  o   For best absorption
      - Take with vitamin C or water
      - Take at bedtime
      - Avoid caffeine, black teas
  o   Common side effects include:
      - GI upset, constipation or diarrhea
      - Nausea
      - Heartburn

Follow-up Care:

Follow-up Measures to Consider

- Document
  o   Findings
  o   Education
  o   Plan for continued care
- Parameters for consultation
- Return for care
  o   Repeat H&H 4-6 weeks after initiating therapy
  o   Add indices for persistent anemia

Collaborative Practice:

Criteria to Consider for Consultation or Referral

- For abnormal indices or elevated serum ferritin
- For anemia resistant to conventional therapy
- For concern regarding cause of anemia

Care of the Pregnant Woman with Fetal Demise

Key Clinical Information

Fetal demise may occur at any stage of pregnancy. No matter when it occurs, a common response for the woman is to wonder what she did wrong. Some fetal or placental conditions are incompatible with life, while other fetal demises may be due to maternal illness, or unknown factors.

Fetal demise is associated with an increased likelihood of developing disseminated intravascular coagulation (DIC). Onset of labor may be spontaneous or may be induced using a variety of measures. Emotional support and grief counseling may be helpful to parents. Genetic investigation and counseling may be useful for exploring potential causes in case where unknown factors are the cause of fetal demise, but often no cause can be determined.

Client History:

Components of the History to Consider
- LMP/EGA
- Regression of signs of pregnancy
  o Previous HCG results
  o Absence of fetal activity
  o Absence of fetal heart tones
- Precipitating event(s)
  o Idiopathic
  o Trauma/physical abuse
  o Substance abuse

Physical Examination:

Components of the Physical Exam to Consider
- Maternal vital signs
- Abdominal exam
  o Fundal height
  o Uterine tenderness
  o Absence of FHTs
- Cervical status
  o Bishops score

Clinical Impression:

Differential Diagnoses to Consider
- Fetal demise related to
  o Cord accident
  o Chromosomal anomalies
  o Congenital anomalies
  o Ectopic pregnancy
  o Blighted ovum
  o False pregnancy

Diagnostic Testing:

Diagnostic Tests and Procedures to Consider
- Maternal blood work
  o Kleinhauer-Betke
  o Hbg A1C
  o RPR/VDRL
  o Serum/urine toxicology screen
- Ultrasound
  o Absent fetal heart beat (verified by 2 examiners)
  o Overlapping of fetal cranial bones: Spalding sign
  o Presence of gas in fetal abdomen: Robert sign
- Fetal evaluation
  o Cord blood
  o Placenta to pathology
  o Skin biopsy
  o Fetal autopsy, per parents request
  o Genetic testing if indicated
    ▪ Anomalies

  ▪ Family history
  ▪ Recurrent fetal losses

Providing Treatment:

Therapeutic Measures to Consider
- Surgical D&E for early pregnancy
- Induction of labor
  o Prostin E2 suppositories
  o Misoprostol 50-100 mg per vagina or po
  o Oxytocin drip after 32 weeks gestation

Providing Treatment:

Alternative Measures to Consider
- Await onset of spontaneous labor
  o Emotionally difficult
  o Increased risk of DIC
- Natural remedies to stimulate labor
  o Blue/black cohosh
  o Castor oil
  o Homeopathic Caulophyllum Thal.

Providing Support:

Education and Support Measures to Consider
- Options for birth
- Discussion regarding labor initiation
  o Maternal preferences
  o Parameters for consultation
  o Therapeutic measures to initiate labor
- Location for birth
- Anticipated course of events
- Cause of death if known
- Care of the body
  o May vary with gestational age
  o Family time
  o Autopsy or testing
  o Burial
  o Cremation
  o Hospital disposal
  o Funeral
- Postpartum period
  o Lochia
  o Lactation
  o Depression
- Support groups/community resources

Follow-up Care:

Follow-up Measures to Consider
- Document
  o Findings
  o Education

- o   Plan for continued care
- o   Maternal response
  - ▪   Birth of babe
  - ▪   Anomalies if any
  - ▪   Care and arrangements for the babe
  - ▪   Placental disposition
  - ▪   Planned follow-up
- •   Follow-up care
  - o   1-6 weeks
  - o   Frequently by phone, home or office visit
  - o   Results of any testing
  - o   Evaluation of emotional status
  - o   2-6 weeks for
    - ▪   Postpartum check

- ▪   Initiation of birth control prn
- ▪   Support

Collaborative Practice:

Criteria to Consider for Consultation or Referral

- •   For fetal demise >12 weeks gestation
- •   For evidence of DIC
- •   For mother who prefers surgical D&E in early pregnancy
- •   For induction of labor
  - o   As indicated by midwifery scope of practice
  - o   Maternal preference
  - o   Per collaborative practice agreement

Care of the Pregnant Woman Exposed to Fifth's Disease

Key Clinical Information

Fifth's disease is caused by the Parvo B19 virus. It causes childhood erythema infectiosum. It is spread by droplet, most often in the springtime. Viremia occurs 7 days after inoculation, and lasts 4 days. It is common to have women who are school teachers find that their students have Fifth's disease. Fortunately, most women contracted Fifth's disease as children, and are no longer at risk for primary infection.[2]

---

[2]Division of Maternal-Fetal Medicine, MMC Ob/Gyn Associates. (Dec. 1997). I am a schoolteacher and there is fifth's disease in the school system: What do I do? Division of Maternal-Fetal Medicine Newsletter, 2, 1-2.

Client History:

Components of the History to Consider

- History of recent outbreak with close contact, i.e.
  - School teachers
  - Healthcare workers

Physical Examination:

Components of the Physical Exam to Consider

- Routine prenatal surveillance
  - Evaluate for rash
  - Rash
    - Occurs 16 days post inoculation
    - 5 days post disappearance of the virus
    - Children with rash are no longer infectious

Clinical Impression:

Differential Diagnoses to Consider

- Fifth's disease
- Viral exanthema
- Allergic rash

Diagnostic Testing:

Diagnostic Tests and Procedures to Consider

- Serologic testing for Parvo B19 indicated for
  - Post-exposure
  - Positive clinical signs and symptoms
  - Fetal non-immune hydrops
  - AFP
- Level II ultrasound
  - Cardiac evaluation
  - Fetal hydrops

Providing Treatment:

Therapeutic Measures to Consider

- None available

Providing Treatment:

Alternative Measures to Consider

- For possible exposure consider
  - Immune support
  - Rest
  - Whole foods diet, avoiding processed foods
  - Echinacea tincture 10 gtts tid x 10 days followed by 5-10 gtts daily

Providing Support:

Education and Support Measures to Consider

- Reassure: most adults are immune
- Potential for fetal
  - Demise
  - Hydrops
  - Anemia
- Explain screening and management plan
- Warning signs
  - Report rash if it occurs
  - Decreased fetal movement
- Effects of fetal infection
  - May have no effect
  - May cause spontaneous abortion in 1st trimester
  - May cause fetal death or stillbirth in 2nd trimester (3-6 weeks post maternal infection)
  - Non-immune hydrops
  - Severe anemia
  - Viral-induced cardiomyopathy
- May cause elevated AFP
- No association of Parvo B19 and birth defects

Follow-up Care:

Follow-up Measures to Consider

- Document
  - Findings
  - Education
  - Discussions with client
  - Results of testing
  - Plan for continued care
- Return for care
  - 2-3 weeks post-exposure
  - Mother with acute illness
- Follow for hydrops
  - Weekly ultrasound x 12 weeks

Collaborative Practice:

Criteria to Consider for Consultation or Referral

- Active infection with Parvo B19
- Fetus with evidence of
  - Hydrops
  - Anemia
  - Cardiomyopathy
- Fetal demise

Care of the Pregnant Woman with Gestational Diabetes

Key Clinical Information

Gestational diabetes occurs in 2-3% of all pregnant women in the U.S. There is s significant increase in fetal malformations in pregnant women with persistently elevated glucose levels. This risk is noted to be higher for women with Hgb A1c levels that are elevated early in pregnancy compared to those pregnant women whose Hgb A1c levels are normal in spite of abnormal glucose metabolism. Fructosamine shows control from the previous 2-4 weeks, while hemoglobin A1c shows control for previous 2-3 months.

It is especially important to enlist the participation of the mother when gestational diabetes presents. Daily attention to diet is imperative, with food sources providing excellent nutrition and a balance of proteins, fats, and complex carbohydrates. A food diary can be very helpful in determining what foods are preferred by the client, and making recommendations for changes that are culturally and financially reasonable.

Screening and Diagnostic Testing for Gestational Diabetes

Time	Whole Blood	Plasma
Fasting	90 gm/dl	105 gm/dl
1 Hr Glucose Challenge Test (GCT)	N/A	130-140 gm/dl
1 Hr. Glucose Tolerance Test (GTT)	165 gm/dl	190 gm/dl
2 Hr Glucose Tolerance Test (GTT)	145 gm/dl	165 gm/dl
3 Hr Glucose Tolerance Test (GTT	125 gm/dl	145 gm/dl

Client History:

Components of the History to Consider

- Identify risk factors for GDM
  - Maternal age > 35
  - Obesity
  - Previous GDM
  - Previous infant weighing > 4,100 g
  - Previous unexplained fetal demise
  - Family history of diabetes
  - Glycosuria
  - Polyhydramnios
  - Previous birth of a child with a congenital anomaly
  - Signs and symptoms of diabetes
  - Preeclampsia or chronic hypertension
  - Polyhydramnios

Physical Examination:

Components of the Physical Exam to Consider

- VS, including weight
- Weight/height
- Weight gain
- Monitor fundal heights for fetal macrosomia

Clinical Impression:

Differential Diagnoses to Consider

- Gestational diabetes
- Abnormal glucose metabolism
- Diabetes mellitus
- Fetal macrosomia secondary to
  - Gestational diabetes
  - Constitutionally large fetus
  - Polyhydramnios

Diagnostic Testing:

Diagnostic Tests and Procedures to Consider

- Dip U/A at each prenatal visit
- Serum screening
  - With risk factors screen at
    - First visit or first trimester
    - 24-28 weeks
    - 34-36 weeks
  - No risk factors screen at
    - 24-28 weeks
- Testing with indications only
  - Prior history of gestational diabetes
  - Obesity
  - Prior baby > 9 lbs.
  - Family history
- Screening methods
  - Fasting blood sugar
  - One or two hour glucose challenge test
  - If either screen is elevated obtain GTT

- Consider fructosamine or Hgb A1c
- Diagnosis
  - Elevated fasting *and* 1 or 2 hour glucose
  - Elevated 3 hour GTT
- Maternal assessment
  - Hgb A1C or fructosamine monthly
  - Hgb A1C
    - Normal range: 4.0-8.2%
    - <6% preferable in pregnancy
  - Frucosamine
    - Normal range: 205-285 micromol/L
  - Glucose monitoring (whole blood with glucometer)
    - Fasting 70-80 mg/dL
    - 1 hr post prandial <120 mg/dL
- Fetal assessment
  - Ultrasound
    - 12-24 weeks for fetal anomalies
    - 35 weeks: begin weekly U/S
    - Biophysical profile
    - Fetal size
  - NST: twice weekly beginning at 35 weeks
  - Fetal kick counts

Providing Treatment:

Therapeutic Measures to Consider

- Diet
  - Caloric intake by weight
  - Underweight - 40 Kcal/Kg/day
  - Average weight - 30 Kcal/Kg/day
  - Overweight – 24 Kcal/Kg/day
  - Carbohydrates 55-60% of diet
  - Protein 12-20% of diet
  - Fat for the remainder
  - 6 small meals daily
- Insulin, begin for FBS > 105
- Consider induction of labor at 37-38 weeks
  - Insulin required
  - Fetal macrosomia
  - Poor or marginal control
  - Based on tests for fetal well-being
- Plan birth at facility with newborn special care
  - Anticipate RDS

Providing Treatment:

Alternative Measures to Consider

- Macrobiotic or whole food diet
- Herbs
  - Chicory,
  - Dandelion,
  - Nettle
  - Red raspberry tea
  - Onion

Providing Support:

Education and Support Measures to Consider

- Risks and benefits of options for care
- Diabetic education
- Dietary recommendations
  o Provide information on balanced diet for GDM
  o Nutritionist or dietician referral
- Blood glucose testing
  o Home testing (fingerstick)
  o Office testing (fingerstick)
  o Lab testing (venipuncture)
- Maternal and fetal evaluation
- Increased risks related to GDM
- Provide instruction related to
  o Fetal surveillance
  o Blood sugar testing
  o Medication use
- Social services as indicated

Follow-up Care:

Follow-up Measures to Consider

- Document
- Findings
  o Lab results

o Maternal & fetal evaluation
- Patient discussions
  o Patient preferences
  o Midwifery plan of care
  o Parameters for consultation
  o Follow-up care
- Return visits weekly
  o Review/evaluation of blood sugars
  o Interval fetal growth
  o Maternal compliance with recommendations
  o Maternal and fetal well-being
- Blood sugars
  o Monitor weekly
  o Fasting
  o 2 hr post prandial
  o Bedtime
  o Fasting blood sugar at 6 weeks post-partum
    ▪ >126 mg/dL diagnostic of DM

Collaborative Practice:

Criteria to Consider for Consultation or Referral

- Gestational diabetic not controlled by diet
- Ongoing insulin dosage requirements
- Fetal macrosomia or anomalies

Care of the Pregnant Woman with Hepatitis B

Key Clinical Information

Hepatitis B is a viral illness that is transmitted via blood or body fluids. It may be vertically transmitted to the fetus during pregnancy. Infected women may become acutely ill, or may become a chronic carrier, that is asymptomatic, but able to transmit the infection. Individuals who have been immunized may not always develop immunity, and the immune response may diminish over time.

Client History:

Components of the History to Consider

- LMP, EDC, gestational age
- Immunization status
- Risk factors for any form of hepatitis
  o Health care professional
  o History of IV drug use, shared needles
  o Multiple sex partners for self or partner
  o Presence of tattoos
  o Ingestion of raw shellfish
  o Liver or gallbladder disease
- Presence, onset and duration, and severity of symptoms
  o Malaise and lethargy
  o Pale colored stools
  o Dark urine
  o Anorexia
  o Nausea/vomiting and/or diarrhea

Physical Examination:

Components of the Physical Exam to Consider

- VS, including weight
- Interval
  o Weight gain
  o Fundal height growth
- Examine for evidence of jaundice

o Skin
  o Mucous membranes
  o Sclera
- Palpate and percuss for
  o Liver margins
  o Splenomegaly
  o RUQ pain

Clinical Impression:

Differential Diagnoses to Consider

- Hepatitis B
- Hepatitis A
- Hepatitis C
- Obstructive cholelithiasis
- Other liver disorders

Diagnostic Testing:

Diagnostic Tests and Procedures to Consider

- Hepatitis B surface antibody; immunized individuals
- Hepatitis B surface antigen; non-immunized individuals
- Hepatitis profile
  o Hepatitis B
  o Hepatitis A
  o Hepatitis C
- Liver function testing (LFTs)
  o SGOT, SGPT

- o   ↑ during acute phase
- Ultrasound, RUQ
  - o   Gallbladder

Providing Treatment:

Therapeutic Measures to Consider

- Supportive therapy for mother
- Medical therapies as prescribed by PCP
- Administer to infant following birth
  - o   Hepatitis B immune globulin
  - o   Hep-B-Gammagee 0.5 ml
    - ▪   IM in anterior thigh at birth
  - o   Hepatitis B vaccine
    - ▪   Engerix-B 10 mcg/0.5ml
    - ▪   Recombivax HB 5 mcg/0.5ml
    - ▪   IM in anterior thigh at birth
    - ▪   Repeat in 1 and 6 mo.

Providing Treatment:

Alternative Measures to Consider

- Whole foods diet with minimum of toxins
- Herbs
  - o   Milk thistle tea
  - o   Silymarin 420 mg (from milk thistle) tid x 6 weeks
- Adequate rest

Providing Support:

Education and Support Measures to Consider

- Provide information about hepatitis
  - o   Transmission
  - o   Prevention
  - o   Medication recommendations for infant
  - o   Breastfeeding

- ▪   Not contraindicated for immunized infant
- ▪   Not recommended for non-immunized infant
- Discussion regarding
  - o   Options for care of self and infant
  - o   Disease
  - o   Medications
  - o   Location for birth
  - o   Parameters for referral

Follow-up Care:

Follow-up Measures to Consider

- Document
  - o   History
  - o   Physical findings
  - o   Laboratory results
  - o   Discussions with patient/family
  - o   Patient preferences
  - o   Midwifery plan of care
- Return for care
  - o   Per routine for carrier
  - o   Weekly for acute phase of infection
    - ▪   Periodic LFTs
    - ▪   Fetal evaluation with acute illness

Collaborative Practice:

Criteria to Consider for Consultation or Referral

- Acute hepatitis, any type
- Pediatric care provider consult
  - o   Prior to birth
  - o   Collaborative plan for newborn care
- Hepatitis C to hepatitis specialist for consideration of medication regimen postpartum

Care of the Pregnant Woman with Herpes Simplex Virus

Key Clinical Information

Infection of the infant with the herpes simplex virus (HSV) varies with the incidence of primary versus secondary infection. When primary infection with HSV occurs during pregnancy the perinatal infection rate may be as high as 50%. With secondary, or recurrent, HSV infection during pregnancy the perinatal infection rate diminishes to approximately 4%. Up to 60% of infants who are infected as a result of primary maternal infection will die from severe neonatal HSV, and the mother may be asymptomatic in up to 70% of instances where the infant is infected.[3]

---

[3] Emmons, L., Callahan, P., Gorman, P., Snyder, M. (1997) Primary care management of common dermatologic disorders in women. Journal of Nurse-Midwifery, 42, 228-253.

Client History:

Components of the History to Consider

- LMP, EDC, gestational age
- Current sexual history
- Previous history of
  - o Genital or oral herpes
  - o Other STIs
- Duration and quality of present symptoms
  - o Presence of vesicular lesions
  - o Location
    - ▪ Oral
    - ▪ Genital
  - o Number
  - o Symptoms
    - ▪ Pain
    - ▪ Tingling
    - ▪ Dysuria
    - ▪ Headache
    - ▪ Photophobia
- Primary infection associated with
  - o Fever
  - o Headache
  - o Malaise
  - o Aseptic meningitis

Physical Examination:

Components of the Physical Exam to Consider

- VS, including temperature
- Physical evaluation with emphasis on
  - o Oral examination
  - o Inguinal lymph nodes
    - ▪ Enlargement
    - ▪ Tenderness
  - o External genitalia, buttocks and pelvic region
    - ▪ Characteristic lesions
    - ▪ Vesicles
    - ▪ Shallow ulcers
  - o Speculum exam
    - ▪ Presence of other STD symptoms
    - ▪ Cervical discharge
    - ▪ Cervical or uterine motion tenderness

Clinical Impression:

Differential Diagnoses to Consider

- Herpes simplex infection (HSV)
  - o Primary
  - o Recurrent
- Other STI
- Genital trauma

Diagnostic Testing:

Diagnostic Tests and Procedures to Consider

- Culture lesions for HSV
- Consider serum testing for HSV antibody titer
  - o Documents primary infection
  - o Repeat 7-10 days
  - o Four-fold increase = primary infection
- Other SDI testing
  - o With symptoms
  - o As indicated by history

Providing Treatment:

Therapeutic Measures to Consider

- Valtrex (valacyclovir hydrochloride)
  - o Pregnancy category B
  - o Pregnancy registry 1-800-722-9292 ext. 39437
  - o Dose: 500 mg bid x 5 d
  - o Begin medication within 24 hours of first symptom
- Famvir (famciclovir)
  - o Pregnancy category B
  - o Dose: 125 mg bid x 5 d
  - o Begin medication within 6 hours of first symptom
- Zovirax (Acyclovir)
  - o Pregnancy category C
  - o Pregnancy registry 1- 800-722-9292 ext. 58465
  - o Topical ointment 5%
    - ▪ Apply 3 x day x 7d
  - o Initial outbreak
    - ▪ 200 mg po 5 x day x 10 days
  - o Recurrent outbreak
    - ▪ 200 mg po 5 x day x 7 days
    - ▪ Repeat treatment prn
  - o Suppression or severe recurrent outbreaks
    - ▪ 400 mg po bid x 6-12 mo.
- Tylenol for pain relief

Providing Treatment:

Alternative Measures to Consider

- Lysine
  - o 1000 mg po bid x 3 months
  - o Begin with first sign of an outbreak
- Echinacea
  - o Tea, tincture, tablets or capsules t
  - o Tid x 2 weeks
- Sitz bath or salve made with:
  - o Lemon balm
  - o Calendula
  - o Comfrey

Providing Support:

Education and Support Measures to Consider

- Information about herpes (HSV) infection
- Effect of infection on
  - o Pregnancy
  - o Baby
  - o Labor and birth plans
    - ▪ Anticipated location for birth
    - ▪ Potential for Cesarean birth
- Discussion regarding
  - o Treatment options
  - o Labor and birth options
  - o Maternal preferences
  - o Midwife recommendations
- Dietary recommendations
  - o *Include* foods high in lysine
    - ▪ Brewer's yeast
    - ▪ Potatoes
    - ▪ Fish
  - o *Avoid* foods high in arginine
    - ▪ Chocolate
    - ▪ Cola
    - ▪ Peanuts, cashews, pecans, almonds
    - ▪ Sunflower and sesame seeds
    - ▪ Peas and corn
    - ▪ Coconut
    - ▪ Gelatin.
- Rest and comfort measures
  - o With initial outbreak
  - o To enhance immune response

Follow-up Care:

Follow-up Measures to Consider

- Document
  - o History
  - o Physical findings
  - o Laboratory results
  - o Discussions
    - ▪ Patient preferences
    - ▪ Informed consent, prn

- o   Midwifery plan of care
- Return for care
  - o   Per routine with history of herpes
  - o   For culture with active lesion
  - o   Primary herpes
    - ▪   If symptoms persist > 10 days
    - ▪   Worsening symptoms i.e.
      - •   Stiff neck
      - •   Unremitting fever
      - •   Inability to urinate

- Care of patient with active herpes
  - o   During pregnancy
    - ▪   For medication, based on
      - •   Client preference
      - •   Midwife scope of practice
    - ▪   For discussion regarding
      - •   Potential for Cesarean birth
  - o   Onset of labor
    - ▪   In presence of active lesion

Collaborative Practice:

Criteria to Consider for Consultation or Referral

- For symptoms of herpes meningitis

Care of the Pregnant Woman who is HIV Positive

Key Clinical Information

HIV testing is recommended for every pregnant woman whose current HIV status is unknown. Early testing allows for prompt evaluation and the potential for anti-retroviral medication which may decrease the incidence of perinatal transmission of the infection considerably. Many women feel threatened by the thought of HIV testing. Many states require HIV specific pre-test counseling and documentation of informed consent prior to test specimen collection.

Client History:

Components of the History to Consider

- LMP, EDC, gestational age
- GYN & Sexual history
  - o   Current sexual practices
  - o   Previous sexual practices
  - o   Number of sexual partners
  - o   Partner(s) sexual practices
  - o   Abnormal pap smears
- Self and/or partner(s)
  - o   STIs
  - o   Substance abuse
  - o   IV drug use
  - o   Other substance use
  - o   Blood transfusions
  - o   History of opportunistic infections
- Current symptoms
  - o   Fever
  - o   Cough
  - o   Skin lesions

Physical Examination:

Components of the Physical Exam to Consider

- VS, including temperature
- HEENT
  - o   Fundoscopic exam
  - o   Oral exam for thrush or lesions
- Skin lesions
- Respiratory system
  - o   Cough
  - o   Adventitious breath sounds
  - o   SOB
- Liver margins
- Lymph nodes
  - o   Characteristics of enlarged nodes

- o   Location(s) of enlarged nodes
- Pelvic exam
  - o   Internal or external lesions
  - o   Symptoms of STIs

Clinical Impression:

Differential Diagnoses to Consider

- HIV infection
- AIDS
- STIs
- Monilia, secondary to
  - o   Antibiotic use
  - o   Diabetes

Diagnostic Testing:

Diagnostic Tests and Procedures to Consider

- Pap smear
- Wet mount
- Toxoplasmosis titer
- CMV titer
- Herpes culture
- CD4 and viral load q trimester
- Liver function tests
- PPD

Providing Treatment:

Therapeutic Measures to Consider

- Antiretroviral therapy (See current facility guidelines for medication regimen)
- Other therapies based on diagnosis

Providing Treatment:

Alternative Measures to Consider

- Supportive measures
- Most immune stimulating herbs *not* recommended

- Cautious use of herbals/homeopathic remedies for
  - o Appetite stimulation
  - o Skin integrity
  - o Emotional & spiritual balance

Providing Support:

Education and Support Measures to Consider

- Information, listening & discussion regarding
  - o HIV and AIDS
  - o Prevention and transmission
  - o Benefits of testing
  - o Viral load evaluation & significance
  - o Potential effects on baby
  - o Medication and treatment options
    - Perinatal transmission
    - Antiretroviral medication (for self and/or baby)
      - Benefits
      - Risks
      - Side effects
      - Alternatives
  - o Lifestyle issues
  - o Patient/family preferences
  - o Local resources
    - Support groups
    - Clean needle programs
    - Substance abuse treatment options
    - Victim advocacy groups
- Encourage
  - o Abstinence, or
  - o Consistent condom use
  - o Avoid shared needles

Follow-up Care:

Follow-up Measures to Consider

- Antiretroviral Pregnancy Registry (Glaxo-Smith-Kline)1-800-722-9292

- Document
  - o History
  - o Risk factors
  - o Review of systems
  - o Physical findings
  - o Consent for testing, prn
  - o Clinical impression
  - o Laboratory results
  - o Midwifery plan of care
  - o Maternal response to diagnosis or treatment recommendations
  - o Discussions
  - o Patient preferences
  - o Consultations & referrals
- Follow-up care
- Planned location for birth
- Pediatric consult
- Return visits
- As indicated by prenatal course & gestation
- For support

Collaborative Practice:

Criteria to Consider for Consultation or Referral

- For all newly diagnosed HIV positive women
- For any HIV positive women with
  - o Onset of infection
  - o Decrease CD4 cell counts (Co-ordinate testing with primary care provider/site)
  - o For initiation of antiretroviral regimen
- As indicated for
  - o Social service referrals
  - o Drug rehabilitation center referrals
  - o Mental health referrals

Inadequate Weight Gain

Key Clinical Information

Inadequate weight gain may be an indicator for a number of medical problems. The most common cause, however, is inadequate nutrition, which may be related to poverty, substance abuse, or mental illness. Women with a history of anorexia or bulimia may have difficulty maintaining adequate intake to support growth of a healthy baby. Overweight women may require fewer calories during pregnancy, while still demonstrating adequate fundal growth. Adequate fetal growth is the most reassuring parameter of fetal well-being when maternal weight gain is modest.

Client History:

Components of the History to Consider

- LMP, EDC, gestational age
- Accuracy of LMP
- Physical health issues
  - o Preferred diet
  - o Food sources available
  - o Activity level and general metabolic rate
- Presence of other symptoms i.e.
  - o Nausea & vomiting
  - o Constipation
    - o Abdominal pain
    - o Pica
- Prior health history
  - o Presence of maternal illness or infection
  - o Hyperthyroid
  - o TORCH
  - o Hepatitis
- Emotional & spiritual health issues
  - o Stress levels & coping skills
  - o Family & personal support for pregnancy
  - o Mental illness
  - o Social living conditions

- o   Prior history of anorexia or bulimia
- Substance abuse

Physical Examination:

Components of the Physical Exam to Consider

- VS
- Physical exam with focus on
  - o   Weight & its distribution
  - o   Pre-pregnancy weight
  - o   Interval gain
  - o   Fundal heights
    - For gestation
    - Fundal height growth curve
  - o   Dental/oral evaluation
    - Caries
    - Abscess
- Evaluation of other symptoms

Clinical Impression:

Differential Diagnoses to Consider

- Intrauterine growth retardation
  - o   Note secondary cause if known
  - o   PIH
  - o   Eating disorder
  - o   Mental illness
  - o   Substance abuse
  - o   Social issues leading to malnutrition
    - Homeless
    - Physical abuse
    - Poverty
- Small for gestational age baby
- Constitutionally small baby

Diagnostic Testing:

Diagnostic Tests and Procedures to Consider

- Labs
  - o   PIH labs
  - o   Toxicology if drug use suspected
  - o   Cotenine levels (smokers)
  - o   TSH
  - o   Serum albumin
  - o   Hepatitis screen
  - o   TORCH screen
- Fetal kick counts
- Ultrasound for
  - o   Gestational age
  - o   AFI
  - o   Evidence of IUGR
  - o   Interval fetal growth

Providing Treatment:

Therapeutic Measures to Consider

- Diet & nutrition counseling
- Minimum of 1000 cal/day up to 2400 cal/day
- Dietary supplements
  - o   Ensure
  - o   Boost
  - o   Slim-fast
- Hospitalization for
  - o   Anorexia or bulimia
  - o   Malnutrition
  - o   Significant mental illness

Providing Treatment:

Alternative Measures to Consider

- Dietary supplements
  - o   Spirulina
  - o   Smoothies
- Homeopathic Pulsatilla
  - o   For persistent nausea
  - o   Intolerance of fatty foods

- Herbal appetite stimulants
  - o   May be combined for flavor and effectiveness
  - o   Alfalfa 500 mg daily (avoid with lupus or allergies to pollen)
  - o   Dandelion root tea 1 cup bid (avoid with hx gallstones)
  - o   Hops tea 1-2 cups daily
  - o   Chamomile tea 1-2 cups daily

Providing Support:

Education and Support Measures to Consider

- Concern about weight gain/fetal growth pattern
- Anticipated weight gain for gestation
- Importance of
  - o   Fundal/fetal growth over weight gain
  - o   Maternal and fetal well-being
  - o   Dietary needs during pregnancy
  - o   Small frequent meals
  - o   Balanced selection of food choices
  - o   Adequate caloric intake
- Potential effect on
  - o   Planned location for birth
  - o   Need for pediatric care at birth
- Provide information about
  - o   IUGR babies
  - o   Small for gestational age babies
  - o   Constitutionally small babies
  - o   Fetal kick counts
- Warning signs
  - o   Decreased fetal motion
  - o   PIH signs and symptoms
- Provide support
- Develop plan *with* patient
- Address patient/family concerns

Follow-up Care:

Follow-up Measures to Consider

- Document
  - o   Relevant history
  - o   Physical findings
  - o   Diagnostic testing
  - o   Patient concerns and preferences
  - o   Clinical impression
  - o   Discussions with patient
- Midwifery plan of care
  - o   Parameters for consultation or referrals
  - o   Anticipated follow-up
- Return for care
  - o   Re-evaluate weekly or bi-weekly for
    - Interval fetal growth
    - Signs and symptoms of PIH
    - Nutritional counseling
    - Emotional issues

Collaborative Practice:

Criteria to Consider for Consultation or Referral

- Persistent poor weight gain accompanied by
  - o   Lagging fetal growth
  - o   Asymmetric fetal growth
  - o   Evidence of malnutrition
  - o   Suspected or documented
    - Mental health issues
    - PIH
    - Medical illness
    - Drug abuse
- Social service referral
- Nutritional counseling
- For transfer of care or change planned location of birth

Pregnancy Induced Hypertension

Key Clinical Information

Pregnancy induced hypertension is a broad category that includes hypertension, severe hypertension, gestational hypertension, pre-eclampsia, eclampsia, and HELLP syndrome. Differential diagnosis can be challenging as PIH may present with an uncommon array of symptoms. Lab testing is the most reliable way to assess a woman's potential for development of PIH. Onset of clinical signs and symptoms suggesting PIH should prompt careful evaluation in order to have the opportunity to institute early treatment. Treatment improves the likelihood of having a healthy mother, healthy baby, and increases the mother's chance for a vaginal birth.

Client History:

Components of the History to Consider

- LMP, EDC, gestational age
- Presence, onset & durations of symptoms
  - o Edema
  - o Headache
  - o Fatigue
  - o Epigastric or right upper quadrant pain
- Evaluate for risk factors
  - o History of essential hypertension
  - o Hydatidiform mole (10x risk)
  - o Fetal hydrops (10x risk)
  - o Primigravida (6-8x risk)
  - o Hypertension in previous pregnancy
  - o Diabetes
  - o Collagen vascular disease
  - o Renal vascular disease
  - o Renal parenchymal disease
  - o Multiple gestation (5x risk)
  - o African-American heritage
  - o Age < 20 & > 35
  - o Social habits
    - ▪ Smoking
    - ▪ Alcohol use
    - ▪ Excessive salt intake
    - ▪ Current vasoactive drug use
    - ▪ Nasal decongestants
    - ▪ Cocaine
  - o Prior use of anti-hypertensive medications
  - o Other complicating medical factors
  - o Family history

Physical Examination:

Components of the Physical Exam to Consider

- Vital signs including BP & weight
- Weight: patterns of gain
- Blood Pressure
  - o At least two occasions > 4 hours apart
  - o Allow a 'rest' period following
    - ▪ Anxiety
    - ▪ Pain
    - ▪ Smoking
    - ▪ Exercise
  - o Equipment of correct size should be used
  - o Use same maternal position for each BP
  - o Arm should be supported at level of the heart
- Extremities for

  - o Presence or absence of edema
  - o Deep tendon reflexes
- Abdominal exam
  - o Fundal heights for evaluation of fetal growth
  - o Liver margins
  - o Epigastric pain
- Monitor pulmonary status

Clinical Impression:

Differential Diagnoses to Consider

- Pre-existing hypertension
- PIH superimposed on chronic hypertension
- Pregnancy induced hypertension (PIH)
- Pre-eclampsia
- Eclampsia
- HELLP syndrome

Diagnostic Testing:

Diagnostic Tests and Procedures to Consider

- Baseline PIH labs
  - o Urine analysis for protein by dip
  - o Hematocrit (normal range10.5-14 G/dL)
  - o Platelet count (normal range 130,000-400,000/ml)
  - o Liver function tests
    - ▪ SGOT (normal range 0-35U/L)
  - o Coagulation studies
  - o Kidney function tests
    - ▪ Serum uric acid (normal range 1.2-4.5 mg/dL)
    - ▪ Serum albumin (normal range 2.5-4.5 G/dL)
    - ▪ Serum creatinine (normal range <1.0 mg/dL)
    - ▪ BUN
- 24 hour urine for protein and creatinine when dip U/A shows > 1+ protein
- Fetal evaluation
  - o Fetal kick counts
  - o NST
  - o Ultrasound if IUGR is suspected
  - o Periodic biophysical testing

Providing Treatment:

Therapeutic Measures to Consider

- Increase calcium intake (1200 mg daily)
- Limit activity
- Consider hospitalization
- Medications
  - o MGSO4
  - o 4 Gm IV bolus

o Followed by 2 G/hr
o Titrated to renal output & reflexes
- Monitor intake and output
- Delivery if no improvement or condition worsens

Providing Treatment:

Alternative Measures to Consider
- Balanced nutrition
- No salt restriction
- Whole foods diet
- Adequate protein intake
- Garlic, 1 clove or the equivalent daily
- Cucumbers, 1 daily
- Hops tea, 1 cup night in last month of pregnancy
- Hawthorn berries
- Best for chronic hypertension
- Infusion: 1 cup daily
- Tincture: 15 drops tid

Providing Support:

Education and Support Measures to Consider
- Discussion with client/family regarding
  o PIH
  o Treatment options/recommendations
  o Smoking cessation
  o Drug treatment plans, if indicated
  o Attention to
  o Diet
  o Rest
  o Low-key exercise with mild PIH
  o Potential need for
    ▪ Hospitalization
    ▪ OB/GYN consultation/referral
    ▪ Change planned location for birth

- Pediatric care at birth
- Newborn special care after birth
- Indications for immediate care
  o Epigastric pain
  o Scotomata
  o Visual disturbance
  o Severe headache

Follow-up Care:

Follow-up Measures to Consider
- Document
  o Chief complaint
  o Review of systems
  o Physical findings
  o Lab results
  o Discussion with patient/family
  o Clinical impression
  o Midwifery plan of care
    ▪ Parameters for consultation & referral
    ▪ Update plan weekly or as indicated
    ▪ Return visit
- Increased frequency of return visits
  o Bi-weekly in compliant patient
  o Early hospitalization for non-compliant patient
  o Fetal surveillance testing
  o Maternal evaluation/labs

Collaborative Practice:

Criteria to Consider for Consultation or Referral
- For chronic hypertensive in pregnancy
- With diagnosis of preeclampsia or PIH
- For abnormal lab values (consider HELLP)
- IUGR

Pruritic Urticarial Papules & Plaques of Pregnancy (PUPPP)

Key Clinical Information

Puritic uticarial papules and plaques of pregnancy most commonly appears in the third trimester. It generally resolves within 7 days of the birth. There are no systemic disorders associated with PUPPP, therefore treatment is aimed at relieving symptoms.

Client History:

Components of the History to Consider
- LMP, EDC, gestational age
- Onset, duration and severity of symptoms
- Location of initial eruptions
- Pattern of spread
- Medication history
- Presence of allergies
- Immune titers
- Exposure to viral infections, including
  o Herpes
  o Rubella
  o Measles
  o Chicken Pox
- Exposure to topical irritants
  o Detergents
  o Fleas
  o Plant material

- Self-help remedies and their effects

Physical Examination:

Components of the Physical Exam to Consider
- VS, including temperature
- FHR
- Location and appearance of lesions
  o Appear initially on abdomen
  o May spread to
    ▪ Thighs
    ▪ Buttocks
    ▪ Chest
  o Appearance of lesions
    ▪ Erythematous, edematous papules
    ▪ Urticarial plaques
    ▪ May form papulovesicular lesions

Clinical Impression:

Differential Diagnoses to Consider
- PUPPPs

- Erythema multiforme
- Allergic/drug reaction
- Viral exanthema
- Scabies
- Herpes gestationis
- Poison ivy

Diagnostic Testing:

Diagnostic Tests and Procedures to Consider

- PIH testing
- Culture of vesicular lesions
  - o Herpes
  - o Impetigo
- Immune titers
  - o Rubella
  - o Rubeola
  - o Varicella

Providing Treatment:

Therapeutic Measures to Consider

- Topical corticosteroids
  - o Pregnancy category C
  - o Rule out viral cause before using
  - o Alclometasone dipropionate 0.05%
  - o Aclovate cream or ointment
  - o Hydrocortisone 1%
  - o Cortisporin cream
  - o Hytone cream, lotion or ointment
  - o Triamcinolone acetonide 0.025%, 0.1%, 0.5%
  - o Aristocort cream
  - o Kenalog cream, lotion or ointment
- Topical antipuritic lotions
  - o Calamine, caladryl (OTC)
  - o Doxepin HCL 5% cream (Cat. B)
- Oral antihistamines
  - o Diphebhydramine HCL (Benadryl)
  - o 25-50 mg q 4-6 hrs
  - o Preg. Cat. B in third trimester
  - o Loratadine (Claritin)
  - o 10 mg daily
  - o Preg. Cat. B in third trimester
  - o Cetirizine HCL (Zyrtec)
  - o 5-10 mg daily
  - o Preg. Cat. B in third trimester

Providing Treatment:

Alternative Measures to Consider

- Topical relief of itching
  - o Colloidal oatmeal baths
  - o Calendula cream
- Herbal support
  - o Yellow dock root
  - o Dandelion root
- Homeopathic support
  - o Cantharis
  - o Rhus. Tox.
  - o Urticaria

Providing Support:

Education and Support Measures to Consider

- PUPPP not associated with fetal jeopardy
- Call if symptoms persist or worsen
- Address patient concerns
- Treatment options
- Medication instructions
  - o Topical steroids
  - o Apply thin film only
  - o Do not cover or occlude
  - o May be systemically absorbed

Follow-up Care:

Follow-up Measures to Consider

- Document
  - o Chief complaint
  - o Review of systems
  - o Physical findings
  - o Lab testing
  - o Clinical impression
  - o Midwifery plan of care
- Return for care
  - o Per routine for prenatal care
  - o If symptoms worsen or additional symptoms develop

Collaborative Practice:

Criteria to Consider for Consultation or Referral

- No relief of symptoms with treatment
- Rash accompanied by
  - o Fever
  - o Malaise
  - o Rising titers
  - o Elevated liver function tests

Care of the Woman who is Rh Negative

Key Clinical Information

Rh isoimmunization or ABO incompatibility can have devastating results on both mother and baby. Infants become at-risk when there is feto-maternal bleeding that initiates the process of Rh or ABO incompatibility, or if the mother became sensitized previously following blood transfusion. This may result from an Rh positive infant that is born to an Rh negative mother, a baby with type A or B blood born to a mother with type O blood, a baby with type B or type AB blood born to a mother with type A blood, or a baby with type A or AB blood born to a mother with type B blood.

Often the baby who is being carried when the feto-maternal bleed occurs may not have a problem, but the mother becomes sensitized. The problem will manifest itself in a subsequent pregnancy when maternal antibodies attack the fetal blood. This may have devastating results on the fetus.

Client History:

Components of the History to Consider
- Previous blood transfusions
- Prior obstetrical history
  - Unexplained fetal losses
  - Stillborn
  - Miscarriage,
  - Ectopic pregnancy or t
  - Termination of pregnancy at >8 since LMP
- Indications for Rh immune globulin administration in an unsensitized Rh negative woman include any procedure or trauma that may cause maternal/fetal bleeding, such as:
  - Amniocentesis
  - Chorionic villus sampling
  - External version
  - Trauma, such as with a car accident
  - Placenta previa
  - Abruptio placenta
  - Fetal death
  - Multiple gestation
  - Cesarean section
  - 28 weeks gestation prophylaxis if father of baby is Rh positive or his Rh status is unknown
  - Accidental transfusion of Rh-positive blood to an Rh-negative person

Physical Examination:

Components of the Physical Exam to Consider
- Routine prenatal surveillance

Clinical Impression:

Differential Diagnoses to Consider
- Rh negative mother
- Rh sensitized mother
- ABO sensitized mother

Diagnostic Testing:

Diagnostic Tests and Procedures to Consider
- Maternal – 1st prenatal and repeat at 24-28 weeks for Rh-negative mothers
  - Type and Rh factor
  - Antibody screen (Indirect Coombs)
  - Antibody ID for positive antibody screen
  - Antepartum RhIG for amnio or threatened SAB with give positive titer at 24-28 week screen
- Maternal Test Results
- Titer < 1:8 anti-D – suggests passive immunity from RhIG
- Titer > 1:8 – suggests active immunization due to Rh incompatibility
- If mother is Rh(D)-negative, or Type O
- Newborn
  - Type and Rh
  - Direct Coombs
  - Bilirubin levels
- Maternal testing postpartum
  - Type and Rh
  - Antibody screen (Indirect Coombs)
  - Antibody ID for positive antibody screen

- Fetal red cell screen
- Kleihauer-Betke quantitative testing
  - Determine volume of fetal blood in maternal system and dosage of Rh IG to give mother
  - Performed when high-risk of feto-maternal hemorrhage
    - Previa
    - Abruption
    - Abdominal trauma
    - Hydrops
    - Sinusoidal fetal heart rates
    - Unexplained fetal demise

Providing Treatment:

Therapeutic Measures to Consider
- Offer Rh Immune Globulin for (Pregnancy Category C)
  - Threatened or spontaneous miscarriage < 12 weeks give 50 or 300 µg IM
  - Procedures or trauma give 300 µg IM
  - 28-36 week prophylaxis give 300 µg IM with negative 28 week antibody screen
  - Postpartum give 300 µg IM
  - Provide to unsensitized Rh-negative mother with Rh-positive infant
  - Give ASAP after birth, preferably within 72 hours postpartum
- Adjust dose for large feto-maternal transfusion based on lab results
  - IV administration
    - 9 µg/ml whole blood or 18 µg/ml of RBCs
    - 800 µg q 8 hrs until total dose delivered
  - IM administration
    - 12µg/ml whole blood or 24µg/ml of RBCs
    - 1200 µg q 12 hrs until total dose delivered

Providing Treatment:

Alternative Measures to Consider
- Work to maintain a healthy pregnancy & placenta
- Well balance diet
- Decrease or eliminate fluoride intake (may interfere with placental attachment)
- Ensure adequate trace mineral intake
  - Sea vegetables
  - Mineral supplement
- Avoid invasive procedures
- Avoid traumatic placental delivery

Providing Support:

Education and Support Measures to Consider
- Provide information about
  - Rh and blood type status
  - Rh immune globulin
  - Prophylaxis and desired result
  - Potential risks with Rh immune globulin
    - Transfusion-type adverse reactions
    - Mercury sensitivity or reaction with RhoGAM® (mother or fetus w/ prophylactic dose)

- o   Potential risks without Rh immune globulin
  - Maternal sensitization
  - Fetal hydrops or other complications with future pregnancy
  - Difficulty cross-matching blood for woman in future, i.e., following accident or surgery
  - Potential for jaundice in infant due to Rh or ABO incompatibility

Follow-up Care:
Follow-up Measures to Consider

- Document
  - o   Indication for RhIG
  - o   Negative Rh and antibody status
  - o   Client education, discussion, and preferences
  - o   Administration of medication
    - Dose
    - Lot #

- Expiration date
- o   Observe for potential blood transfusion-type reactions
  - Warmth at injection site
  - Low-grade fever
  - Flushing
  - Chest or lumbar pain
  - Poor clotting
- Anticipated follow-up
- Indications for consultation or referrals

Collaborative Practice:
Criteria to Consider for Consultation or Referral

- For Rh-negative mother with positive antibody screen
- Evidence of large feto-maternal bleed
- Transfusion-type reactions

Size-Date Discrepancy

Key Clinical Information

Size-date discrepancy has a multitude of potential contributing factors, with the most common causes including intrauterine growth retardation and gestational diabetes. Many babies may, however, simply be constitutionally small or large. Evaluation of overall interval fetal growth as well as the symmetry of growth can help determine the correct diagnosis.

Client History:
Components of the History to Consider

- LMP, EDC
- Verify gestational age
  - o   Estimated date of conception
  - o   Size at first visit
  - o   Date of quickening
  - o   Early U/S report
- Diet history
- Tobacco, alcohol or drug use
- Birth weights of prior infants
- Personal or family Hx diabetes
- Other preexisting disease
- Psycho-social factors

Physical Examination:
Components of the Physical Exam to Consider

- Vital signs including BP & weight
- Weight gain/loss & pattern
- Presence/absence of edema
- General appearance/well-being
- Reflexes
- Palpation of thyroid
- Abdominal exam
  - o   Fundal height
  - o   Interval growth
  - o   Fetal lie
  - o   FHR
- Physical evidence of substance abuse
- Pelvic exam
  - o   Station of presenting part
  - o   Evidence of ROM

Clinical Impression:
Differential Diagnoses to Consider

- Small for dates
  - o   Incorrect dates
  - o   Intrauterine growth retardation
  - o   Small for gestational age
  - o   Oligohydramnios
  - o   Constitutionally small infant
  - o   Congenital malformations
- Large for dates
  - o   Incorrect dates
  - o   Large for gestational age
  - o   Gestational or maternal diabetes
  - o   Multiple pregnancy
  - o   Polyhydramnios
  - o   Constitutionally large infant
  - o   Fibroid uterus
- IUGR (Intrauterine growth retardation)
  - o   Symmetric vs. asymmetric IUGR secondary to:
    - Hypertension
    - Underlying maternal disease or infection
    - Poor nutrition
- SGA (Small for gestational age)
  - o   May be constitutionally small infant
  - o   May be incorrect EDC
  - o   May be IUGR
- LGA (Large for gestational age)
  - o   May be constitutionally large infant
- May be incorrect EDC
- May be gestational diabetes
- May be multiple gestation

Diagnostic Testing:

Diagnostic Tests and Procedures to Consider

- Labs
  - o Dip U/A
  - o Diabetes screen
  - o MSAFP (may be ⇑ in early pregnancy)
  - o Toxicology
  - o Maternal drug screen
- Symmetric IUGR
  - o Fetal karyotype
  - o TORCH titers
  - o PIH labs
- Ultrasound evaluation
  - o Verify singleton pregnancy
  - o EDC by U/S parameters
  - o Fetal growth – may be done serially
  - o Schedule at least 3 weeks apart
  - o Abdominal circumference
    - ▪ Decreased in asymmetric IUGR
  - o Umbilical arterial flow studies
  - o AFI for oligo- or polyhydramnios
  - o Anomaly study
  - o Presence of fibroids
  - o Placenta previa
- Fetal surveillance for IUGR
  - o Begin as early as IUGR suspected
  - o Weekly NST
  - o Consider OCT or CST if NST non-reactive
  - o AFI – weekly, should be >6

Providing Treatment:

Therapeutic Measures to Consider

- Treatment of any underlying medical condition
- Consider delivery if fetal compromise evident
- Substance abuse treatment
- IUGR
  - o Decrease maternal activity
  - o Left lateral position to ⇑ placental blood flow
  - o Ensure adequate nutrition and oxygenation

Providing Treatment:

Alternative Measures to Consider

- Nutritional counseling & surveillance
  - o Evaluation of intake
  - o Adequate hydration
  - o Careful food choices for maximum nutrition

Providing Support:

Education and Support Measures to Consider

- Discussion & information about
  - o Clinical impression
    - o Options for treatment
    - o Parameters for intervention
    - o Induction
    - o Change in location or providers for birth
    - o Labor evaluation of fetal well-being
- Provide support
- Address patient/family concerns

Follow-up Care:

Follow-up Measures to Consider

- Document
  - o Relevant history
  - o Physical findings
  - o Results of diagnostic testing
  - o Clinical impression
  - o Discussions with client/family
  - o Midwifery plan of care
  - o Indications for consultation/referral
- Anticipated follow-up
  - o Update plan weekly or as indicated
  - o Anticipate potential need for
    - ▪ Pediatric care at birth
    - ▪ Anticipate need for birth before term with
      - • Positive OCT or CST
      - • Oligohydramnios
      - • U/S documentation of limited cranial growth
  - o LGA infant anticipate potential for
    - ▪ Shoulder dystocia
    - ▪ Newborn resuscitation
      - • In utero
      - • Post delivery

Collaborative Practice:

Criteria to Consider for Consultation or Referral

- As indicated for
  - o Transfer of care
  - o Change in planned location for birth
- For documented IUGR
  - o Prenatal consultation
  - o Potential referral to high-risk OB service
  - o Arrange pediatric coverage at delivery
- For anticipated LGA infant
  - o If induction considered
  - o As needed for birth
- Social services as indicated
  - o Tobacco, drug or ETOH use
  - o Anticipated preterm infant
  - o Poor support systems

Toxoplasmosis

Key Clinical Information

Acute primary maternal infection with toxoplasmosis puts the unborn baby at risk for congenital toxoplasmosis infection. The risk of congenital fetal infection rises during pregnancy from 15% in the first trimester, to 30% during the second trimester, and peaking at 60% during the last trimester. Complications of maternal infection with toxoplasmosis include spontaneous abortion or miscarriage, fetal demise, fetal microcephaly, chorioretinitis, cerebral calcifications, and abnormalities of the cerebral spinal fluid.

Client History:

Components of the History to Consider

- LMP, EDC
- Query regarding contact with
  - Cat feces, fur and bedding
  - Raw or rare meat
- Onset, duration, severity of symptoms
- Presence of symptoms
  - Fever
  - Exhaustion
  - Sore throat

Physical Examination:

Components of the Physical Exam to Consider

- VS, including temperature
- General physical exam with focus on
- Swollen lymph nodes

Clinical Impression:

Differential Diagnoses to Consider

- Toxoplasmosis
- Influenza
- Viral illness

Diagnostic Testing:

Diagnostic Tests and Procedures to Consider

- Toxoplasmosis testing
  - Pre-conception
  - If negative and at risk
  - Re-test each trimester
- Types of tests
  - ELISA
  - IFA
- If titers exceed 1:512 recent acute infection is likely
- Possible exposure
  - IgG & IgM negative = no infection
  - IgG positive & IgM negative = previous infection
  - IgM positive = possible acute infection
    - Recheck IgM in 3 weeks
    - If titers rising acute infection likely

Providing Treatment:

Therapeutic Measures to Consider

- Maternal spiromycin & pyrimethamine therapy per perinatologist
- PUBS for fetal IgM & culture
- Ultrasound for anomaly screen

Providing Treatment:

Alternative Measures to Consider

- Maintain quality diet

- Immune support
  - Echinacea
  - Emotional support & reassurance

Providing Support:

Education and Support Measures to Consider

- Prevention measures
  - Avoid
    - Contact with cats, cat feces, cat bedding
    - Travel to areas with endemic toxoplasmosis
    - Handling raw meat whenever possible
  - Do
    - Careful handwashing with soap and water
    - Use gloves when gardening or cleaning
    - Cook meat to at least 150° F
    - Clean surfaces after processing raw meat
- Information and discussion about
  - Test results & diagnosis
  - Options for care
  - Recommended plan

Follow-up Care:

Follow-up Measures to Consider

- Document
  - Physical findings
  - Laboratory results
  - Clinical impression
  - Discussion with client regarding:
    - Testing
    - Results
    - Options for care
  - Midwifery plan of care
    - Location for birth
    - Pediatric involvement
    - Consultations
- Referral/consultation for positive titer
- Return for care
  - Per prenatal routine
  - Ultrasound at 20-22 weeks for fetal anomalies
  - Serial ultrasounds as indicated by results
- Evaluation of the newborn for congenital infection
- Provide ongoing support

Collaborative Practice:

Criteria to Consider for Consultation or Referral

- Diagnosis of acute toxoplasmosis refer to
  - Perinatology
  - Genetic counseling
  - Counseling or support group

Urinary Tract Infection in Pregnancy

Key Clinical Information

Urinary tract infection during pregnancy may have a variety of presentations. *Asymptomatic bacteriuria* is common in pregnancy, and acute *pylonephritis* will occur in up to 30% of women. with previously untreated asymptomatic bacteriuria. Simple *cystitis* may occur during pregnancy and is extremely painful. *Renal calculi* may present as flank pain, accompanied by blood or leukocytes in the urine. Urinary tract infections may lead to renal damage, severe pain, and may increase risk of preterm labor.

Client History:

Components of the History to Consider

- LMP, EDC
- Current symptoms
  - o Onset, duration, severity
  - o Urinary urgency, frequency, burning
  - o Fever/chills
  - o Nausea/vomiting
  - o Flank pain
  - o Colicky pain
- Previous history of
  - o UTIs
  - o Renal calculi
- Voiding and fluid intake habits
- Presence of contractions
- Fetal movement (>20 weeks gestation)

Physical Examination:

Components of the Physical Exam to Consider

- Vital signs, including temp
- CVA tenderness
- Abdominal evaluation
  - o FHT
  - o Presence of contractions
  - o Suprapubic tenderness
  - o Guarding or rebound tenderness
- Signs & symptoms of renal involvement
  - o Fever
  - o CVA tenderness
  - o Pyuria
  - o Positive dip U/A
- Pelvic exam
  - o Presence of contractions
  - o Evaluate cervical length, consistency and dilation

Clinical Impression:

Differential Diagnoses to Consider

- Asymptomatic bacteriuria
- Cystitis
- Pylonephritis
- Renal calculi
- Appendicitis
- Pregnancy induced hypertension
- Ectopic pregnancy
- Preterm labor

Diagnostic Testing:

Diagnostic Tests and Procedures to Consider

- For suspected UTI
  - o Urinalysis
  - o + Nitrates
  - o + Leukocytes
  - o + Blood
- Urine culture and sensitivity

- o + Urinalysis
- o Hx UTI
- o Sickle trait
- o Diabetes
- o Chronic renal disease
- o Hypertension
- o Test of cure following treatment & q 6-12 weeks
- For complicated UTI (pylonephritis, calculi)
  - o CBC
  - o Electrolytes
  - o BUN, creatinine
  - o Renal ultrasound
  - o Strain all urines
  - o Fetal surveillance
    - ▪ Monitor FHR
    - ▪ Monitor for uterine contractions
    - ▪ Evaluate for cervical changes
- Ultrasound to evaluate for
  - o Hydronephrosis
  - o Calculi
  - o Fetal status
- For recurrent UTI screen for
  - o Sickle cell
  - o G6PD
  - o Diabetes
  - o Kidney function
  - o BUN
  - o Creatinine/ 24 hour creatinine clearance
  - o Total protein

Providing Treatment:

Therapeutic Measures to Consider

- Ampicillin 500 mg
  - o Pregnancy category B
  - o 1 PO qid x 7-10 days
- Sulfa trimethoprim DS
  - o Pregnancy category C
  - o 1 (400/80mg) PO bid x 7-10 days
  - o Do not use before 13 or after 36 weeks gestation
  - o Do not use with G6PD anemia
- Macrobid
  - o Pregnancy category B
  - o 100 mg PO bid x 7-10 days
  - o Suppressive therapy
    - ▪ 50-100 mg daily
- Keflex
  - o Pregnancy category B
  - o 500 mg PO q 12 hr x 7-10 days, or
  - o 250 mg PO QID x 7-10 days
- Pyridium, for dysuria
  - o 200 mg tid after meals
  - o Maximum 6 doses
  - o Pregnancy category B
- Pylonephritis
  - o Hospitalization

- o   IV hydration
    - ▪   200 ml/hr
    - ▪   Balanced electrolyte solution
- Antibiotics
    - o   IV Cefoxitin 1-2 g q 6 hrs
    - o   Other cephalosporins
    - o   Change to PO when afebrile x 24 hours
- Pain control
    - o   PCA
    - o   Demerol
    - o   Morphine

Providing Treatment:

Alternative Measures to Consider

- May be used in combination with antibiotics
    - o   Uva-ursi infusion 1 cup q 4-6 hours
    - o   Cranactin tablets 1-2 tablets q 4-6 hours with fluid
- Homeopathic remedies
    - o   Aconitum (renal discomfort, fever & chills)
    - o   Cantharis (painful urination, urgency & frequency)

Providing Support:

Education and Support Measures to Consider

- Medication instructions
- Review warning signs of progression
    - o   Fever & chills
    - o   Flank pain
    - o   Urinary urgency, burning
- Review perineal hygiene
    - o   Void after intercourse
    - o   Blot after voiding
    - o   Wipe front to back after BM
- When to call or come in for care
    - o   Symptoms
        - ▪   Do not resolve within 24 hrs
        - ▪   Worsen
        - ▪   Recur
    - o   Indications for
        - ▪   Hospitalization
        - ▪   Consult or referral

- Encourage
    - o   Increased frequency of voiding
    - o   Increased fluid intake
        - ▪   Water preferable
        - ▪   Cranberry juice/tea
        - ▪   1 cup/hr while awake
- Avoid
    - o   Caffeine
    - o   Excess vitamin C
    - o   Sugars

Follow-up Care:

Follow-up Measures to Consider

- Document
    - o   Chief complaint
    - o   Physical findings
    - o   Lab results
    - o   Clinical impression
    - o   Midwifery plan of care
- U/A each visit for blood, nitrites, leukocytes
- Culture each trimester
- Maternal/fetal surveillance
    - o   Observe for improvement
    - o   Change antibiotics based on sensitivities
    - o   Hospital discharge after
        - ▪   24 hours on PO antibiotics
        - ▪   Afebrile
        - ▪   Calculi passed
        - ▪   No signs or symptoms of preterm labor
- Suppressive therapy after 2 positive cultures

Collaborative Practice:

Criteria to Consider for Consultation or Referral

- o   Pylonephritis
- o   Renal calculi
- Pain control
- Threatened preterm labor
- Recurrent cystitis or asymptomatic bacteria

Vaginal Bleeding, First Trimester

Key Clinical Information

While vaginal bleeding in the first trimester is a relatively common occurrence, it must be considered serious until all potential abnormal caused have been effectively ruled out. The precipitating cause may not readily present itself, and may take some investigation to identify. Serial evaluation of quantitative β-HCG levels may assist in evaluation, as may ultrasound.

Client History:
Components of the History to Consider
- LMP, estimated gestational age
- Date of conception if known
- Onset, duration, severity of bleeding
- Color, amount, and characteristics of discharge
- Precipitating events if any
- Presence of cramping or abdominal pain
- Exposure to
  - o Sexually transmitted infections
  - o Viral infections
  - o Physical abuse or trauma
- OB/GYN history
  - o Previous pregnancy losses
  - o Risk factors for ectopic pregnancy
    - PID
    - IUD
    - Adnexal surgery
  - o History of abnormal pap smears
- Fever or flu-like symptoms

Physical Examination:
Components of the Physical Exam to Consider
- Vital signs including temperature
- FHR
- Bimanual evaluation for
  - o Uterine size for dates
  - o Uterine tenderness
  - o Presence of adnexal mass or pain
  - o Cervical evaluation for
    - Dilatation
    - Presence of products of conception at os or in vaginal vault
    - Presence of erosion, polyps or other cervical cause of bleeding

Clinical Impression:
Differential Diagnoses to Consider
- Implantation bleeding
- Spontaneous abortion
- Threatened spontaneous abortion
- Inevitable spontaneous abortion
- Incomplete spontaneous abortion
- Complete spontaneous abortion
- Missed spontaneous abortion
- Ectopic pregnancy
- Molar pregnancy
- Cervicitis

- Cervical polyps
- Cervical trauma
- Cervical cancer

Diagnostic Testing:
Diagnostic Tests and Procedures to Consider
- Labs
  - o Quantitative β-HCG x2 48 hrs apart
  - o Hematocrit &/or hemoglobin
  - o Type and Rh status
  - o Coagulation studies if missed abortion suspected
    - Prothrombin time
    - Partial prothrombin time
    - Fibrinogen level
    - Platelets
- Ultrasound for
  - o Viability
  - o Dating
  - o Placenta previa
  - o Ectopic

Anticipated β-HCG Levels	
Weeks Post-LMP	**Anticipated HCG Level**
4 weeks	Up to 425 mIU/ml
5 weeks	18-7,350 mIU/ml
6 weeks	1,080-56,500 mIU/ml
7-8 weeks	7,650-230,000 mIU/ml
9-12 weeks	25,700-288,000 mIU/ml
13-16 weeks	13,500-253,000 mIU/ml
17-24 weeks	4,060-65,500 mIU/ml

Providing Treatment:
Therapeutic Measures to Consider
- Referral for D&C as indicated or desired
- Methotrexate for ectopic pregnancy
- Rh immune globulin for Rh negative mother
- Iron replacement therapy

Providing Treatment:
Alternative Measures to Consider
- Await spontaneous resolution to SAB
- Encourage expulsion of products of conception with
  - o Blue or black cohosh tincture
  - o Homeopathic caulophyllum
- Promote healing following SAB
  - o Homeopathic arnica
  - o Rescue remedy
  - o Herbal combinations which may include

- ▪ Red raspberry leaf
- ▪ Vitex berries
- ▪ Black haw root
- Bleeding during pregnancy with rising HCG levels
  - o Red raspberry leaf
  - o False unicorn root
  - o Wild yam root
  - o Crampbark
  - o Lemon balm

Providing Support:
Education and Support Measures to Consider

- Provide emotional support
- Discuss
  - o Potential for miscarriage
  - o Options for care
  - o Expectant care
  - o Tests available
  - o Potential findings
  - o RhIG for Rh negative mother
  - o Threatened SAB
  - o Pelvic rest
  - o Avoid heavy lifting
  - o Call if bleeding increases or is accompanied by pain
- If awaiting spontaneous resolution of SAB at home
  - o Call or seek care immediately if h
    - ▪ Heaving bleeding with pain x 1 ½ hrs
    - ▪ Faintness or weakness
    - ▪ Adnexal pain
    - ▪ Fever
- Prior to next pregnancy
  - o Use multivitamin with folic acid daily
  - o Improve nutrition if indicated
  - o Avoid cigarettes, drugs and alcohol
- Abstain from intercourse x 2 weeks
- Bleeding may last 7-10 days
- Discuss birth control if desired

Follow-up Care:
Follow-up Measures to Consider

- Document
  - o Presenting complaint
  - o Related history
  - o Physical findings
  - o Results of diagnostic testing
  - o Clinical impression
  - o Discussions with patient
  - o Patient preferences for care

- o Midwifery plan of care
- Subchorionic bleed on ultrasound
  - o Follow-up ultrasound for anomalies
  - o Follow HCG levels
- Follow-up β-HCG
  - o 48-96 hours if threatened SAB
  - o 4-6 weeks post SAB at home
    - ▪ ☙Rule out
      - • Molar pregnancy
      - • Choriocarcinoma
      - • Ectopic pregnancy
      - • Incomplete SAB
  - o Follow-up ultrasound 2-7 days
  - o Refer for D&C prn
- No IUP seen on ultrasound
  - o Serial HCGs
  - o Continued + or ⇑ HCG
  - o ☙Suspect ectopic pregnancy
  - o Repeat U/S 2-7 days
- Post spontaneous abortion
  - o Exam in 2-4 weeks
  - o Evaluate return to non-pregnant state
  - o Assess emotional status
  - o Initiate birth control if desired

Collaborative Practice:
Criteria to Consider for Consultation or Referral

- Clients requiring physician intervention
  - o Excessive bleeding
  - o Ectopic pregnancy
  - o Patient preference for D&C
  - o No IUP seen on U/S
  - o Molar pregnancy
  - o Cervical lesion or suspected cervical cancer
- Other referrals prn
- Evaluation for other medical problems which can lead to SAB
  - o Maternal disease (lupus, listeria, syphilis)
  - o Congenital anomalies of the genital tract
  - o Previous cervical surgery
  - o Hormonal imbalances
  - o Fibroids
- Mental health
- Social services
- Genetic counseling

References

1. Bakerman, S., (1994). <u>Bakerman's ABC's of Interpretive Laboratory Data.</u> Myrtle Beach, SC: Interpretive Laboratory Data, Inc.

14. Barger, M. K. Ed. (1988). <u>Protocols for Gynecologic and Obstetric Health Care.</u> Philadelphia, PA: W. B. Saunders.

15. Briggs, G.G., Freeman, R. K., Yaffe, S. J. (1994) <u>Drugs in Pregnancy and Lactation</u> (4th Ed.). Philadelphia, PA: Williams & Wilkins.

16. Burkhart, C. G., (2000). Dermatology Clinic: Itching to have a baby. <u>The Clinical Advisor.</u> March 25, 2000, 93-94.

17. Engstrom, J.L., & Sittler, C. P., (1994) Nurse-midwifery management of iron deficiency anemia during pregnancy. <u>Journal of Nurse-Midwifery, 39.</u> 20s-34s.

18. Enkin, M., Keirce M., Renfrew, M., Neilson, J. (1995). <u>A Guide to Effective Care in Pregnancy and Childbirth</u> (2nd Ed.). New York, NY: Oxford University Press.

19. Fennell, E. (1994). Urinary tract infections during pregnancy. <u>The Female Patient, 19</u> (11), 27-35.

20. Foster, S. (1996). <u>Herbs for Your Health.</u> Loveland, CO: Interweave Press.

21. Frye, Anne. (1998). <u>Holistic Midwifery</u>. Portland, OR. Labrys Press

22. Frye, Anne. (1997). <u>Understanding Diagnostic Tests in the Childbearing Year.</u> (6th Ed.) Portland, OR. Labrys Press

23. Gordon, J. D., Rydfors, J. T., et al. (1995) <u>Obstetrics, Gynecology & Infertility</u> (4th Ed.) Glen Cove, N.Y., Scrub Hill Press.

24. Murphy, J. L., Ed. (2002). <u>Nurse Practitioner's Prescribing Reference.</u> New York, NY. Prescribing Reference, Inc.

25. Murray, M. (1997) <u>Advanced Fetal Monitoring;</u> Antepartal & intrapartal assessment and intervention. Program presented Milwaukee, WI 6/98.

26. Myles, M.F., (1985). <u>Textbook for Midwives</u> (10th ed.). Edinburg: Churchill Livingstone.

27. Nolan, T. E., (1994) Chronic hypertension in pregnancy, <u>The Female Patient, 19</u> (12), 27-42.

28. Phelan, J. P. (1997, October). <u>Intrauterine Fetal Resuscitation; Betamimetics & Amnioinfusion.</u> Presented at Issues & Controversies in Perinatal Practice, Bangor, ME.

29. Roberts, J. (1994). Current perspectives on preeclampsia. <u>The Journal of Nurse-Midwifery, 39,</u> 70-90.

30. Scoggin, J., Morgan, G., (1997). <u>Practice Guidelines for Obstetrics and Gynecology.</u> Philadelphia, PA, Lippincott.

31. Scott, J. R., Diasaia, P.J., et al. (1996). <u>Danforth's Handbook of Obstetrics and Gynecology.</u> Philadelphia, PA, Lippincott - Raven.

32. Smith, T., (1984). <u>A Woman's Guide to Homeopathic Medicine.</u> New York, NY, Thorsons Publishers Inc.

33. Soule, D. (1996). <u>The Roots of Healing.</u> Secaucus, NJ: Citadel Press.

34. Speroff, L., Glass, R. H., Kase, N. G. (1994) <u>Clinical Gynecologic Endocrinology and Infertility</u> (5th Ed.) Philadelphia, PA, Williams & Wilkins.

35. Varney, H., (1997). <u>Varney's Midwifery</u> (3rd ed.). Boston, MA: Jones and Bartlett.

36. Weed, S. (1985). <u>Wise Woman Herbal for the Childbearing Year.</u> Woodstock, NY: Ashtree Publishing

Care of the Woman During Labor and Birthing

Care of women in labor is the hallmark of midwifery care, and remains the essence of being 'with woman'.

Women in labor are at their most vulnerable. Not only do they have to expend an incredible amount of energy in the process of laboring and bringing for their children, but they also must be vigilant in protecting their birth experience, and navigating the health care system. Few women have the resources to do both at once. One component of being 'with woman' is to foster an environment where women may give birth and feel supported.

In many settings the conditions under which women give birth is not ideal. This is true throughout the world. In the United States, women from many nations and all walks of life come to midwives for care. Women look to midwives for safe, compassionate, maternity care. They do not hold the expectation that midwives can change the healthcare system during the course of their pregnancy, labor or birth. As midwives who focus on 'woman-centered' care, it is easy to feel frustration at the system we work within. It is essential to learn the ways of our local health care systems in order to determine how we can best meet the needs of each woman who comes to us for care.

Expectations and standards for midwifery care vary geographically in the U.S., as well as by birth location. Familiarity with state, regional and local standards for birthing care can ease the way for negotiation when adopting an innovative or unfamiliar practice. Use of sound scientific resources is useful in developing midwifery policy, but it should not supersede the centuries of sound midwifery care that has served women so well. Nowhere in the life of a woman is individualized care more important than during labor and birthing.

During labor and birth the midwife must pay attention to verbal and non-verbal cues to evaluate the woman's response to labor. In the setting where the midwife cares for women she or he has not met previously, where there are language or cultural barriers, or other developmental or social obstacles to communication providing sensitive care can be difficult. Midwives should explore the options and avenues open to them for overcoming these challenges, so that they may continue to be 'with woman'.

Initial Midwifery Evaluation of the Laboring Woman

Key Clinical Information

Evaluation of the woman in labor is an essential midwifery skill. Evaluation of the woman in labor encompasses not only physical evaluation of both mother and baby, but also meticulous assessment of the woman's coping skills and strengths that she brings to the task of bringing forth her child.

Client History:
Components of the History to Consider
- Verify LMP, EDC, anticipated gestational age
- Determine
  - Onset of labor
  - Frequency, length, duration of contractions
  - Status of membranes
  - Presence of meconium
  - Presence of bloody show
  - Recent nutritional intake
- Review OB history for risk factors
  - Current pregnancy course
    - GBS status
    - Rh status
    - Hepatitis status
    - HIV status
    - Other risk factors
  - Previous OB history
- Review of systems (ROS)
  - Genitourinary system
  - Respiratory system
  - Circulatory system
  - Gastrointestinal system
  - Nervous system
  - Musculoskeletal system
- Review past medical and surgical history
- Maternal and fetal well-being
  - Fetal motion patterns
  - Support for labor
  - Coping mechanisms for labor
  - Preferences for labor and birth

Physical Examination:
Components of the Physical Exam to Consider
- Evaluate maternal:
  - Vital signs
  - Abdominal exam
    - Contraction pattern: frequency, duration, strength
    - Fetal lie, presentation, position and variety
  - Pelvic exam
    - Dilation and effacement
    - Station
    - Status of membranes
    - Presence of bleeding or show
    - Presence of amniotic fluid
      - Nitrazine
      - Ferning
      - Meconium-staining
  - Extremities:
    - Reflexes
    - Edema
  - Cardiopulmonary status
  - Developmental/emotional status

- Evaluate additional body systems as indicated by
  - History
  - Client presentation
  - Physical exam
  - Diagnostic testing
- Evaluate fetal
  - Lie, presentation, position and variety
  - Heart rate and rhythm
    - Auscultation, or
    - Electronic fetal monitoring
    - Baseline heart rate
    - Beat to beat variability
    - Periodic changes
  - Estimated fetal weight

Clinical Impression:
Differential Diagnoses to Consider
- Uterine contractions, without cervical change
- Uterine irritability, secondary to…
- Onset of labor at term
  - Prodromal labor
  - Early labor
  - Active labor
- Spontaneous rupture of membranes
- Onset of labor, complicated by…

Diagnostic Testing:
Diagnostic Tests and Procedures to Consider
- As indicated by history, risk factors & facility or practice parameters
- Urinalysis
  - Dip for protein and sugar
  - Microscopic prn
- CBC
- Type and screen/cross
- Other screening as indicated by history & physical
  - PIH labs
  - Hepatitis profile
  - Chlamydia & gonorrhea cultures
  - GBS testing
  - HIV
  - RPR/VDRL
  - Rubella titers
  - Ultrasound
    - Amniotic fluid index (AFI)
    - Biophysical profile
    - Fetal presentation
    - Placental location & integrity

Providing Treatment:
Therapeutic Measures to Consider
- None, or
- As indicated by mother's history or facility protocol
  - Saline lock for venous access

o   IV fluids for hydration, or venous access
  ▪   GBS antibiotic prophylaxis (see GBS)
  ▪   PIH magnesium sulfate (see PIH)
  ▪   GDM on insulin (see GDM)
o   Medications as indicated by
  ▪   Maternal history
  ▪   Fetal status

Providing Treatment:

Alternative Measures to Consider
- Watchful waiting
- Oral hydration and nutrition
- Ambulation
- Hydrotherapy
- Support people present

Providing Support:

Education and Support Measures to Consider
- Labor evaluation process
- Expected care during labor and birth
  o   Hydration options
  o   Activity options
  o   Pain relief options
    ▪   Non-pharrmaceudical
    ▪   Pharmaceudical

o   Artificial rupture of membranes
o   Internal exams
o   Positions for birth
o   Role of birth professionals
o   Progress updates
- Provide encouragement and support
- Provide information for informed decision-making
- Monitor client responses to
  o   Support people
  o   Unfamiliar care providers
  o   Labor progress and information

Follow-up Care:

Follow-up Measures to Consider
- Re-evaluate for presence of progress every 4-6 hours
- Document in admission H&P
  o   All findings
  o   Plan for care
  o   Anticipated progression
  o   Consultations or referrals

Collaborative Practice:

Criteria to Consider for Consultation or Referral
- For deviations from norm
- For admission per facility guidelines

Care of the Woman in First Stage Labor

Key Clinical Information

On-going evaluation of the woman in labor provides the midwife with necessary information for determining maternal and fetal well-being during labor. Individual progress during labor may vary widely even within the same woman. The midwife plays a critical role is providing support and reassurance while at the same time remaining vigilant for subtle variations that may indicate developing or the potential for problems. Early identification of actual or potential problems allows problem-solving measures, and treatments to be initiated before emergency conditions exist.

Client History:

Components of the History to Consider
- Gravida, parity
- LMP, EDC, gestational age
- Prior labor and birth history
- Prenatal course
- Birth plan or preferences
- Interval history since admission, at least q 4-6 h
  o   Frequency, length, duration of contractions
    ▪   Pattern of labor
    ▪   Maternal coping ability
    ▪   Presence of pelvic pressure
  o   Internal exam
    ▪   When last assessed
    ▪   Cervical dilation, effacement
    ▪   Presenting part & station
    ▪   Status of membranes
  o   Recent fetal and maternal vital signs
  o   Deviations from anticipated labor course

Physical Examination:

Components of the Physical Exam to Consider
- Maternal and fetal vital signs

o   Maternal BP, pulse, and temp
o   Fetal heart rate and rhythm
- Evaluation of fetal response to labor
  o   Fetal heart tones:
    ▪   At least q 30 min
    ▪   Immediately after ROM
    ▪   Following pain medication
    ▪   At medication peak
    ▪   With change in contraction pattern
    ▪   As indicated by course of labor
  o   Auscultation with doppler or fetoscope
  o   Electronic fetal monitoring
    ▪   External fetal monitoring
    ▪   Internal scalp electrode
- Evaluation of maternal response to labor
  o   Contraction pattern
  o   Duration
  o   Frequency
  o   Strength
    ▪   Evaluate by
      ·   Palpation
      ·   External toco
      ·   Intrauterine pressure catheter

- Pelvic exam
  - Cervical dilation/effacement
  - Status of membranes
  - Presenting part
  - Station
  - Position
  - Reevaluate pelvimetry
  - Assess soft tissues for distensibility
- Urinary system
  - Bladder distention
  - Urine: protein & ketones
  - Output
- Hydration and nutrition
  - Fluid intake
  - Nutritive intake
  - Nausea & vomiting
- Energy level
- Coping abilities
- Maternal support
- Evaluate for changes in cervical status &/or fetal descent
  - Less than 4 exams π risk of endometritis
  - With change in maternal behavior
  - Prior to administration of pain medication
  - With urge to push
  - PRN for ongoing evaluation of labor progress

Clinical Impression:

Differential Diagnoses to Consider

- Progressive labor
- False or prodromal labor
- Labor dystocia, secondary to
  - Cephalopelvic disproportion
  - Dysfunctional labor
    - Hypotonic
    - Hypertonic
  - Persistent posterior presentation
  - Obstructed labor
- Abnormal fetal heart rate patterns in labor

Diagnostic Testing:

Diagnostic Tests and Procedures to Consider

- Dip urine for protein & ketones
- As indicated by labor status & risk factors
  - CBC
  - Type & screen
  - PIH labs (*see* Pregnancy Induced Hypertension)

Providing Treatment:

Therapeutic Measures to Consider

- False or prodromal labor
  - Reassurance
  - Medications
    - Morphine 10-20 mg IM, with
    - Vistaril 25 mg IM
    - Consider add'l 10 mg MS if no sleep in 1-2 hours
  - Seconal 100 mg PO - false labor
- Hypertonic uterine dysfunction
  - Reassurance
  - Rest
  - Morphine 10-20 mg IM as above
- IV access
  - If indicated by patient history
  - If required by facility
  - Consider saline lock vs. IV
  - Consider IV start kit on hand for prn use

- **Pain relief**
- Analgesic medications:
  - May decrease newborn respiratory drive
  - **Nembutal** 100 mg IM – early labor

  - **Vistaril** 50 mg IM - early or active labor
  - **Phenergan** 25-50mg IM or IV – early or active labor, nausea and vomiting
  - **Stadol** 0.5 - 2.0 mg IM or IV - active labor
  - **Nubain** 10-20 mg SQ or IM or IV - active labor
  - **Demerol** 50 mg IM – active labor
  - **Demerol** 12.5-25 mg IV – active labor
- Regional anesthetic:
  - Requires IV hydration
  - May decrease placental perfusion secondary to hypotension
  - **Epidural**
    - Continuous infusion possible
    - May diminish urge to push
  - **Intrathecal** Usually one-time dose
    - Lasts 2-4 hrs
- Hydration
  - Oral fluid intake
  - IV fluids
- Consider IV access for the following conditions
  - P5 or greater
  - Over-distended uterus (i.e. twins, polyhydramios, etc.)
  - Oxytocin administration
  - History of postpartum hemorrhage
  - Maternal dehydration or exhaustion
  - Fetal distress with fatigued mother
  - Any condition that is potentially life threatening (i.e. pre-eclampsia)
  - LR, D5W or D5LR or similar fluid at 100-200 ml/hr
  - Fluid bolus, 300-1000 ml, prior to regional anesthesia
- Desultory labor
  - IV oxytocin (see Augmentation of labor)
  - Nipple stimulation
  - Enema
  - AROM if vertex well applied and station 0 or below
- Catheterize prn for distended bladder if unable to void

Providing Treatment:

Alternative Measures to Consider

- Pain relief:
  - Hydrotherapy
    - Shower
    - Tub
  - Acupressure
  - Hypno-birthing
  - Massage
    - Effleurage
    - Lower back
    - Neck & shoulders
  - Ice packs
  - Hot packs
  - Frequent voiding
  - Position changes
    - Birth ball
    - Rocking chair
    - Hands & knees
    - Squatting
    - Side lying
    - Walking
  - Doula or support person

Providing Support:

Education and Support Measures to Consider

Information and discussion regarding

- Fetal and maternal well-being
- The progress of labor
- The process of labor
- Any imposed limits, or medical therapies, with rationale
  - Maternal concerns
  - Fetal concerns

- o   Facility policy
- Any anticipated procedures
  - o   Indications
  - o   Process
  - o   Anticipated results
  - o   Risks & benefits
  - o   Alternatives
- Address patient/family concerns
- Emotional support
  - o   Presence of support people
  - o   Access to midwife prn
  - o   Familiar environment or objects
  - o   Reassurance of labor as normal physiologic process
  - o   Maternal control of
    - ▪   Food and fluid as desired
    - ▪   Position changes as desired
    - ▪   Frequent voiding

Follow-up Care:

Follow-up Measures to Consider

- Document
  - o   Results of each assessment performed in labor
  - o   Discussions regarding treatments or therapies
  - o   Alternative therapies used and results obtained
  - o   Medical therapies used and results obtained
  - o   Maternal response to labor or treatments
  - o   Continued plan for care
  - o   Anticipated course of labor
- Re-evaluate q 1-4 hours in active labor

Collaborative Practice:

Criteria to Consider for Consultation or Referral

- For Rx not within the scope of the midwife's practice
- For deviations from the norm
- As indicated by collaborative practice agreements

Care of the Woman in Second Stage Labor

Key Clinical Information

During second stage the fetus must traverse the bony confines of the birth canal before he or she can emerge from the womb as a newborn. The baby's position as s/he enters the pelvis contributes to the duration and difficulty of second stage labor. Prenatal evaluation of the internal pelvic diameters, known as *pelvimetry*, can be very useful in anticipating the course of second-stage labor, and offering suggestions for maternal positioning to facilitate fetal descent.

Client History:

Components of the History to Consider

- Review progress of first stage
- Previous OB history
  - o   Previous infant's weights
  - o   Second stage length
  - o   Previous shoulder dystocia
  - o   Previous operative deliveries
    - ▪   Forceps
    - ▪   Vacuum extractor
    - ▪   Cesarean delivery
- Documented pelvimetry
- Estimated fetal weight

Physical Examination:

Components of the Physical Exam to Consider

- Abdominal and or pelvic examination for evaluation of
  - o   Fetal descent
    - ▪   Abdominal contour
    - ▪   Location of FHR
    - ▪   Bulging of perineum
    - ▪   Fetal position
    - ▪   Molding
  - o   Assess rate of progress
  - o   Fetal well-being
  - o   Frequent FHTs
    - ▪   FHR may π in mid-pelvis
    - ▪   Head compression may πFHR
    - ▪   FHR should return to >100 between pushes
    - ▪   FHR <90 anticipate resuscitation
- Determine maternal well-being

- o   Vital signs
- o   Assess hydration
- o   Evaluate her energy level
- o   Determine her coping ability
- o   Assess for bladder distention
  - ▪   May cause second stage obstruction
- o   Perineal tissue elasticity
- Evaluate for signs or symptoms of:
  - o   Lack of descent
  - o   Slow descent
  - o   Caput formation
  - o   Fetal distress
  - o   Maternal exhaustion
  - o   Perineal edema

Clinical Impression:

Differential Diagnoses to Consider

- Progressive second stage
  - o   Spontaneous vaginal birth
    - ▪   No lacerations
    - ▪   First or second degree lacerations
    - ▪   Episiotomy
- Progressive second stage, complicated by
  - o   Precipitous birth
  - o   Meconium stained fluid
  - o   Nuchal cord, state number of loops
  - o   True knot in cord
  - o   Third or forth degree laceration
  - o   Fetal distress
- Slowly progressive second stage, complicated by
  - o   Shoulder dystocia
  - o   Cephalopelvic disproportion
  - o   Meconium stained fluid

- o   Fetal distress
- Failure to descent during second stage
- Fetal distress during second stage

Diagnostic Testing:

Diagnostic Tests and Procedures to Consider

- None

Providing Treatment:

Therapeutic Measures to Consider

- Perineal massage and or support
- Local or other anesthesia if episiotomy performed
- Catheterization if bladder distended and unable to void
- Assisted birth
  - o   Manual assistance (*see:* Shoulder Dystocia)
  - o   Vacuum extraction (*see:* Vacuum Extraction)
- Clamping and cutting of the umbilical cord
  - o   Before birth of the shoulders for nuchal cord
  - o   When cord had stopped pulsing
  - o   Immediately following birth
  - o   Following birth of placenta for waterbirth
  - o   Family member may wish to cut cord
  - o   Collect cord blood sample
    - ▪   For Rh negative mother
    - ▪   Per facility or practice routine
    - ▪   As indicated by history

Providing Treatment:

Alternative Measures to Consider

- Positioning for second stage and birth
  - o   Semi-sitting
  - o   Left lateral
  - o   Squatting
  - o   Hand & knees
  - o   Birthing stool
  - o   Lithotomy for persistent posterior or slow descent
- Water birth
- Perineal management
  - o   Hot packs to perineum
  - o   Perineal massage
  - o   Perineal support
- Family participation in birth

Providing Support:

Education and Support Measures to Consider

- Pushing
  - o   Allow for natural expulsive efforts
  - o   Direct pushing efforts when needed
  - o   Remind about pelvic pressure
  - o   Instruct when not to push
- Immediate care after birth
  - o   Discuss plan for newborn handling
    - ▪   Newborn to mother
    - ▪   Newborn to warming unit
    - ▪   Initial evaluation process for baby
    - ▪   Cord cutting

- Remind about third stage

Follow-up Care:

Follow-up Measures to Consider

- Document all pertinent birth information:
  - o   Vital information
    - ▪   Time of birth
    - ▪   Sex of infant
    - ▪   Apgar score
    - ▪   Weight
  - o   Labor and birth summary
    - ▪   Length of labor
    - ▪   Length of second stage
    - ▪   Position of baby at birth
    - ▪   Position of mother for birth
    - ▪   Delivery of placenta
    - ▪   Examination of placenta
    - ▪   Estimated blood loss
  - o   Procedures
    - ▪   For complications
    - ▪   Vacuum extraction
    - ▪   Management of shoulder dystocia
    - ▪   Newborn resuscitation
    - ▪   Management of placenta/post-partum hemorrhage
  - o   Episiotomy or lacerations
    - ▪   Extent and location(s)
    - ▪   Repair, if performed
    - ▪   Anesthesia
    - ▪   Suture used
  - o   Medications for late labor and second stage
    - ▪   Analgesia
    - ▪   Anesthesia
    - ▪   Oxytocin
    - ▪   Methergine
    - ▪   IV fluids
    - ▪   Blood or crystalloid
  - o   Maternal and newborn condition following birth
    - ▪   EBL
    - ▪   Bonding
    - ▪   Breastfeeding
    - ▪   Fundal and flow evaluation
- Determine maternal stability
- Provide for on-going care post-partum

Collaborative Practice:

Criteria to Consider for Consultation or Referral

- For Rx or procedures not within the midwife's scope of practice
- For deviations from the norm
  - o   Maternal
  - o   Fetal
  - o   Newborn
- As indicated by collaborative practice agreements

Care of the Woman in Third Stage Labor

Key Clinical Information

Birth of the placenta signals the end of labor, and the beginning of the post-partum period. Significant blood loss may occur prior to, or following the birth of the placenta. Active management of the third stage of labor may result in decreased blood loss. Evaluation of the placenta should include manual palpation of the maternal surface as well as visual inspection of both sides of the placenta for areas of fragmentation, divots, or torn blood vessels that may indicate retained placental parts.

Client History:

Components of the History to Consider

- Previous obstetrical history
- Risk factors for postpartum hemorrhage
    - Over-distended uterus
    - Large infant
    - Prolonged first or second stage
    - Cervical manipulation
    - Anemia
    - Course of labor and birth

Physical Examination:

Components of the Physical Exam to Consider

- Vital signs
- Evaluate for tears or lacerations
    - Vagina
    - Peri-urethral area
    - Rectum
    - Cervix
- Evaluate for placental separation
    - Lengthening cord
    - Globular fundus
    - Gush of blood
- Gross exam of the placenta after delivery
    - Verify placenta is intact
        - Visual exam
            - Maternal surface
            - Fetal surface
        - Tactile exam of maternal surface
    - Cord insertion and vessel pattern
    - Look for gross pathological changes
    - Examine for # cord vessels (2 arteries, 1 vein)

Clinical Impression:

Differential Diagnoses to Consider

- Third stage labor
- Intact placenta, normal appearance
- Intact placenta with unusual cord insertion
    - Marginal cord insertion
    - Velementous insertion of the cord
- Post-partum hemorrhage
- Retained placenta
    - Fragments
    - Accreta
    - Percreta
    - Increta

Diagnostic Testing:

Diagnostic Tests and Procedures to Consider

- Placenta to pathology for evaluation
    - Maternal indications
        - Diabetes
        - Chronic hypertension or PIH
        - Preterm delivery (<35 weeks)
        - Post-term delivery (.42 weeks)
        - Unexplained fever
        - Previous poor Ob history
        - No or minimal prenatal care
        - Substance abuse
        - Unexplained elevation of α-fetal protein
    - Fetal indications
        - Stillbirth

- Neonatal death
- Multiple gestation
- Intrauterine growth retardation
- Congenital anomalies
- Hydrops fetalis
- Admission to neonatal intensive care
- Low 5-minute Apgar(<6)
- Umbilical artery pH (<7.20)
- Meconium stained fluid
- Polyhydramnios or oligohydramnios

- Fetal cord blood testing
    - Cord blood type and Rh
    - Cord blood gasses

Providing Treatment:

Therapeutic Measures to Consider

- Collect cord blood sample
- Use gentle traction to *guide* placenta
- Place one hand on symphysis to guard uterus
- ***DO NOT PULL ON THE CORD***
- Oxytocin administration:
    - After delivery of the anterior shoulder
    - After delivery of placenta
    - Defer unless boggy uterus or excessive flow
    - 10 units IM or 10-20 units in IV fluids
- Tease membranes out as necessary
- Manual removal of placenta
- Repair of episiotomy or any lacerations
- Excessive bleeding (*see:* PPH)
    - IV access
    - Oxytocin 20 units in 1000ml IV fluids
    - Methergine
        - 0.2 mg IM
        - May continue PO q 6hr x 1-7 D
    - Cytotec
        - 200-400 mcg rectally
    - Hemabate
- Pain medication, as needed for after pains

Providing Treatment:

Alternative Measures to Consider

- Baby to breast to stimulate uterine contractions
- Herbal formulas to stimulate uterine contractions
    - Blue or black cohosh tincture
    - Shepherd's purse tincture
- Leave cord intact until placenta births
- Allow placenta to come naturally
- Ice to perineum after birth

Providing Support:

Education and Support Measures to Consider

- Encourage mother/baby contact
- Encourage breastfeeding of baby
- Be gentle
- Provide information about
    - Third stage
    - Lacerations
    - Need for repair, if any
    - Interventions, if indicated
- Show placenta at client request
- Show client firm fundus

- Advise to notify midwife or support staff if
  - o Fundus boggy
  - o Flow excessive
  - o Concerns about baby

Follow-up Care:

Follow-up Measures to Consider

- Document
  - o Mechanism of delivery of placenta
  - o Number of cord vessels
  - o Estimated blood loss (EBL)
  - o Lacerations and repairs
  - o Medications given
    - ▪ Rationale
    - ▪ Dose
    - ▪ Effect
- Post-partum evaluation
  - o Vital signs
  - o Fundal/flow checks

  - o 1-2 hours after birth or until stable
  - o Evaluate maternal/infant bonding
- Follow-up evaluation within 12-24 hours

Collaborative Practice:

Criteria to Consider for Consultation or Referral

- For excessive bleeding uncontrolled by
  - o Oxytocin, methergine or cytotec
  - o Bi-manual compression
- As needed for
  - o Vaginal lacerations
  - o Rectal lacerations
  - o Cervical lacerations
- For suspected retained placental parts
- For placenta that is undelivered
  - o >30-60 minutes after birth of infant
  - o Accompanied by vaginal bleeding

Amnioinfusion

Key Clinical Information

Amnioinfusion has mixed results in the medical literature based. The intention of amnoinfusion is to either decrease cord compression related to oligohydramnios, or to dilute the concentration of meconium in an effort to decrease risk of meconium aspiration syndrome. Some studies suggest that amnioinfusion may decrease the incidence of meconium noted below the level of the vocal cords, and may decrease the rate of Cesarean birth for fetal distress by decreasing the frequency and severity of variable decelerations, and improving umbilical cord pH. [4]

Amnioinfusion is not without risk. It has been associated with overdistention of the uterus resulting in increased basal uterine tone and sudden deterioration of the fetal heart rate pattern[5] In one 2000 study, amnioinfusion did not result in a any decrease in the incidence of meconium aspiration syndrome or other respiratory disorders. [6] Clinical indications and use of amnioinfusion vary widely from facility to facility.

---

[4] Paszkowski, T. (1994). Amnioinfusion; a review. The Journal of Reproductive Medicine, 39, 588-594.

Phelan, J. P. (1997, October). Intrauterine Fetal Resuscitation; Betamimetics & Amnioinfusion. Presented at Issues & Controversies in Perinatal Practice, Bangor, ME.

[5] ACOG. (2001). Compendium of selected publications, pp 165-166.

[6] Wiswell, T.E., et al. (2000). Delivery room management of the apparently vigorous meconium-stained neonate: Results of the multicenter, international collaborative trial. Pediatrics 105, 1-7.

Client History:

Components of the History to Consider

- LMP, EDC, gestational age
- Maternal vital signs, including temp
- Cervical status
- Fetal presentation
- Status of membranes
- History of low AFI
    o By ultrasound
    o By clinical exam
    o PROM
- Severe variable decelerations
- Fetal distress associated with cord compression
- Passage of meconium-stained fluid
- Presence of amnionitis

Physical Examination:

Components of the Physical Exam to Consider

- Maternal vital signs, including temp
- Vaginal exam
    o Status of membranes: amniotomy must be performed if SROM has not occurred
    o Dilation, effacement and station: delivery should not be imminent
    o Verify presenting part
    o Place intrauterine pressure catheter
- Abdominal exam
    o Singleton fetus, vertex lie
    o Evaluation of FHR
        ▪ Variable decelerations presenting prior to 8-9 cms most common with oligohydramnios
    o Presence of abdominal tenderness
        ▪ Amnioinfusion contraindicated in the presence of amnionitis

Clinical Impression:

Differential Diagnoses to Consider

- Amnioinfusion for treatment of
    o Fetal distress, secondary to oligohydramnios
    o Meconium stained amniotic fluid
- Bolus amnioinfusion
- Continuous amnioinfusion

Diagnostic Testing:

Diagnostic Tests and Procedures to Consider

- Pre-op labs
- Ultrasound
    o AFI before amnioinfusion
    o AFI after bolus

Providing Treatment:

Therapeutic Measures to Consider

- Insert IUPC if not already in place
- Use double lumen IUPC if available
- Internal fetal scalp lead or external doppler
- Procedure
    o Infuse sterile saline or Ringer's lactate into the intra-amniotic space
    o Warmed solution not necessary

---

    o Bolus infusion
        ▪ 250-1000 ml at rate of 10-15 ml/min
        ▪ Usual bolus +/- 500ml in 30 min
        ▪ May follow with bolus of 250ml after decel resolves
    o Continuous infusion
        ▪ 10ml/min for 1 hour
        ▪ Maintenance rate of 3ml.min
- May take 20-30 minutes to see effect
- ☛Do not delay Cesarean birth while performing amnioinfusion
- Management of fetal distress
    o Maternal position changes
    o Oxygen therapy
    o Terbutaline therapy
- Emergency C-section
- Pediatric support with meconium stained fluid

Providing Treatment:

Alternative Measures to Consider

- Expectant management

Providing Support:

Education and Support Measures to Consider

- Provide information regarding
    o Concerns
    o Goal of procedure
- Address patient/family concerns
    o Informed consent
    o Risks, benefits and alternatives
    o Client requirements
        ▪ Positioning for procedure
        ▪ Confined to bed post-procedure
        ▪ Continuous fetal and maternal monitoring

Follow-up Care:

Follow-up Measures to Consider

- Document procedure
    o Indications
    o Informed consent
    o Volumes infused
    o Maternal & fetal response
    o On-going plan for care
- Observe for complications
    o Deterioration of FHRUterine hypertonus
    o Cord prolapse
    o Uterine scar separation
    o Amniotic fluid embolism
    o Placental abruption
    o Signs or symptoms of infection
- Monitor and document maternal and fetal response
- Monitor and document progress of labor

Collaborative Practice:

Criteria to Consider for Consultation or Referral

- With indications for amnioinfusion
    o For potential surgical consult
    o For pediatric coverage
- In the presence of complications related to amnioinfusion

Assisting with Cesarean Section

Key Clinical Information

Assisting with Cesarean birth is included as an expanded role of the midwife[7]. By first assisting during Cesarean birth the midwife may provide greater continuity of care to women, and greater versatility within her or his clinical practice. Care must be taken, however, not to lose sight of the midwifery model of care when one is working in the highly medical environment of the Operating Room. Skills for first assisting may also enhance the midwife's ability to perform repairs of perineal lacerations or episiotomy.

---

[7] ACNM, (1998). Position Statement: The Certified Nurse-Midwife/Certified Midwife As First Assistant at Surgery, Author.

Client History:

Components of the History to Consider

- Complete OB history on chart
  - o Prenatal labs
  - o Admission labs
  - o History of labor
  - o Indication for C-section
    - ▪ Maternal
    - ▪ Fetal
    - ▪ Urgent vs scheduled
- Medical history on chart
  - o Allergies
  - o Medication or herb use
  - o Medical conditions
    - ▪ Asthma
    - ▪ Cardiac dysfunction
    - ▪ Respiratory disorders
    - ▪ Scoliosis
    - ▪ Back surgery
  - o Previous surgeries
  - o Response to anesthesia
    - ▪ General
    - ▪ Regional
- Review of systems
- Social history on chart
  - o Support systems
  - o Smoking
  - o Alcohol or drug use
  - o Client concerns

Physical Examination:

Components of the Physical Exam to Consider

- General maternity admission physical
  - o Cardiorespiratory system
  - o GI system
  - o Fetal presentation, EFW
- Pre-operative considerations
  - o Mobility of
    - ▪ Jaw
    - ▪ Neck
    - ▪ Back
  - o Body mass index
  - o Positioning limitations

Clinical Impression:

Differential Diagnoses to Consider

- Primary Cesarean section for
  - o Maternal indication
  - o Fetal indication
- Repeat Cesarean section
  - o Scheduled
  - o In labor
  - o Following VBAC attempt

Diagnostic Testing:

Diagnostic Tests and Procedures to Consider

- Pre-op labs (see Preparing for Cesarean section)
- Fetal and maternal vital signs

Providing Treatment:

Therapeutic Measures to Consider

- Ensure IV patency
- Ensure airway patency
- Assist with induction of general or regional anesthesia prn
- Assist surgeon with
  - o Prep
  - o Draping
  - o Hemostasis
  - o Retraction
  - o Suctioning
    - o Follow suture
    - o Extraction of infant,
- Procedure
- Abdomen opened in layers
  - o Skin
  - o Subcutaneous fat
  - o Fascia
  - o Muscle
  - o Peritoneum
- Bladder flap created
- Uterine incision made
  - o Follow scalpel with suction
  - o Rotate bladder blade to provide exposure
- Incision extended with scissors or bluntly
- Rupture of membranes
- Remove bladder blade
- Head/ buttocks delivered
  - o Manually
  - o Vacuum extractor
  - o Pipers for after-coming head
- Fundal pressure for birth of body
- Suction mouth and nares
- Clamp and cut cord
- Collect cord blood
- Administration of medications prn
  - o Oxytocin
  - o Antibiotics
  - o Anxiolytics
  - o Narcotics
  - o Antiemetics
- Placenta
  - o Spontaneous removal
    - ▪ πrisk infection
    - ▪ π blood loss
  - o Manual removal of placenta
    - ▪ Identification of attachment location
    - ▪ Opportunity to learn skill
    - ▪ Surgeon preference
- Uterus inspected and cleared of debris
- Uterus closed in layers
- Inspection of other organs; ovaries, tubes, appendix
- Closure of layers per surgeon preference
- Sterile dressing applied

Providing Treatment:

Alternative Measures to Consider

- Allow/encourage support person(s)
  - o Pre-op area
  - o Holding area
  - o Operating room
  - o Recovery room (PACU)
- Encourage mother to hold baby after initial evaluation
- Allow support person(s) to care for infant until mother able

Providing Support:

Education and Support Measures to Consider

- Provide emotional support
  - o During anesthesia
  - o During surgery
  - o Following surgery
- Advise client of routines related to
  - o Anesthesia
  - o C-section procedure
  - o Newborn care
    - ▪ In OR
    - ▪ Special care
  - o Recovery room
  - o Return to post-partum unit

- o   Post-operative course
- Listen
    - o   Address patient/family concerns

Follow-up Care:

Follow-up Measures to Consider

- Provide and document routine post-op care
    - o   Cardio pulmonary system
        - ▪   CBC
        - ▪   Physical exam
        - ▪   Incentive spirometry
    - o   GI system
        - ▪   Auscultate for bowel sounds
        - ▪   Passage of flatus
        - ▪   Passage of stool
    - o   Urinary system
        - ▪   Ensure voiding post catheter removal
        - ▪   Assess for signs or symptoms of
            - •   Post-void residual
            - •   Urinary tract infection

- Bladder injury
- Bladder spasms
    - o   Evaluate client's emotional response to
        - ▪   Procedure
        - ▪   Infant
        - ▪   Parenting
        - ▪   Evaluation for postpartum depression risk
- Ensure adequate pain control
    - o   Patient controlled analgesia (PCA)
    - o   IM narcotics
    - o   PO narcotics
    - o   PO NSAIDs
- Advance diet as tolerated
- DC IV/saline lock when taking PO fluid well

Collaborative Practice:

Criteria to Consider for Consultation or Referral

- Presence of intra-operative or post-op complications
- For routine post-op care per practice setting

Caring for the Woman Undergoing Cesarean Birth,

Key Clinical Information

In many settings the midwife may help prepare the client who will have her child born via Cesarean. This provides a wonderful opportunity to provide women with education and support. The mother who was anticipating a planned birth center or home birth may need additional assistance in coping with the disappointment of the unexpected change in birth plans, and in assimilating the procedure and its outcome. Any mother who undergoes Cesarean delivery may have conflicted feelings about her labor and birth experience.

Client History:

Components of the History to Consider

- See First assisting with Cesarean section
- Complete maternity admission history
    - o   Maternity history
    - o   Medical and surgical history
    - o   Review of systems
    - o   Social history on chart
- Interval labor history as indicated

Physical Examination:

Components of the Physical Exam to Consider

- Complete maternity admission physical
- Physical examination related to indication for Cesarean

Clinical Impression:

Differential Diagnoses to Consider

- Cesarean section
    - o   Primary, secondary to
        - ▪   Note indication(s)
    - o   Repeat, secondary to
        - ▪   Patient preference
        - ▪   Previous incision type
        - ▪   Onset of labor
        - ▪   Following VBAC attempt
            - •   Note secondary indication(s)
    - o   Fetal indications
        - ▪   CPD
        - ▪   Fetal distress
        - ▪   Malpresentation

- ▪   Multiple gestation
- ▪   Congenital anomalies
- ▪   Preterm birth
    - o   Maternal indications
        - ▪   Dysfunctional labor
        - ▪   Pregnancy induced hypertension
        - ▪   Diabetes mellitus
        - ▪   Preterm labor
        - ▪   Placenta previa
        - ▪   Placental abruption
        - ▪   Uterine rupture

Diagnostic Testing:

Diagnostic Tests and Procedures to Consider

- Urinalysis
- CBC
- Type and screen or type and cross
- Other necessary labs as indicated by maternal/fetal status
    - o   PIH labs
    - o   Clotting studies
    - o   Antibody identification

Providing Treatment:

Therapeutic Measures to Consider

- NPO
- IV fluids
    - o   LR, D5LR, NS or similar balanced electrolyte solution
    - o   14-20 gauge IV catheter
    - o   Rate150 ml/hr
    - o   Bolus of 500-1000 ml if regional anesthesia anticipated
    - o   IV fluids per anesthesia request

- Foley catheter
  - o May insert in OR following regional anesthesia
- Notify appropriate personnel of pending surgery
  - o OB/GYN
  - o Nursing or OR supervisor
  - o Anesthesia
  - o Pediatrics
- Medications per anesthesia request
- Continuous maternal and/or fetal monitoring as indicated

Providing Treatment:

Alternative Measures to Consider

- Provide emotional support
- Allow/encourage family or support person(s) in OR

Providing Support:

Education and Support Measures to Consider

- Discuss indication(s) for Cesarean birth
- ⊕Provide interpreter as necessary
- Obtain informed consent
  - o Risks
    - ▪ Infection
    - ▪ Bleeding
    - ▪ Injury
      - • Bowel or bladder
      - • Fetus
      - • Uterus
    - ▪ Blood loss
  - o Benefits
    - ▪ Delivery in controlled environment
    - ▪ Expedited delivery
    - ▪ C/S *may* decrease risk to mother or baby, based on indication for Cesarean birth, i.e.:
      - • Breech/transverse lie
      - • CPD
      - • Severe PIH
      - • Preterm fetus
  - o Alternatives to procedure
    - ▪ Continued labor
    - ▪ Vaginal birth, based on indications, i.e.:
      - • VBAC
      - • Breech
      - • Preterm
- Discuss recommendations and process with family
  - o Unless time is critical allow for maternal input

- o Maternal participation in decision-making may impact
  - ▪ Feelings about surgical delivery
  - ▪ Bonding with baby
  - ▪ Self-image as woman
- Considerations for client and family education
  - o Time in OR
  - o If support person(s) can stay with mother
  - o Expected care for baby flowing birth
    - ▪ Routine care
    - ▪ Special care
    - ▪ Procedures
  - o Anticipated post-operative care
    - ▪ Recovery
    - ▪ Post-partum hospital stay
- Provide emotional support related to
  - o Indication for Cesarean birth
  - o Change in
    - ▪ Birth plans
    - ▪ Birth attendant
    - ▪ Birth location

Follow-up Care:

Follow-up Measures to Consider

- Document
  - o Relevant history and physical findings
  - o Indication for Cesarean delivery
  - o Consultations and referrals
    - ▪ OB
    - ▪ Pediatrics
  - o Midwifery plan of care
    - ▪ Transfer of care to physician
    - ▪ Collaborative care with physician
    - ▪ Anticipated midwifery follow-up
    - ▪ Assist at surgery if qualified (see Assisting with C-section)
  - o Remain with client if possible
  - o Review experience with client postpartum

Collaborative Practice:

Criteria to Consider for Consultation or Referral

- o Anticipating potential for Cesarean birth
- o As indicated by
  - ▪ The midwife's scope of practice
  - ▪ Practice setting
  - ▪ Client preference
- o Development of complications post-operatively

Caring for the Woman with Umbilical Cord Prolapse

Key Clinical Information

Cord prolapse is a clinical emergency. Unless compression is removed from the cord the fetus will be deprived of oxygen and may suffer brain and organ damage. While Cesarean birth is one method of resolving cord prolapse, maternal positioning, and manual replacement of the cord may help diminish cord compression. Cord prolapse is more common in women who have polyhydramnios, a fetal presentation other than vertex, and during spontaneous, or artificial, rupture of the membranes when the head or presenting part is not engaged in the pelvis

Client History:

Components of the History to Consider

- LMP, EDG, gestational age
- ❡Identify risk factors for cord prolapse
- Amniotic fluid index (AFI), if known
- Status of membranes
- Fetal heart rate
  - o Previously documented FHR/FHT
  - o Fetal heart rate changes
- Maternal medical or obstetric problems

Physical Examination:

Components of the Physical Exam to Consider

- Diagnosis and prevention
  - o Avoid ROM unless presenting part is engaged
  - o Evaluate FHR following ROM
    - ▪ Severe bradycardia = likely cord prolapse
    - ▪ Severe FHR drop with resolution = potential occult cord or true knot in cord
- Abdominal exam
  - o Evaluation of fluid volume
  - o Determination of fetal lie, and presentation
  - o Estimation of fetal weight
- Vaginal exam
  - o Determine presenting part(s)
  - o Station, cervical dilation
  - o Risk for cord prolapse
    - ▪ Floating presenting part
    - ▪ Bulging bag of waters
    - ▪ Ballooning or hourglass membranes
  - o In presence of suspected cord prolapse
    - ▪ Elevation of presenting part off of cord
    - ▪ Continuous evaluation of fetal heart rate

Clinical Impression:

Differential Diagnoses to Consider

- Cord prolapse, secondary to
  - o Polyhydramnios
  - o Compound presentation
  - o Malpresentation
- Fetal distress, secondary to
  - o Cord prolapse

Diagnostic Testing:

Diagnostic Tests and Procedures to Consider

- Pre-op labs STAT
  - o CBC
  - o Type and screen/cross
  - o Urinalysis

Providing Treatment:

Therapeutic Measures to Consider

- Terbutaline
  - o 0.25 mg sq., or
  - o 0.125-0.25 mg IV,
  - o To decrease contractions and uterine tone
- O2 by mask at 6-8 lpm
- Discontinue any oxytocin if running
- Trendelenberg position with left lateral tilt
- Consider amnioinfusion for cord compression (i.e. occult cord prolapse)

- If infant continues to deteriorate
  - o Multip with active labor
    - ▪ May attempt rapid vaginal birth if fully dilated
    - ▪ Vacuum extraction
  - o Transport if out of hospital
  - o Maintain elevation of presenting part until delivery
  - o Cesarean section for delivery
  - o Pediatric care for birth
  - o Plan for newborn resuscitation

Providing Treatment:

Alternative Measures to Consider

- Knee chest position
- Attempt to reduce prolapse
  - o Manually lift presenting part
  - o Attempt to reinsert cord into uterus
  - o Evaluate for fetal response
  - o Maintain knee chest position until presenting part is well applied to cervix or engaged
- If unable to reduce cord prolapse
  - o Keep cord warm and moist
  - o Maintain knee chest position
  - o Arrange for surgical delivery
- Rescue Remedy at pulse points

Providing Support:

Education and Support Measures to Consider

- Education
  - o Include cord prolapse in informed consent
    - ▪ Breech births
    - ▪ Polyhydramnios
- During emergency
  - o Provide emotional support
  - o Briefly explain to nature of emergency
  - o Keep patient/family advised of what is happening
- Following emergency
  - o Compassionate listening
  - o Information about the emergency
  - o Support groups when needed

Follow-up Care:

Follow-up Measures to Consider

- Evaluate FHR continuously following treatment
  - o Auscultation
  - o Electronic fetal monitoring
- Following delivery
  - o Reassure patient that cord prolapse occurs by chance
  - o Review what happened and allow patient to verbalize feelings, understanding
- Document, as soon as possible after delivery
  - o Identification of problem
  - o Diagnosis
  - o Treatment
  - o Maternal and fetal outcomes
- Consider peer review if poor outcome occurs

Collaborative Practice:

Criteria to Consider for Consultation or Referral

- Suspected or confirmed cord prolapse
- Fetal distress responsive to therapy

Care of the Woman with Failure to Progress in Labor

Key Clinical Information

Failure to progress is a common diagnosis that may have multiple components. Delay in progression may be related to the effectiveness of uterine contractions, the size of the mother's pelvis in relation to the baby, fetal position or anatomy, or psychosocial factors that inhibit labor progress. The challenge to the midwife is to identify and treat the specific component(s) causing the delay.

In many instances fetal size or positioning will slow the progression of labor, while the uterus works hard to literally push past the difficulty. Time and patience may be rewarded with slow but steady progress. When the uterus is not working efficiently, as in desultory labor, augmentation of labor via oxytocin may help prevent prolonged labor, and avoid unnecessary Cesarean birth.

Client History:
Components of the History to Consider
- G, P, LMP, EDC, gestational age
- Review of labor
  - Onset of labor
  - Progress of labor
  - Fetal response to labor
  - Maternal response to labor
  - Status of membranes
    - Color of fluid
    - Length of rupture
  - Oral intake of food or fluids
  - Positions used and results
- Estimated fetal weight
- Previous clinical evaluation of fetal lie
- Previous labor and delivery history
- Inquiry into potential barriers to labor progress
  - Cultural
  - Developmental
  - Emotional/social
  - Physical
    - Hydration
    - Nutrition
    - Voiding

Physical Examination:
Components of the Physical Exam to Consider
- Maternal vital signs and evaluation
  - Evaluate for signs of exhaustion
  - Maternal attitude
    - Fear or anxiety
    - Tension
- Abdominal exam
  - Fetal lie, presentation, position, EFW, engagement
  - Uterine contractions; frequency, duration, intensity
  - Bladder distension
- Pelvic exam
  - Cervical dilation and effacement
  - Edema of asymmetry of cervix
  - Station
  - Application of presenting part to the cervix
  - Reassess pelvimetry
  - Fetal position and variety
  - Synclitism/asynclitism

- Caput formation and/or molding
- Fetal vital signs
  - FHR/FHT; short- and long-term variability
  - Fetal activity
  - Fetal response to stimulation

Clinical Impression:
Differential Diagnoses to Consider
- Labor dystocia
  - Protraction of dilation
  - Protraction of descent
  - Arrest of dilation
  - Arrest of descent
- Failure to progress in labor, secondary to
  - Fetal presentation or position
  - Cephalopelvic disproportion
  - Inadequate contractions
  - Feto-pelvic dystocia
  - Maternal emotional response to labor

Diagnostic Testing:
Diagnostic Tests and Procedures to Consider
- Urine for ketones
- Uterine pressure catheter to evaluate uterine contractions
- Pre-op labs if consideration for potential C-section

Providing Treatment:
Therapeutic Measures to Consider
- Hydration, PO or IV
  - Bolus of 500 ml IV LR, D5LR, or other solution suitable for labor
  - Maintain at 125-200 ml/hr
- Rest, if maternal and fetal status is stable
  - Consider MS 10-20 mg IM (see Management of Labor)
  - Have Narcan immediately available
- Antibiotic prophylaxis
  - Not indicated with negative GBS
  - ROM > 24 hours or per facility recommendations
  - Maternal fever or ↑WBC
- Consider measures to stimulate uterine contractions
  - Oxytocin (see induction/augmentation of labor)
  - Amniotomy
  - Empty bladder – Foley catheter
  - Pain relief to facilitate rest/relaxation

Providing Treatment:

Alternative Measures to Consider

- Discuss emotional issues that may interfere with labor
  - o Fear
  - o Previous trauma, such as rape, abortion
  - o Family issues (i.e. gender of infant, history of abuse)
  - o Deadlines related to
    - Labor management
    - Interventions
- Position changes
  - o Side lying
  - o Walking
  - o Rocking chair
  - o Semi-sitting
  - o Flat on back encourages descent
    - Opens pelvic inlet
    - Legs flexed
    - Arms pull
    - Move upright once vertex descends
  - o Avoid upright positions until head enters pelvis
  - o Squatting
    - Squatting bar
    - Birth stool
  - o Standing
  - o Sitting
    - Birth ball
    - Bed
    - Chair
    - Toilet
- Sleep
  - o Early labor
  - o Active labor
    - If contractions slow secondary to fatigue
    - Mother & fetus are both stable
  - o Hydrotherapy
    - Tub
    - Whirlpool
    - Shower
  - o Empty bladder, bowels
- Assess maternal environment for stress factors
  - o Light
  - o Noise
  - o Family or staff members
- Allow more time if mother and fetus stable
- Nipple stimulation
- Herbal remedies(see induction/augmentation of labor)

Providing Support:

Education and Support Measures to Consider

- Discuss
  - o Findings with client, family
  - o Options available
    - Rest
    - Time
    - Pain control
    - Amniotomy
    - Augmentation
- Address patient/family concerns
- Formulate plan with patient
  - o Potential need to transport if out-of-hospital
  - o Recommendations for midwifery care
  - o Increased potential for augmentation with
    - Prolonged ROM
    - Desultory labor
  - o Increased potential for c-section
    - Active labor with
    - Failure to progress
    - Failure to descend
    - Fetal stress

Follow-up Care:

Follow-up Measures to Consider

- Follow-up care, reassess
  - o At least every 1-3 h
  - o Following institution of treatment measures
  - o With maternal or fetal indication
- Update plan after each assessment
  - o Maternal and fetal response
  - o Interval change
  - o Clinical impression
  - o Discussions with patient/family
  - o Consultations
  - o Interval midwifery plan of care

Collaborative Practice:

Criteria to Consider for Consultation or Referral

- Dysfunctional labor
  - o For augmentation
  - o In spite of augmentation
  - o For transport
- For persistently non-progressive labor
  - o Dilation
  - o Descent
  - o Suspected CPD
  - o Fetal malposition
- For fetal or maternal distress

Group B Strep

Key Clinical Information

An average of 10-30% of women are colonized, either vaginally or rectally, with Group B Streptococcus (GBS). GBS may cause maternal urinary tract infection, amnionitis, post-partum endometritis, and wound infections. As many as 50% of infants born to colonized mothers may become colonized with GBS, and 4% of those babies colonized will develop serious complications related to the infection.[8]

Early onset GBS disease is most likely in the presence of both maternal colonization and additional risk factors for GBS disease. The rate of early-onset GBS disease has diminished significantly since the institution of antibiotic prophylaxis in the early 1990's. Late onset GBS disease has not diminished during this time Complications of neonatal GBS infection includes meningitis, pneumonia, and sepsis. There is an associated newborn mortality rate of up to 22%.

---

[8] CDC. (2002) Perinatal Group B Streptococcal Disease: Background, Epidemiology, and overview of revised CDC prevention guidelines. Avvailable as a slide show on-line at www.cdc.gov/groupbstrep/docs/GBS.slideset.DEC2.forweb.ppt

Jolivet, RR (2002). Early-onset neonatal group B streptococcal infection: 2002 guidelines for prevention. Journal of Midwifery & Women's Health 47:435-446.

Client History:

Components of the History to Consider

- G, P
- Ethnic & racial background
- Medication allergies
  - o PCN allergy
    - Not at risk for anaphylaxis
      - Cefazolin
    - High risk for anaphylaxis
      - Clindamycin
      - Erythromycin
      - Vancomycin
- Review prenatal course
- GBS status known
  - o Culture at 35-37 weeks (
    - Distal vagina rectum, through anal sphincter
    - Self-collect an option
    - Use selective broth medium for GBS
  - o Urine culture
- GBS status unknown
  - o Evaluate risk factors
  - o Use risk-based strategy
- Identify risk factors for neonatal sepsis
  - o African American women
  - o Non-smokers
  - o + GBS culture
  - o GBS bacteriuria in pregnancy
  - o Previous infant with GBS sepsis
  - o Previous amnionitis
  - o PPROM
  - o Prolonged ROM
  - o Maternal fever (>38°C/100.4°F) in labor
  - o Preterm birth/ low birth weight

Physical Examination:

Components of the Physical Exam to Consider

- Vital signs, including
  - o Maternal temp & pulse
  - o Fetal heart rate
- Routine maternal & fetal labor evaluation
- Evaluate for symptoms of chorioamnionitis
  - o Febrile patient
  - o Significant & persistent fetal tachycardia

Clinical Impression:

Differential Diagnoses to Consider

- Group B Strep
  - o Colonization
  - o Infection
  - o Amnionitis
- Consider other organism causing
- Maternal fever of unknown origin
- Fetal distress

Diagnostic Testing:

Diagnostic Tests and Procedures to Consider

- CBC
- Maternal blood cultures if no GBS results available
- Cultures at delivery
- Amnion/placenta
- Baby; axilla groin or behind ear

Providing Treatment:

Therapeutic Measures to Consider

- GBS negative - no treatment
- GBS unavailable - offer treatment if
  - o Delivery at <37 weeks gestation
  - o Intrapartum fever (>38°C/100.4°F)

- o ROM > 18 hours
- GBS positive - offer treatment for
  - o Positive culture this pregnancy
  - o Previous infant with GBS disease
  - o GBS bacteriuria in current pregnancy
  - o Labor onset at < 37 weeks gestation
- Intrapartum prophylaxis *not* indicated
  - o Previous pregnancy with positive GBS culture
  - o Planned Cesarean without labor or ROM
  - o Negative culture this pregnancy, regardless of risk factors
- Allow time for 2 doses of antibiotics prior to delivery
- Penicillin G
  - o 5 million U IV followed by
  - o 2.5 million U q 4 hours until delivery
- Ampicillin
  - o 2 g IV followed by
  - o 1 g q 4 hours until delivery
- For PCN allergy
- Clindamycin
  - o 900 mg IV q 8 hours until delivery
- Erythromycin
  - o 500 mg IV q 6 hours until delivery
- Oral therapy for expectant management of ROM
  - o Not current CDC recommendations
  - o < 37 weeks gestation
  - o Amoxicillin
    - 500 mg TID
    - Begin at 18 hours ROM
  - o Clindamycin
    - For PCN allergy
    - 300 mg q 6 hrs
  - o Patient obtains temp q 4-6 hours while awake
    - Call with temp > 37.8°C
  - o Change to IV chemoprophylaxis
    - Onset of active labor
    - Temp > 38°C

Providing Treatment:

Alternative Measures to Consider

- Expectant management with or without screening
- Evaluation and treatment of symptomatic infants

Providing Support:

Education and Support Measures to Consider

- Practice routine regarding GBS screening
- Treatment options if GBS +
- Provide information to allow informed decision-making
  - o Current CDC recommendations
  - o Risks & benefits of antibiotics
  - o Individual risk for GBS disease in infant
  - o Alternatives to current recommendations
- Provide information regarding neonatal sepsis
  - o May occur from birth through 28 days of life
  - o Seek care immediately if any symptoms develop
    - Symptoms
    - Lethargy
    - Pallor
    - Poor feeding
    - Fever
    - Abnormal cry

Follow-up Care:

Follow-up Measures to Consider

- Document all discussions regarding
  - o GBS culture results
  - o Treatment plan options
  - o Client preferences for care
  - o Risk factors for GBS infection

- Schedule regular infant assessment

Collaborative Practice:

Criteria to Consider for Consultation or Referral

- Maternal conditions
  - Women with intrapartum fever (>38°C/100.4°F)
  - Women with + GBS and preterm labor or PROM

  o   Transfer of care or birth location due to GBS status or symptoms
- Newborn conditions
  - Symptomatic infants
  - Infant whose mothers have received antibiotic

Induction or Augmentation of Labor

Key Clinical Information

Induction or augmentation of labor may be initiated for a wide variety of indications. Practices vary tremendously toward the approach to induction and augmentation. Maternal involvement in the decision-making process is essential, as stimulation of labor may contribute to maternal feelings of failure or success based on maternal motivation and attitude toward the induction or augmentation process.

Bishops Score	0	1	2	3
Dilation (cms)	0	1-2 cms	3-4 cms	5-6 cms
Effacement	0-30%	40-50%	60-70%	80+%
Station	-3	-2	-1/0	+1/+2
Consistency	Firm	Medium	Soft	N/A
Position	Posterior	Mid-position	Anterior	N/A

Client History:

Components of the History to Consider

- Verify
  - LMP, EDC, gestational age
  - Estimated fetal weight
- Identify indication for induction/augmentation
  - Desultory or non-progressive labor
  - PROM
    - Temperature rising
    - + BGS culture
  - Time limits post SROM for delivery
  - Chorioamnionitis
  - Post-term pregnancy (ƒ42 weeks)
  - Moderate or severe PIH
  - Maternal diabetes mellitus
  - Maternal medical problems
  - Fetal risk in utero
  - Fetal demise
- OB history that would demonstrate contraindication
  - Abnormal lie
  - Placenta previa
  - Vasa previa
  - Classical uterine incision
  - Active genital herpes
  - Invasive cervical cancer
- Cytotec contraindications
  - VBAC
  - Asthma
- Obtain general labor admission history

Physical Examination:

Components of the Physical Exam to Consider

- Maternal & fetal vital signs
- Pelvic exam
  - Pelvimetry to rule out CPD

  o   Bishop's score
- Labor evaluation
  - Fetal & maternal well being
  - Contraction status
    - Frequency, duration, strength
    - Palpation
  - External or internal monitoring
  - Pelvic exam
    - Cervical status
      - Effacement
      - Dilation
      - Consistency
    - Status of membranes
    - Descent of presenting part

Clinical Impression:

Differential Diagnoses to Consider

- Induction or augmentation of labor for
- Dysfunctional labor
- PROM
- Chorioamnionitis
- Post-term pregnancy (ƒ42 weeks)
- Severe PIH
- Maternal diabetes mellitus
- Maternal medical problems
- Fetal risk in utero
- Fetal demise

Diagnostic Testing:

Diagnostic Tests and Procedures to Consider

- Fetal evaluation
  - NST
  - Biophysical profile
  - Amniotic fluid index
  - Intermittent auscultation of FHT

- o   Continuous fetal monitoring
- Pre-op labs
  - o   CBC
  - o   Urinalysis
  - o   Type and screen (or red top tube to hold)

Providing Treatment:

Therapeutic Measures to Consider

- Cervical ripening
  - o   Prostin E2
  - o   Prepidil
  - o   Cervidil
  - o   Hospital compounded prostin E2 gel 5mg
  - o   Cytotec (may result in induction)
    - ▪   25-50 mcg po or in posterior vaginal fornix
    - ▪   Repeat doses q 3-6 hours
  - o   Laminaria
  - o   Foley catheter balloon
- Induction/augmentation
  - o   Amniotomy
  - o   Oxytocin infusion
    - ▪   10 units oxytocin/1000 ml IV solution such as LR
    - ▪   Titrate to 3 contractions q 10 minutes
    - ▪   Rates vary, examples include
    - ▪   0.5 to 2 mU/min
    - ▪   Increase 1-2 mU/min q 15-60 min
  - o   Maximum dose 20-40 mU/min
  - o   Complications
    - ▪   Over-stimulation of the uterus
    - ▪   Fetal distress
    - ▪   Under-dosing and resultant exhaustion
    - ▪   Water intoxication
    - ▪   Nausea and vomiting
    - ▪   Lethargy
    - ▪   Headache
    - ▪   Confusion
    - ▪   Convulsions
    - ▪   Coma
    - ▪   Hypotension
    - ▪   Cardiac arrhythmias

Providing Treatment:

Alternative Measures to Consider

- Repeated fetal surveillance and patience
- Cervical ripening/initiation of labor
  - o   Nipple stimulation
  - o   Sexual intercourse
  - o   Castor oil 2 oz PO
  - o   Stripping of membranes
  - o   Herbs
    - ▪   Evening primrose oil
    - ▪   Blue/black cohosh
  - o   Homeopathic remedies
    - ▪   Caulophyllum
    - ▪   Cimicifuga

- ▪   Pulsitilla

Providing Support:

Education and Support Measures to Consider

- Outline recommendations
  - o   Indication for induction or augmentation
  - o   Informed consent
  - o   Risks: maternal & fetal
  - o   Benefits: maternal & fetal
  - o   Alternatives: risks & benefits
  - o   Potential for
    - ▪   Transport if out-of-hospital
    - ▪   IVs
    - ▪   Fetal monitoring
    - ▪   Potential restrictions
      - •   NPO
      - •   Clear liquids
      - •   Bedrest, etc.
    - ▪   IV oxytocin
    - ▪   Electronic fetal monitoring
    - ▪   Limited mobility
    - ▪   Operative assistance at birth
    - ▪   Vacuum extraction
    - ▪   Forceps
    - ▪   C-section
  - o   Patient/family preferences
  - o   Provide support

Follow-up Care:

Follow-up Measures to Consider

- Document
  - o   Relevant history
  - o   Indication for induction or augmentation
  - o   Physical findings
  - o   Test results as applicable
  - o   Clinical impression
  - o   Discussion with patient/family
  - o   Patient preferences & informed consent
  - o   Consultation/referral
  - o   Midwifery plan of care
- Follow-up care
  - o   Evaluate maternal/fetal status at regular intervals
    - ▪   Evaluate for progress
    - ▪   Per indication for induction/augmentation
  - o   Update plan after each evaluation
  - o   Ensure access to emergency services prn
  - o   Allow client to express feelings and concerns about induction/augmentation

Collaborative Practice:

Criteria to Consider for Consultation or Referral

- As needed for transport
- Prior to induction or ripening per practice agreement
- Onset of complications
- Women requiring c-section or other assisted birth

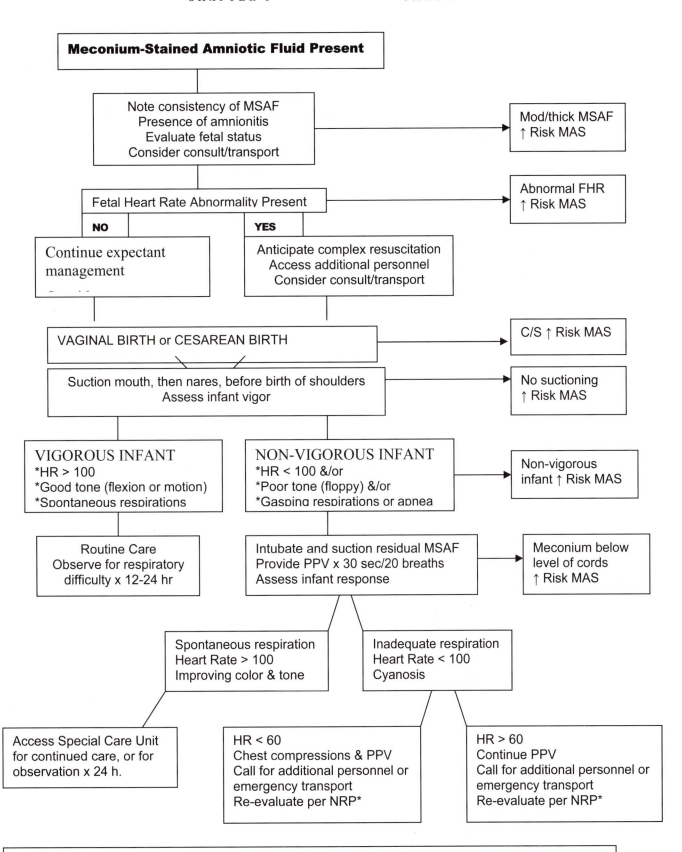

Meconium-Stained Amniotic Fluid Present

Note consistency of MSAF
Presence of amnionitis
Evaluate fetal status
Consider consult/transport

→ Mod/thick MSAF
↑ Risk MAS

Fetal Heart Rate Abnormality Present

→ Abnormal FHR
↑ Risk MAS

NO — Continue expectant management

YES — Anticipate complex resuscitation
Access additional personnel
Consider consult/transport

VAGINAL BIRTH or CESAREAN BIRTH

→ C/S ↑ Risk MAS

Suction mouth, then nares, before birth of shoulders
Assess infant vigor

→ No suctioning
↑ Risk MAS

VIGOROUS INFANT
*HR > 100
*Good tone (flexion or motion)
*Spontaneous respirations

NON-VIGOROUS INFANT
*HR < 100 &/or
*Poor tone (floppy) &/or
*Gasping respirations or apnea

→ Non-vigorous
infant ↑ Risk MAS

Routine Care
Observe for respiratory
difficulty x 12-24 hr

Intubate and suction residual MSAF
Provide PPV x 30 sec/20 breaths
Assess infant response

→ Meconium below
level of cords
↑ Risk MAS

Spontaneous respiration
Heart Rate > 100
Improving color & tone

Inadequate respiration
Heart Rate < 100
Cyanosis

Access Special Care Unit
for continued care, or for
observation x 24 h.

HR < 60
Chest compressions & PPV
Call for additional personnel or
emergency transport
Re-evaluate per NRP*

HR > 60
Continue PPV
Call for additional personnel or
emergency transport
Re-evaluate per NRP*

NRP: American Heart Association & American Academy of Pediatrics Neonatal Resuscitation Program
recommendations from the Neonatal Resuscitation Textbook (2000).

Meconium-Stained Amniotic Fluid

Key Clinical Information

Meconium-stained amniotic fluid occurs in approximately XX% of pregnancies. It is more common in the post-dates pregnancy, but it can also occur in preterm pregnancies. Meconium-aspiration syndrome may occur when the fetus born through meconium-stained breathes the meconium in to the lungs, but it occurs more often as a prenatal occurrence in the compromised fetus. Suctioning of the mouth and nose, after the birth of the head and before the birth of the shoulders, is the single most important action to prevent meconium aspiration syndrome in the healthy newborn. Identification of the fetus at risk for meconium-aspiration syndrome should prompt availability of pediatric care at birth.

Client History:

Components of the History to Consider

- Verify EDC, gestational age
- Presence of recent fetal activity
- Characteristics of meconium in fluid
  o Thin
  o Moderate
  o Thick
  o Particulate
- Risk factors for meconium [9]
  o Maternal factors
    ▪ <5 prenatal visits
    ▪ Oligohydramnios
    ▪ Term or post-term pregnancy
  o Labor risk factors
    ▪ Consistency of meconium
    ▪ Abnormal FHR patterns
    ▪ Precipitous birth
    ▪ Cesarean delivery
  o Fetal factors
    ▪ Advancing gestational age
    ▪ Lack of suctioning before birth of shoulders
    ▪ Apgar of <7 (1 or 5 minutes)

Physical Examination:

Components of the Physical Exam to Consider

- Abdominal exam for:
  o FHT in relation to contractions
  o Fetal mobility or fluid adequacy (thick meconium is often associated with oligohydramnios)
  o Frequency, duration and strength of contractions
  o Fetal lie, presentation (meconium common with breech)
- Pelvic exam for:

---

[9] Hernández C, Little BB, Dax JS, Gilstrap LC, Rosenfield CR. Prediction of the severity of meconium aspiration syndrome. Am J Obstet Gynecol 169;1:61-70.

Wiswell TE, Gannon CM, Jacob J, Goldsmith L, Szyld E, Weiss K, et al. Delivery room management of the apparently vigorous meconium-stained neonate: Results of the multicenter, international collaborative trial. Pediatrics 2000:105:1; 1-7

- Cervical status
- Confirmation of presentation
- Station of presenting part
- Fetal position

Clinical Impression:

Differential Diagnoses to Consider

- Meconium stained amniotic fluid
  o Thin, watery
  o Thick, particulate
- Term fetus with normal bowel function
- Fetal distress
- Fetus at risk for meconium-aspiration syndrome

Diagnostic Testing:

Diagnostic Tests and Procedures to Consider

- Evaluation of fetal status
  o Intermittent auscultation
  o Electronic fetal monitor
    ▪ External
    ▪ Internal
- Ultrasound
  o Amniotic fluid index
  o Fetal presentation
- Pre-operative labs
  o Persistent or worsening fetal distress
  o Arrest of dilation or descent
  o Per facility standard

Providing Treatment:

Therapeutic Measures to Consider

- Evaluate fetal well being
- Consider amnioinfusion
- Birth in gravity neutral position
- Upon birth of the head suction
  o Nares
  o Mouth
  o Pharnyx
- Prepare for potential
  o Intubation of infants who are
    ▪ Not vigorous
    ▪ Initially vigorous but develop respiratory distress
  o Neonatal resuscitation
  o Neonatal transport

Providing Treatment:

Alternative Measures to Consider

- Expectant management
- Atraumatic birth

Providing Support:

Education and Support Measures to Consider

- Advise patient of risks with meconium
  o Meconium aspiration syndrome
  o Trauma potential with intubation
  o No treatment increases risk for
    ▪ Severe respiratory disorders
    ▪ Newborn death
- Encourage maternal participation in prevention
  o No pushing until mouth & nose are suctioned
  o Gravity neutral positioning for birth
  o No stimulation until airway is ensured
  o Importance of maternal attention to newborn
- Advise of potential for interventions
  o Amnioinfusion
  o Intubation of newborn
  o Oxygen for newborn
  o Transport if out-of hospital birth planned
  o Newborn special care
  o Antibiotic therapy for infant
- Provide ongoing information

  o In labor
  o At birth
  o If newborn needs special care

Follow-up Care:

Follow-up Measures to Consider

- Assure professional skilled in intubation is available
- Have all resuscitation equipment on hand and tested
- Document:
  o Consistency and amount of meconium
  o Therapeutic measures instituted
  o Maternal and fetal response to treatment
  o Parents preferences for infant care
  o Consultations obtained

Collaborative Practice:

Criteria to Consider for Consultation or Referral

- Abnormal FHR patterns
- Thick or particulate meconium
- Documented or suspected oligohydramnios
- For change in planned location of birth
  o Consider hospital birth in presence of
    ▪ Meconium-stained amniotic fluid, and
      • Post-dates pregnancy, *or*
      • Abnormal FHR pattern
- Respiratory distress in neonate

Caring for the Woman with Multiple Pregnancy

Key Clinical Information

Midwives may attend women with multiple pregnancies in some settings. Early identification of the multiple pregnancy may provide the opportunity to address potential complications before they arise. In the home birth setting, the midwife assumes the responsibility for advising parents of the increased risk of adverse outcomes with multiple pregnancy when birth occurs in the home.[10] Regardless of planned birth location, the midwife must have a mechanism to provide access to obstetrical or pediatric care should it be indicated. Incidence of multiple gestation may be as high as 3%, and is associated with increased risk for preterm labor, preterm rupture of membranes, intrauterine fetal growth retardations, twin to twin transfusion and other less common problems

---

[10] Mehl-Madrona, L., Medrona, M. M.(1997). Physician and midwife attended home births; Effects of breech, twin, and post-dates outcome data on mortality rates. *Journal of Nurse-Midwifery*, 42, 91-98.

[10] ACOG (2002). Educational Bulletin No. 253, Nov. 1998, in: Compendium of selected publications, ACOG, Washington, DC.

Client History:

Components of the History to Consider

- LMP, EDC
- Contributing factors for multiple gestation
  - Family history of multiples
  - Personal history of multiples
  - Use of fertility drugs
  - In vitro fertilization
- History suggestive of multiple gestation
  - Fundal growth pattern
    - Size > dates by exam
  - Fetal motion not detected by 18-20 weeks size
  - Elevated AFP results
- Individual client risk assessment
  - Fetal anomaly v preterm labor
  - Uterine irritability
  - Cervical status
  - Other pregnancy complications
  - Rh status
  - Medical conditions
  - Social support
  - Nutrition status
  - Working or living conditions
  - Response to multiple gestation

Physical Examination:

Components of the Physical Exam to Consider

- Size greater than dates on two or more occasions
- Two fetal hearts heard via Doppler or fetoscope
- Interval fundal growth pattern
- Cervical length and dilation
- Interval weight gain

Clinical Impression:

Differential Diagnoses to Consider

- Multiple pregnancy, with increased risk for
  - Structural anomalies
  - Chromosomal anomalies
  - Preterm labor
  - Preterm rupture of membranes
  - Fetal discordance

Diagnostic Testing:

Diagnostic Tests and Procedures to Consider

- Alfa fetal protein testing
- Amniocentesis
- Ultrasound evaluation for
  - Gestational age
  - Presence of multiple gestation
  - Presence of anomalies
  - Amniocentesis
  - Placenta(s) & membranes
    - Monochorionic
    - Dichorionic, diamniotic
  - Fetal gender(s)
  - Interval growth
  - Cervical evaluation
    - Width
    - Length
    - Funnelling
- Antepartum surveillance
  - Not indicated for uncomplicated multiple gestation[11]

---

[11] AGOC, Ibid.

- For complications of multiple gestation
  - IUGR
  - Abnormal AFI
  - Discordant fetal growth
  - PIH
  - Fetal anomalies
  - Monoamniotic twins
  - Non-stress testing
  - Biophysical profile

Providing Treatment:

Therapeutic Measures to Consider

- Not recommended per ACOG
  - Cervical cerclage
  - Bedrest
- Selective fetal termination
  - Common with in vitro fertilizaton
  - May pose ethical challenges
- Preterm labor (see Preterm Labor)
- Preterm ROM (see PROM)
- Vertex - Vertex twins
  - Anticipate vaginal birth
  - C/S for same indications with singleton birth
- Vertex - Non-vertex twins
  - Consider vaginal birth for second twin over 1500 g
  - Consider Cesarean birth based on
    - Fetus weight (under 1500 g)
    - Maternal preference
    - Clinician skill & experience
- Non-vertex first twin
  - Cesarean delivery is usual
  - Vaginal delivery of non-vertex first twin has not been studied
  - Potential for locked twins with breech-vertex twins
- Ongoing evaluation of second fetus following first birth
  - Ultrasound
  - Electronic fetal monitoring
  - Close observation for complications
    - Cord prolapse
    - Placental abruption
    - Abnormal fetal heart rate pattern
  - Oxytocin stimulation or augmentation of labor
  - Amniotomy
  - For deteriorating fetal status
    - Internal podalic version
    - Breech extraction

Providing Treatment:

Alternative Measures to Consider

- Diagnosis of twins via clinical exam
- Out of hospital birth
  - Uncomplicated multiple gestation
  - Maternal preference
  - Informed choice considerations
    - Risk factors for individual
    - Midwife skill and experience
    - Distance/time to emergency care
    - Multiple births hold increased risk regardless of birth location
    - Poor outcomes at home birth may hurt home birth
    - Freedom of choice includes ready access to care as needed
- In hospital birth
  - Vaginal birth
    - Birth room

- Minimum of people
- Opportunity to meet staff before hand
- Negotiation of preferences
- Ability to see & touch babies immediately
- Care provided in family's presence
- Rooming in and breastfeeding fostered
  o Cesarean birth
    - Support people present
    - Ability to see & touch babies immediately, if stable
    - Care provided in family's presence
    - Rooming in an breastfeeding fostered

Providing Support:
Education and Support Measures to Consider
- Discussion and education re: multiple gestation
- Anticipated care during pregnancy
- Information on testing or surveillance
  o Procedures
  o Results
  o Implications
  o Options for on-going care
- Listening to client
  o Individual needs
  o Preferences
  o Collaborative planning of care
- Options for high-risk care as indicated

Follow-up Care:
Follow-up Measures to Consider
- Increase frequency of prenatal visits

  o By gestational age
  o As indicated by results of testing
  o In presence of any complicating factors
  o As term approaches (third trimester)
- Detailed documentation of
  o Diagnosis of multiple gestation
  o Client preferences
    - Prenatal care
    - Labor & birth
    - Infant feeding
    - Home care, prn
  o Plan for care
    - On-going evaluation
    - Identification of risk factors
    - Treatments & results
    - Consultations
    - Update plan as changes occur

Collaborative Practice:
Criteria to Consider for Consultation or Referral
- For all multiple pregnancies per midwife scope of practice
- For multiple gestation with complications
  o Maternal complications
  o Fetal complications
  o Triplet or greater
- Maternal preference
- As indicated for labor, birth and newborn care

Caring for the Woman with a Non Vertex Presentation

Key Clinical Information

Breech presentation is the most common non-vertex presentation, occurring in 3-4% of term singleton pregnancies. Breech and other non-vertex presentations carry an increased risk of complications over a vertex presentation. The relative safety of breech birth may be affected by the skill and experience of the birth attendant. Women's preferences for care should be taken into account during discussions of options.

ACOG recommends external version to convert breech or transverse lie to vertex presentation to decrease the risks associated with non-vertex presentations and avoid unnecessary Cesarean birth[12]. Current recommendations include offering planned Cesarean to women with term breech babies in an attempt to decrease perinatal morbidity and mortality[13]. Planned Cesarean for non-vertex presentation does not apply to those women

---

[12] ACOG (2002). Committee opinion No. 265, Dec. 2001. Mode of term singleton breech delivery. In: Compendium of selected publications. ACOG.

[13] Hannah ME, Hannah WJ, et al. (2000) Planned cesarean section versus planned vaginal birth for breech presentation at term: a randomized multicenter trial. Term Breech Collaborative Group. Lancet, 356:1375-1383.

who refuse surgical delivery, those in advanced labor when birth is imminent at the time of diagnosis, or those whose second twin is a non-vertex presentation.

Client History:

Components of the History to Consider

- LMP, EDC
  o   External version after 36 weeks
- Previous maternity history
  o   Previous breech births
  o   Previous birth weights of children
  o   Presence of uterine scars
- Current pregnancy history
  o   Methods of dating pregnancy
  o   Rh status
  o   Placental location
  o   Presence of labor

Physical Examination:

Components of the Physical Exam to Consider

- Abdominal exam
  o   Leopold's maneuvers
      ▪   Determine fetal presentation lie & variety
      ▪   Estimate fetal weight
  o   Abdominal muscle tone
  o   Uterine tone
  o   Fetal hear rate
- Pelvic exam
  o   Clinical pelvimetry
  o   Cervical status

Clinical Impression:

Differential Diagnoses to Consider

- Pregnancy, non-vertex presentation
  o   Pre-term
  o   Term
  o   Post-term

Diagnostic Testing:

Diagnostic Tests and Procedures to Consider

- Ultrasound
  o   Confirmation of fetal position
  o   Evaluation of placental position
  o   Version may be performed under U/S guidance
- External cephalic version
  o   Fetal evaluation
      ▪   NST or BPP
      ▪   Continuous fetal monitoring during and post procedure
  o   IV access
  o   Pre-operative labs

Providing Treatment:

Therapeutic Measures to Consider

- External cephalic version [14]
  o   Success rates of 35-86%
  o   More successful in
      ▪   Mulitparous women
      ▪   Transverse or oblique lie

---

[14] ACOG. Practice bulletin No. 13, Feb 2000. External Cephalic Version. In: 2000 Compendium of selected publications.

- ▪   Tocolytics
      •   For nulliparous women
      •   For all women
  o   Rh immune globulin
  o   Ready access to emergency Cesarean birth
  o   Method, following fetal evaluation
      ▪   Attempt forward roll using gentle steady pressure
          •   Lift breech from pelvis
          •   Encourage head toward pelvis with gentle pressure & flexion
      ▪   Attempt backward roll if forward roll not successful
      ▪   Two practitioners may work together to encourage fetus to turn
      ▪   Stop in the presence of
          •   Fetal bradycardia
          •   Maternal pain
          •   Unsuccessful version
          •   Successful version
- Vaginal breech birth
  o   More successful in women with
      ▪   Adequate pelvis
      ▪   Previous vaginal birth
      ▪   Skilled birth attendant
  o   Higher risk of perinatal complications vs
      ▪   Vaginal vertex birth post-version
      ▪   Planned Cesarean birth
- Planned Cesarean birth

Providing Treatment:

Alternative Measures to Consider

- Breech tilt position
  o   Use 5 minutes 3-4 times daily
  o   Hips higher than head on tilt board
  o   Music at maternal feet to encourage fetus
- Moxibustion
- Homeopathic remedies

Providing Support:

Education and Support Measures to Consider

- Provide information on risks, benefits and availability of
  o   Vaginal breech birth
  o   External cephalic version
  o   Planned cesarean birth
- Obtain informed consent for planned birth or procedure
  o   Perinatal risk with planned vaginal breech ⪦5%
  o   Perinatal risk with planned cesarean for breech ⪦1.6%
  o   Perinatal risk includes
      ▪   Fetal injury or death
      ▪   Neonatal injury or death
  o   Maternal risk deemed equivalent for C/S vs vaginal breech
- Encourage questions regarding options
- Consider maternal preferences in jointly determining plan for care
- Discuss

Follow-up Care:

Follow-up Measures to Consider

- Reconfirm fetal position prior to birth

- Reconfirm maternal preference for planned birth or procedure
- Persistent breech
  - o   Repeat version attempt
  - o   Reconsider vaginal breech or planned Cesarean
- Document
  - o   All discussions
  - o   Informed consent/informed choice
  - o   Maternal preferences for care
  - o   For planned vaginal breech
    - ▪   Access to emergency care
    - ▪   Estimated fetal weight
    - ▪   Plan of birth

- Number & type of birth attendants
- Presence of resuscitation team for newborn
- Plan for emergency care

Collaborative Practice:

Criteria to Consider for Consultation or Referral

- For all non-vertex presentations
- As indicated by collaborative practice agreement
- For failed version
- For transport for hospital birth

Caring for the Woman with Postpartum Hemorrhage

Key Clinical Information

Postpartum hemorrhage is defined as a blood loss of greater than 500 ml at delivery, or within the first 24 hours following vaginal birth. Postpartum hemorrhage is a leading cause of maternal mortality worldwide. Anemia may be a significant contributor to delayed postpartum healing and predispose to infection. Hemorrhage may be the primary indicator of retained placental tissue, uterine fatigue, lacerations, or disorders of coagulation. The primary cause of postpartum hemorrhage is uterine atony.[15]

---

[15] Long, P Safe management of third stage labor: a technical repost based on review of the current literature.

Client History:

Components of the History to Consider

- Ethnic history
  - Asian
  - Hispanic
- Past OB history
  - Prior history of postpartum hemorrhage
  - Grand multiparity
- Current OB history
  - Length & effectiveness of uterine contractions
  - Oxytocin administration
  - Chorioamnionitis
  - PIH, Hellp syndrome
    - MGSO4 use
    - Low platelets
  - Polyhydramnios
  - Multiple gestation
  - Operative delivery
  - Uterine manipulation, i.e. version
  - Placenta previa or abruption
  - Fetal demise
  - DIC
  - Placental delivery & status
- Medical history
  - Bleeding disorders
  - Asthma (prostin)
  - Hypertension (methergine)

Physical Examination:

Components of the Physical Exam to Consider

- Evaluate bladder, empty prn
- Encourage slow, gentle birth of infant
- Evaluate the uterus for placental separation
  - Uterus globular, firm
  - Fundus rises & is mobile
  - Cord lengthens
- Evaluate the uterus for atony
- If atony present:
  - Massage fundus
  - Bimanual compression
  - Consider retained placental fragments
- If no atony
  - Evaluate for traumatic source of bleeding
  - Cervical lacerations
  - Vaginal lacerations
  - Uterine rupture
- Re-examine placenta for absent fragments
  - Visual exam of maternal & fetal surfaces
  - Tactile exam of maternal surface
  - Uterine exploration for retained placental fragments
  - May need D&E

Clinical Impression:

Differential Diagnoses to Consider

- Postpartum hemorrhage secondary to:
  - Full bladder
  - Rapid labor and birth
  - Prolonged labor and birth
  - Over-distended uterus
  - Retained placental fragments
  - Oxytocin administration
  - MGSO4 administration
  - Grand multiparity
  - Genital tract lacerations
  - Uterine rupture
  - Clotting dysfunction

- HELLP syndrome

Diagnostic Testing:

Diagnostic Tests and Procedures to Consider

- Labs
  - CBC
  - H&H
  - Platelets
  - Type and cross-match
  - Liver function tests
  - PIH labs
  - Labs to confirm suspected coagulopathy
- Ultrasound
  - Evaluation for retained placental fragments

Providing Treatment:

Therapeutic Measures to Consider

- Active management of third stage
  - Slow birth of infant by uterine forces
  - Early cord clamping
  - Verify singleton infant
  - Uterotonic medication with birth of anterior shoulder
  - Drain placental blood, reapply clamp
  - Assess for placental separation
  - When placenta appears separated
    - Provide controlled cord traction
    - Guard uterus with one cupped hand
    - Push uterus toward maternal chest
    - Guide placenta down into vagina
    - When placenta visible guide up to expel
    - Twist to 'rope' membranes
    - Massage uterus until firm
    - Encourage breastfeeding
  - Examine placenta for completeness
- Bimanual compression
  - If uterus fails to contract well
  - Decreases blood supply to large uterine vessels
  - Will not diminish bleeding due to lacerations
  - Technique
    - One hand in vagina against lower uterine segment
    - Second hand on abdomen
    - Bring hands together with uterus in between
- Medications:
  - Oxytocin, 10 units IM, 10-20 units in IV fluids
  - Syntocinon 10 units IM
  - Methergine, 0.2 mg IM, may follow with 0.2 mg PO q6 hrs
  - Hemabate, 250 mcg IM
  - Prostin/15M, 0.25 mg IM
  - Cytotec 100-400 mcg per rectum
- IV therapy
  - Large bore catheter(s)
  - D5LR, LR, Normosol or other similar solution
  - 10 units oxytocin/500ml
  - Blood transfusion
  - Whole blood
  - Packed RBCs
  - Other blood components as indicated
- For shock:
  - Additional IV access
  - O2 by mask
  - Trendelenberg or shock position
  - Foley catheter
- Extreme bleeding
  - Surgical control of bleeding
    - Repair of lacerations

- ▪ Suture ligature of bleeding vessels
- ▪ Dilation & evacuation of retained placenta fragments
- ▪ Hysterectomy or uterine artery ligation in extreme cases
  - o Aortic compression
    - ▪ Emergency measure while awaiting surgical care

Providing Treatment:

Alternative Measures to Consider

- Preventives
  - o Nettle or alfalfa leaf infusion
    - ▪ Given during pregnancy
    - ▪ Immediately following birth of baby
  - o Motherwort tincture
- Allow physiologic third stage
  - o Gentle birth under maternal forces
  - o Avoid clamping cord until pulsations stop
  - o Early breastfeeding
  - o No cord traction
  - o Maternal efforts for expulsion
  - o Allow 30-60 minutes for third stage if
    - ▪ No bleeding
    - ▪ No signs of separation
    - ▪ No maternal pain
- Treatment of hemorrhage due to atony
  - o Shepherd's purse tincture
  - o Tincture of
    - ▪ Blue cohosh
    - ▪ Shepherd's purse
    - ▪ Motherwort
  - o Rescue remedy
  - o Breast feeding
  - o Breast stimulation
  - o Homeopathic arnica

Providing Support:

Education and Support Measures to Consider

- Discuss or arrange transport if out of hospital
- Following resolution of hemorrhage advise patient
  - o Of occurrence of hemorrhage

- o If symptomatic, call for help before arising
- o Take iron replacement therapy as directed
  - ▪ Dietary sources
  - ▪ Supplements
- o Rest and adequate nutrition are essential for healing
- o Reinforce signs and symptoms of infection
  - ▪ How to recognize
  - ▪ When & how to call

Follow-up Care:

Follow-up Measures to Consider

- Document
  - o EBL
  - o Actions and their effectiveness
  - o Medications and their effectiveness
  - o Requests for consult if obtained
  - o Maternal vital signs
  - o Plan for follow-up
  - o Maternal education
- Supervision of activity if symptomatic
  - o Weakness
  - o Dyspnea
  - o Syncope
- H&H
  - o First postpartum day
  - o Repeat if bleeding continues
  - o 4-6 week check

Collaborative Practice:

Criteria to Consider for Consultation or Referral

- With any hemorrhage that does not respond
  - o Immediately to treatment
  - o As expected with appropriate treatment
- Signs and symptoms of shock
- For transport from out of hospital
- For suspicion of
  - o Retained placental fragments
  - o Severe vaginal lacerations
  - o Cervical lacerations
  - o Uterine rupture

Post-Term Pregnancy

Key Clinical Information

Post-term pregnancy is defined as pregnancy that has exceeded 42 completed weeks. There is no evidence that induction is beneficial for the uncomplicated post-term pregnancy. ACOG recommends beginning fetal surveillance by 42 weeks, although they note that many practices begin surveillance prior to 42 weeks gestation.[16] There are no firm guidelines on what constitutes reasonable fetal surveillance in the post-date pregnancy. Induction is indicated for either maternal or fetal indications, but not simply for pregnancy at 42 weeks

[16] ACOG (1997). Practice Patterns, No. 6, Oct. 1997. Management of Post-term Pregnancy. In: 2002 Compendium of Selected Publications. ACOG

gestation. Recent literature review shows a mild rise in perinatal mortality beginning at 43 weeks gestation.[17]

---

[17] Hart, G. (2002). Induction & Circular Logic. Midwifery Today No. 63:24-26, 66.

Client History:

Components of the History to Consider

- Verify EDC
  - LMP
  - B-HCG
  - Uterine size at first visit
  - Initial FHR
    - Fetoscope or stethescope 18-20 wks
    - Doppler 10-14 wks
  - Quickening
  - Fundal height at umbilicus at 20 weeks
  - Early ultrasound
- Evaluate fetal risk status
  - Perinatal mortality risk increases at 43 weeks
  - Review history for additional risk factors

Physical Examination:

Components of the Physical Exam to Consider

- Abdominal examination
  - Assess fetal presentation, position, lie, & variety
  - Evaluation for fetal flexion and engagement
  - Estimate fetal weight
  - Palpate for fluid adequacy
- Pelvic examination
  - Evaluate cervix for
    - Consistency
    - Position
    - Effacement
    - Dilation
  - Station of presenting part
  - Verify presenting part
  - Reassess pelvimetry

Clinical Impression:

Differential Diagnoses to Consider

- Post-term pregnancy (42+ weeks)
- Term pregnancy (<42 weeks)
- Pregnancy with
  - Uncertain dates
  - LGA fetus
  - Decreasing AFI

Diagnostic Testing:

Diagnostic Tests and Procedures to Consider

- Daily fetal kick counts
- Non-stress test
  - Weekly
  - Bi-weekly
- Biophysical profile
  - Weekly
  - Bi-weekly
- AFI as separate indicator
- Contraction stress testing

Providing Treatment:

Therapeutic Measures to Consider

- Cervical ripening
  - As indicated by maternal or fetal status
  - 41 - 43 weeks

- No demonstrated benefit over expectant care
- Prostaglandin E2 effective for ripening
  - Cervidil
  - Prepidil
  - Prostin Gel
- Prosteglandin E1 (Misoprostol)
  - 25 ug recommended dose
- Induction
  - As indicated by maternal or fetal status
  - 41 - 43 weeks
  - See **Induction of Labor**

Providing Treatment:

Alternative Measures to Consider

- Expectant management
- Alternative measures for cervical ripening/induction
- See **Induction of Labor**

Providing Support:

Education and Support Measures to Consider

- Discuss potential risks/benefits of
  - Expectant management
  - Interventions
- Review or teach
  - Post-dates is *after* 42 weeks
  - Fetal kick count
  - Process of labor
  - When to call
- Discuss labor options
  - Expectant care
  - Elective intervention
  - Indicated intervention
  - Any potential change in location or anticipated care for labor and birth
- Listen to and note maternal
  - Preferences
  - Concerns

Follow-up Care:

Follow-up Measures to Consider

- Evaluate fetal status q 4-7 days
- Document ongoing plan
  - Evaluations of fetal & maternal well-being
  - Cervical status
  - Client education and discussions
  - Client preferences for care
  - Midwifery plan of care
  - Consultations/referral
- Anticipate potential for meconium-stained amniotic fluid in labor

Collaborative Practice:

Criteria to Consider for Consultation or Referral

- With pregnancy post 41-43 weeks
- Fetal testing outside the norm
- Cervical ripening or induction
- Concerns regarding reasons for post-dates status
- Change in location of birth due to fetal status/post-dates

Caring for the Woman with Pregnancy-Induced Hypertension in Labor

Key Clinical Information

Approximately 5-7% of pregnant women will develop pregnancy-induced hypertension (PIH). Prompt identification of PIH by the midwife offers women the opportunity for early treatment, which may increase the likelihood of vaginal birth, and decrease the potential for maternal or fetal harm[18]. It is important to note that the woman with PIH may appear well, therefore, systematic evaluation of all women with *any* clinical indicators for PIH is warranted.[19]

PIH frequently causes elevations in maternal BP, proteinuria, and elevations in serum uric acid and liver function test results. The maternal circulating blood volume is diminished resulting in hypovolemia in spite of generalized peripheral edema. Placental and renal blood flow is frequently be diminished. Platelets may fall below well the normal range. HELLP syndrome is associated with a greater incidence of maternal morbidity, including a greater incidence of seizures, epigastric pain, nausea & vomiting, significant proteinuria and stillbirth.[20]

Severe PIH may result maternal or perinatal death.[21] Seizures may be the first sign of PIH, and may occur > 24 hours post partum.[22]

Treatment with magnesium sulfate (MgSO4) may decrease the progression of preeclampsia to eclampsia, but does not appear to slow the progression of the illness. Treatment is geared toward delivery, which resolves preeclampsia in the vast majority of cases.

---

[18] Livingston, JC, et al. (2003). Magnesium sulfate in women with mild preeclampsia: A randomized controlled trial. Obstetrics & Gynecology 101; 217-226.

[19] Roberts J (1994). Current perspectives on preeclampsia. Journal of Nurse-Midwifery; 39, 70-90.

[20] Martin JN, et al (1999). The spectrum of severe preeclampsia: comparative analysis of HELLP syndrome classification. American Journal of Obstetrics and Gynecology; 180: 1373-1384.

[21] Chandrasekhar S, Datta S. (2002) Anesthetic Management of the Preeclamptic Parturient. In Current Reviews for Nurse Anesthetists.

[22] Katz VL, Farmer R, Kuller JA (2000). Preeclampsia into eclampsia: toward a new paradigm. American Journal of Obstetrics and Gynecology; 182, 1389-96.

Evaluation and Diagnosis of Hypertensive Disorders During Pregnancy	Adapted from Roberts & Livingston
Diagnosis	**Criteria for Diagnosis**
Hypertension	Systolic BP ∞ 140, Diastolic BP ∞ 90
Severe Hypertension	Systolic☐P ∞160 mm Hg, Diastolic BP ∞110 mm Hg 2 or more BP readings ∞ 4 hours apart
Gestational Hypertension	Elevated BP without proteinuria, after 20 weeks, or postpartum, OR Hypertension during labor with uric acid ∞ 5.5-6 mg/dl
Preeclamsia	Hypertension [140 mm Hg systolic or 90 mm Hg diastolic] on 2 occasions ∞ 6 hours apart with new onset proteinuria Proteinuria: ∞ 300 mg/24 hours or ∞ 1+ on dip [at least two occasions], absence of UTI
Severe Preeclampsia	Severe hypertension [160 mm Hg systolic or 110 mm hg diastolic] with proteinuria ∞ 5 g/24 hr, or Oliguria 400 ml/24 hr or 30 ml/hr, with symptoms of epigastric pain, scotomata, and/or severe headache [end-organ involvement] OR Hypertension with pulmonary edema or a low platelet count, OR HELLP Syndrome [hemolusis, elevated liver enzymes and low platelets]: hemolysis; ⇑ bilirubin > 1.2 mg/dL, ⇑ serum aspartate aminotransferase > 72 U/L, ⇑ lactate dehydrogenase, and platelet count of 100,000/mm³
Eclampsia	Gestational hypertension with convulsions or coma

Client History:

Components of the History to Consider
- EDC, LMP
- Maternal BP
  - During pregnancy
  - During evaluation
- Review of previous PIH labs
- Symptoms of end-organ involvement
  - Persistent headache
  - Epigastric pain
  - Visual disturbance
  - Persistent nausea & vomiting
- Evaluate for PIH risk factors
  - History of essential hypertension
  - Hydatidiform mole (10x risk)
  - Fetal hydrops (10x risk)
  - Primigravida (6-8x risk)
  - Hypertension in previous pregnancy, other than first
  - Diabetes
  - Collagen vascular disease
  - Renal vascular disease
  - Renal parenchymal disease
  - Multiple gestation (5x risk)
  - African-American and other minority women
  - Age < 20 & > 35
  - Other complicating medical factors
  - Family history
  - Current vasoactive drug use (i.e., nasal decongestants, cocaine)

Physical Examination:

Components of the Physical Exam to Consider
- Pattern of weight gain
- Blood pressure readings
  - Intact equipment of correct size should be used
  - Use same maternal position for each BP
  - Arm should be supported at level of the heart

- Evaluation for pitting edema
  - Face
  - Hands
  - Feet & lower legs
- Deep tendon reflexes
  - Patellar, Achilles
  - 3+ or clonus indicates CNS irritability
- Monitor pulmonary status
- Monitor fetal status
- Optic fundi for evidence of edema or hemorrhage
- Deep tendon reflexes
- Cervical status

Clinical Impression:

Differential Diagnoses to Consider
- Gestational hypertension
- PIH superimposed on chronic hypertension
- Pregnancy induced hypertension (PIH)
- Pre-eclampsia
- Eclampsia
- HELLP syndrome
- Pre-existing undiagnosed essential hypertension

Diagnostic Testing:

Diagnostic Tests and Procedures to Consider
- Baseline PIH lab work
- Urine analysis for protein by dip
- CBC, type and screen or cross
  - Platelet count (normal range 130,000-400,000/ml)
  - Elevated HCT may indicate severity of hypovolemia
- Serum uric acid (normal range 1.2-4.5 mg/dL)
- Renal function testing
  - BUN
  - Creatinine (normal range <1.0 mg/dL)
- Liver function testing (LFTs)
- Coagulation studies, in presence of

- o   Abnormal LFTs
- o   Abruptio placenta
- Fetal surveillance
  - o   Biophysical profile
  - o   Amniotic fluid index
  - o   Fetal monitoring, observe for
    - ▪   π beat to beat variability
    - ▪   Periodic late decelerations

Providing Treatment:

Therapeutic Measures to Consider

- Expectant management
  - o   Preferred for gestation < 34 weeks
  - o   Bed rest with sedation prn
  - o   Monitoring of BP, weight, reflexes
  - o   Serial fetal surveillance
  - o   Serial PIH labs
  - o   Medications as indicated below
- Active management
  - o   Expedite delivery
  - o   Steroids to promote fetal lung maturity
- IV access and fluids
- Medications
  - o   MGSO4, anticonvulsant
    - ▪   4 Gm IV bolus followed by 2 G/hr
    - ▪   Titrat to renal output, reflexes
    - ▪   Have calcium gluconate immediately available
  - o   Oxytocin induction or augmentation of labor frequently necessary
  - o   Antihypertensive meds
    - ▪   Limited benefit
    - ▪   Used to regulate labile BP
    - ▪   170/110 to 130/90 optimum
- Monitor intake and output
  - o   Hourly I&O
  - o   NPO
  - o   Foley catheter
  - o   IV fluids on pump

Providing Treatment:

Alternative Measures to Consider

- Expectant management
- Quiet, dark room
- Rest in left lateral position
- Support people present or available
- Provide calm atmosphere of caring & safety
- Homeopathic Rescue Remedy to pulse points

- Prayer
- Ensure access to medical care

Providing Support:

Education and Support Measures to Consider

- Provide information about
  - o   Diagnosis
  - o   Options for care
  - o   Symptom recognition
  - o   Anticipated course of events
  - o   Need for calm & quiet
- Discussion regarding potential for
  - o   Change in birth plans
  - o   Medical interventions
  - o   Initiation of labor
  - o   Newborn special care
- Address client/family concerns
- Client/family to notify if additional symptoms develop, i.e.
  - o   Epigastric pain
  - o   Scotomata
  - o   Visual disturbance
  - o   Severe headache

Follow-up Care:

Follow-up Measures to Consider

- Follow vital signs/reflexes
  - o   At least q 2-4 hours
  - o   Follow for 24-48 hrs post-partum
- Document
  - o   Relevant history
  - o   Physical findings
  - o   Lab results
  - o   Clinical impression
  - o   Discussions with patient/family
  - o   Consultation/referral
  - o   Midwifery plan of care
  - o   Midwifery role in patient care

Collaborative Practice:

Criteria to Consider for Consultation or Referral

- For all patients in labor with PIH
- For women requiring transport due to PIH
- For PIH patients who appear unstable
- Notify pediatric service of
  - o   Patient's labor status
  - o   Fetal status

Care of the Woman with Preterm Labor

Key Clinical Information

Preterm labor is defined as the onset of uterine contractions that are every 5-8 minutes and consistent in a woman who is between 20-37 weeks gestation, who in addition has either spontaneous rupture of the membranes, or progressive cervical change. Many women who have preterm contractions do not in fact go into preterm labor.

Client History:

Components of the History to Consider

- EDC confirmation:
    o LMP, menstrual cycles
    o Ultrasounds
    o B-HCG
- Prior history of pre-term labor &/or SGA infant
- Determination of labor status
    o Signs and symptoms of pre-term labor
        ▪ Onset and duration of symptoms
        ▪ Precipitating factors
    o Signs and symptoms may be vague
        ▪ Mild or severe cramping
        ▪ Dull backache
        ▪ Suprapubic or pelvic pressure
        ▪ Loose stools
        ▪ Increased or 'different' vaginal discharge
- Presence of infection
    o History or symptoms of urinary tract infections or asymptomatic bacteriuria
    o History or symptoms of vaginal or STD infections
    o History or symptoms of any other infection
    o Group B Strep status

Physical Examination:

Components of the Physical Exam to Consider

- Maternal and fetal vital signs
- Abdominal exam
    o Presence of contractions
    o Uterine tenderness
    o Fetal heart rate
    o Estimated fetal weight for gestational age
    o Fetal presentation, position, lie
- CVA tenderness
- Pelvic exam
    o Cervical changes
    o Rupture of membranes
    o Vaginal discharge
- Evaluation for complications of pregnancy which would favor delivery vs. tocolysis

Clinical Impression:

Differential Diagnoses to Consider

- Pregnancy complicated by:
    o Preterm contractions
    o Preterm labor
    o Multiple gestation
    o Pylonephritis
    o Renal calculi or colic
    o Abruptio placenta
    o Gastritis
    o Appendicitis
    o SGA fetus
    o Inaccurate or unknown dates

Diagnostic Testing:

Diagnostic Tests and Procedures to Consider

- Vaginal/cervical cultures
    o GBS
    o Chlamydia
    o Gonorrhea
- Vaginal fluid
    o Wet mount
    o Ferning, nitrazine testing if SROM suspected
- STAT urinalysis, C&S
- CBC with differential smear

- Additional labs as indicated by client history and presentation
- Ultrasound
    o Determination of approximate gestational age
    o Verify number of fetuses
    o Placental location & status
    o AFI, biophysical profile
    o Amniocentesis for fetal surfactant & L/S ratio

Providing Treatment:

Therapeutic Measures to Consider

- Rest
- Hydration
- Refrain from sexual arousal and intercourse
- Stop breast feeding or other breast stimulation
- Tocolytic medication
    o Use before 34 weeks gestation
    o Dilation less than 4 cms
    o Medications to consider with collaborating physician
        ▪ Terbutaline
        ▪ Ritodrine
        ▪ Magnesium Sulfate
        ▪ Indomethacin
        ▪ Nifedipine
- Elective Cesarean for very preterm infant(s)

Providing Treatment:

Alternative Measures to Consider

- Expectant management
- Neonatal and OB consultants available
- Observe for preterm contractions vs. pre-term labor
- Alternative therapies:[23]
    o False unicorn root tincture
        ▪ 5 drops q 5-15 minutes
        ▪ Taper as contractions diminish
        ▪ Continue for 3-4 days
    o Valerian root tincture, OR
    o Skullcap tincture, OR
    o Cramp bark & wild yam tincture (1:1)
        ▪ ½ dropperful 3 x daily
    o Assessing overall nutritional status, supplement w/
        ▪ Calcium citrate 1000mg daily
        ▪ Magnesium 500 mg daily

Providing Support:

Education and Support Measures to Consider

- If threatened pre-term labor:
    o Limit activity, decrease or stop work, arrange household help
    o Avoid sexual arousal or activity
    o Call if symptoms resume or increase
    o Fetal kick counts
    o Encourage smoking cessation, improvement of nutrition etc. as applicable
- If progressive pre-term labor
    o Advise patient of
    o Delivery routines for pre-term birth
    o Neonatal care for gestational age
- Encourage family/social support involvement

---

[23] Frye, A. (1998) Holistic Midwifery. Labrys Press, Portland, OR.

Follow-up Care:

Follow-up Measures to Consider

- Document, as applicable
  - o Relevant history
  - o Physical findings
  - o Clinical impression
  - o Discussions with client/family
  - o Client preferences
  - o Midwifery plan of care
  - o Consultations
- Threatened pre-term labor
  - o Negative exam & labs
    - ▪ Re-evaluate in 1 week
    - ▪ Sooner if symptoms persist or increase
      - • Decreased fetal motion
      - • Cramping
      - • Pelvic pressure
- Consider serial ultrasound evaluation based on findings
  - o Fetal wellbeing
  - o Cervical length
- Pre-term labor and birth

- o Provide information regarding
  - ▪ Preterm labor & birth
  - ▪ Preterm infant care
  - ▪ Newborn care options locally or regionally
  - o Consider transfer of care to perinatal specialist
- Provide support and reassurance
- Connect with community resources for assistance as indicated, i.e.
  - o Breastfeeding support
  - o Preemie clothing
  - o Rides to neonatal special care unit
  - o Parents of premies support groups

Collaborative Practice:

Criteria to Consider for Consultation or Referral

- For care outside of the scope of the midwife's practice
- For potential preterm labor
  - o Threatened pre-term labor
  - o With evidence of progression
- Consider transfer to
  - o Hospital care
  - o Tertiary care center

Care of the Woman with Prolonged Latent Phase Labor

Key Clinical Information

The latent phase of labor may be considered prolonged when it exceeds approximately 20 hours in nullipara or 14 hours in multipara from the onset of *regular* contractions to the onset of active labor. The latent phase of labor is considered to end with the onset of regular contractions that come at least minutes, last 45 seconds or more, and are at least moderate to palpation. This generally occurs at approximately 3-4 centimeters dilation. Progressive cervical change is the hallmark of labor, persistent uterine contractions in the absence of cervical change should not be considered labor.

Client History:

Components of the History to Consider

- LMP, EDC
- G, P
- Previous labor patterns
- Current labor status
  - o Onset of contractions
  - o Onset of regular contractions
  - o Associated cervical change
  - o Maternal response to labor
  - o Status of membranes

Physical Examination:

Components of the Physical Exam to Consider

- Fetal vital signs & well being
  - o FHT
  - o Fetal motion
- Maternal well being
  - o Vital signs, including temp
  - o Abdominal exam
    - ▪ Estimated fetal weight
    - ▪ Fetal presentation & position
  - o Pelvic exam for progressive changes in

- ▪ Cervical effacement
- ▪ Cervical dilation
- ▪ Descent of presenting part
- ▪ Status of membranes
- ▪ Amniotic fluid volume
- ▪ Pelvimetry
  - o Assess hydration
    - ▪ Urine output, color, sp gravity
    - ▪ Skin turgor
  - o Signs of decreased coping ability
    - ▪ Excessive anxiety
    - ▪ Fear
  - o Tension
- Evaluate for signs of exhaustion

Clinical Impression:

Differential Diagnoses to Consider

- Disordered uterine contractions
  - o False labor
  - o Prodromal labor
  - o Uterine irritability
- Labor complicated by
  - o Uterine inertia
  - o Desultory labor

o   Malpresentation
- Asynclitic presentation
- Persistent occiput posterior
- Face presentation
- Breech presentation

o   Obstructed labor

Diagnostic Testing:

Diagnostic Tests and Procedures to Consider

- Fetal evaluation
  o   Auscultation
  o   EFM
  o   Fetal kick counts
  o   Amniotic fluid color if ROM
- Maternal evaluation
  o   Urine for specific gravity
  o   Evaluation of contractions
  - Palpation
  - External electronic monitoring
  - UPC if membranes ruptured
  o   Pre-op labs if concerned about CPD

Providing Treatment:

Therapeutic Measures to Consider

- Therapeutic rest
  o   Seconal 100 mg PO
  o   Morphine Sulfate 10-20 mg IM or SQ (may combine with Vistaril 50 mg IM)
  o   Benadryl 50 mg PO
  o   Vistaril 50-75 mg IM
  o   Demerol 25-50 mg IM (with or without Phenergan 25 mg)
- Hydration, oral or IV
- Stimulation of labor
  o   Oxytocin stimulation
  o   AROM

Providing Treatment:

Alternative Measures to Consider

- Watchful waiting
- Provide safe environment to allow for
  o   Rest, including intermittent naps
  o   Hydration and adequate nutrition
- Warm bath/hydrotherapy
- Massage
- Strong chamomile tea to facilitate rest
- Labor stimulation
- Nipple stimulation
- Castor oil,
  o   2-4 oz PO

o   Repeat in 1-2 hours if necessary
- Black/blue cohosh tincture,
  o   10 gtt q 10-30 minutes,
  o   Increase dosage as tolerated
- Evening primrose oil
  o   Apply directly to the cervix

Providing Support:

Education and Support Measures to Consider

- Listen to maternal concerns
- Explore fears related to labor, birth, parenting
- Provide reassurance
- Work to provide a safe-feeling birth environment
- Discuss options with woman and her significant other(s)
  o   Review stages of labor
  o   Rest
  o   Stimulation of contractions
  o   Potential change in birth plans
  - Location
  - Provider(s)
  - Support people

Follow-up Care:

Follow-up Measures to Consider

- Document
- Relevant history
- Maternal concerns
- Physical findings
- Diagnostic findings
- Clinical impression
- Discussions with patient/family
- Midwifery plan of care
- Update documentation after each evaluation
- Re-evaluate q 1-2 hours for response to therapy
- If therapeutic rest is not successful
  o   Consider stimulation of labor
  o   Reevaluate potential causes
- If progress does not occur consider
  o   Stimulation of labor
  o   Consultation for collaborative care

Collaborative Practice:

Criteria to Consider for Consultation or Referral

- With diagnosis of prolonged latent phase
- As needed to authorize narcotic (schedule II) administration
- Lack of successful response to therapy
- As needed for change of birth location

Care of the Woman with Premature Rupture of the Membranes

Key Clinical Information

Premature rupture of membranes is defined as ROM that occurs before the onset of labor. 90% of women with PROM will enter labor by 24 hours post-ROM. Complications of premature rupture of the membranes include complications related to preterm birth following PROM, fetal distress related to cord compression and fetal infection. Maternal complications include maternal intra-amniotic infection, increased risk of Cesarean delivery, and post partum endometritis.

Client History:

Components of the History to Consider

- LMP, EDC, gestational age
- Relevant prenatal & OB history
  - GBS status
  - Complications of pregnancy
  - Previous PROM
  - Last pap results
  - STI testing & results
  - New sexual partner(s)
- Current signs & symptoms
  - Onset of ROM
  - Amount, color, consistency of vaginal leakage
  - Fever or chills
  - Palpitations
  - Uterine tenderness
  - Flank tenderness
  - Duration of symptoms
- Presence of risk factors for PROM
  - Previous pregnancy with PROM
  - Amnionitis
  - Polyhydramnios
  - Multiple gestation
  - Vaginal group B strep or other pathogenic vaginal flora
  - Smoking > ½ ppd
  - Nutritional deficiencies
  - Family history of PROM
  - Cervical incompetence

Physical Examination:

Components of the Physical Exam to Consider

- VS with temps q 1-2 hours
  - Maternal fever (temp > 32.2 °C or 99°F)
  - Maternal leukocytosis (WBC > 16,000 with no labor)
  - Maternal or fetal tachycardia (maternal HR > 100, FHR > 160)
- Abdominal exam
  - Palpation for uterine tenderness
  - Presence of contractions
  - Estimated fetal weight
  - Frequent evaluation of fetal well-being
- Sterile speculum exam
  - Visualization of leakage of amniotic fluid
  - Collection of specimen(s) for examination
    - Ferning
    - Nitrazine
- SVE (defer or limit exams)
  - Cervical dilatation
  - Effacement
  - Station
  - Presentation
  - Rule out cord prolapse

Clinical Impression:

Differential Diagnoses to Consider

- Premature rupture of membranes
- Urinary incontinence
  - Physiologic
  - Secondary to urinary tract infection
- Increased vaginal secretions due to
  - Pregnancy
  - Vaginitis
  - Sexually transmitted infection
  - Cervical cancer

Diagnostic Testing:

Diagnostic Tests and Procedures to Consider

- Vaginal fluid evaluation
  - Nitrazine or pH testing (pH 7.0 – 7.7)
  - Ferning
  - Wet Prep and KOH
- Cultures as indicated
  - If expectant management planned
  - GBS culture of vagina and rectum
  - Chlamydia/Gonorrhea status
  - Vaginal
- Ultrasound evaluation
  - Oligohydramnios
  - Biophysical profile
  - Amniocentesis for fetal pulmonary maturity testing
- CBC with differential
- Urine for UA and C&S
  - Clean catch
  - Straight cath specimen
- NST if > 32 weeks gestation
- Daily fetal movement counts

Providing Treatment:

Therapeutic Measures to Consider

- Bedrest if vertex not engaged
- Antibiotic prophylaxis (see **GBS**)
- Fetal surveillance
  - NST
  - Biophysical profile
  - Serial AFI
  - Intermittent auscultation of FHT
  - Continuous fetal monitoring
  - For pre-term PROM consider
  - Amniocentesis for fetal lung maturity
- Cervical ripening or induction of labor (see **induction of labor**)
  - Essential if amnionitis suspected
  - ROM > 24 hrs
- Preterm PROM
  - Glucocorticoids to enhance fetal lung maturity
  - Tocolysis (rarely)
- Transport to center with newborn special care

Providing Treatment:

Alternative Measures to Consider

- Expectant management
  - No internal exams
  - Temps q 2 hours
  - Daily CBC
  - Adequate hydration & nutrition
  - Await inset of labor
- Intervene if signs or symptoms of complications
  - Maternal fever
  - Abdominal tenderness
- Abnormal FHT patterns
  - Tachycardia

- o   Bradycardia
- o   Non-reassuring FHR patterns
- Stimulation of labor with natural remedies (see **induction of labor**)

Providing Support:

Education and Support Measures to Consider

- Significance of PROM
- Potential need to revisit
  - o   Birth plan
  - o   Location of birth
  - o   Birth attendant
- Potential need for medical care
- Anticipated newborn care
- Risks and benefits of options for care
- Anticipated fetal outcome for gestational age
- Signs and symptoms of
  - o   Amnionitis
  - o   Neonatal sepsis
  - o   Postpartum endometritis

Follow-up Care:

Follow-up Measures to Consider

- Document
  - o   Findings
  - o   Client discussion & preferences
  - o   Midwifery plan of care
    - ▪   Consultation

- o   Update plan as changes occur
- Expedite birth if
  - o   Symptoms of infection develop
  - o   Fetal compromise occurs
  - o   Maternal preference
- Evaluate postpartum for
  - o   Endometritis
  - o   Other infection
  - o   Newborn sepsis
- Offer time for discussion and processing
  - o   Labor and birth events
  - o   Outcomes
  - o   Potential effect on future pregnancies

Maternal infection Collaborative Practice:

Criteria to Consider for Consultation or Referral

- OB/GYN consult for patients with
  - o   Documented PROM with
    - ▪   Delay in onset of labor
    - ▪   Signs or symptoms of
      - •   Infection
      - •   Cord prolapse
      - •   Fetal compromise
- Pediatric consult/notification
  - o   Onset of labor
  - o   For birth
  - o   Newborn evaluation

Care of the Woman with Shoulder Dystocia

Key Clinical Information

Shoulder dystocia occurs when there is difficulty birthing the shoulders after the baby's head has already been born. Nearly half of all shoulder dystocias occur in babies that weigh less than 4000 grams, so baby's size alone is not what makes the shoulders get stuck. Rather it is the fit of this particular baby through the pelvis of this particular mother. Studies have been unable to reliably predict which mothers and babies will at risk for shoulder dystocia.[24]

Shoulder dystocia may be anticipated with a long second stage, and the presence of the 'turtle sign' after the head emerges. The head extends with difficulty, and then the chin remains snug against the perineum. Restitution does not occur. The shoulders may be wedged in the pelvis 'tight shoulders', or they may be impacted above the pelvic brim. Prompt identification of shoulder dystocia should result in rapid initiation of the maneuvers to release the baby. Shoulder dystocia may result in significant damage to the infant, such as brachial plexus injury, fracture of the clavicle, hypoxia or death. Traction on the baby has been associated with increased risk of newborn injury.

---

[24] Practice Pattern No. 7: Shoulder Dystocia (1997) in 2002 Compendium of Selected Publications. ACOG.

Client History:

Components of the History to Consider

- LMP, EDC, gestational age
- Maternal height/weight
- Documented clinical pelvimetry
- Potential risk factors for shoulder dystocia:
  - Maternal diabetes
  - History of large infants
  - Maternal obesity
  - Post-date pregnancy
  - Large fetus, by palpation or ultrasound
  - History of prior 'difficult' delivery
  - CPD
  - Desultory labor
  - Prolonged second stage

Physical Examination:

Components of the Physical Exam to Consider

- Abdominal exam in labor
  - Fetal presentation & position
  - Flexion of head at pelvic brim
  - Estimate fetal weight with onset of labor
- Pelvic exam(s) during labor
  - Careful pelvimetry
  - Cervical dilation
  - Descent of presenting part

Clinical Impression:

Differential Diagnoses to Consider

- Shoulder dystocia
- "Tight" shoulders
- Short cord
- Fetal anomaly that prevents descent

Diagnostic Testing:

Diagnostic Tests and Procedures to Consider

- Ultrasound for EFW
- Pre-op labs

Providing Treatment:

Therapeutic Measures to Consider

- Cesarean section for documented macrosomia
  - Not demonstrated to be effective (see ACOG ref.)
- McRobert's maneuver (knees to shoulders)
  - Advantages:
    - Alters angle of inclination of symphysis
    - Gives midwife most room to work
    - Reduces amount of traction required to effect birth
    - May decrease traction-related fetal injury
  - Disadvantages:
    - Requires two assistants
- Request firm supra-pubic pressure
- Encourage maternal pushing efforts
- Attempt birth
  - With *gentle* traction on head
  - With fingers on both shoulders
  - Maintain arms in close contact with trunk
- If birth does not occur
  - Stop maternal pushing eforts
  - With dominant hand in vagina check position of shoulders
    - Place hand on infant's back
      - Palpate anterior axillary crease
      - Do not pull on axilla
  - Use firm traction on the suprascapular bones to

- Attempt to rotate shoulder into the pevis
- Use firm & gentle pressure
- Clockwise for right-handers
- Counterclockwise for lefties
- Rotate shoulders into the oblique
  - As anterior shoulder rotates
    - Move client to hands & knees
    - Bring posterior shoulder into the pelvis
    - Encourage maternal pushing efforts
    - 'Walk' shoulders out using both hands
      - Traction on suprascapular bones
      - Keep arms close to body
      - Use gentle firm traction
      - Rotate baby manually from side to side
      - Back always moving anterior
      - "Corkscrew" the body out.
- For severe unrelieved shoulder dystocia consider:
  - Alternative positioning
  - Call for OB and Pediatric assistance
  - Fracture of clavicle
  - Empty bladder with straight catheter
  - Enlarge or cut episiotomy
  - Rule out other causes of dystocia
    - Direct palpation of pelvic contents
      - Fetal anomalies
      - Extremely short cord
  - Zavenelli maneuver
    - Replacement of head in vagina
    - Reverse process of extension
    - Followed with C-section
- Prepare for
  - Full neonatal resuscitation
  - Immediate postpartum hemorrhage

Providing Treatment:

Alternative Measures to Consider

- Gaskin Maneuver
  - Knee chest position
    - Rotate mother to hands and knees
    - Rotate in direction baby is facing
  - Alters pelvic geometry
  - Advantages:
    - Position change may resolve impaction
    - Gravity may facilitate delivery
  - Disadvantages:
    - Cannot use supra-pubic pressure
    - Limited access to infant
    - May exaggerate impaction
- Squatting
  - Advantages:
    - Position change may resolve impaction
    - Results in a wider pubic (outlet) angle
  - Disadvantages:
    - Cannot use supra-pubic pressure
    - May decrease inlet dimensions
    - Limited access to infant

Providing Support:

Education and Support Measures to Consider

- Discuss
  - Potential of "difficult birth" with mother who has
    - Documented macrosomia
    - EFW more than 1 lb. larger than largest previous infant
- Follow up after birth with discussion

- o   Regarding care given
- o   Infant well-being
- o   Maternal feelings about
  - ▪ Complications
  - ▪ Interventions
  - ▪ Outcomes
  - ▪ About the labor & birth
- Review signs of
  - o   Postpartum endometritis
  - o   Postpartum depression

Follow-up Care:

Follow-up Measures to Consider

- Immediately after birth
  - o   Provide newborn resuscitation as necessary
  - o   Evaluate infant for birth injury
  - o   Observe for PPH following delivery
  - o   Evaluate for maternal injury
- Document:
  - o   Relevant history

- o   Birth details in delivery note ✎
  - ▪ Physical findings at birth
  - ▪ Identification of shoulder dystocia
  - ▪ Maneuvers used and their effects
  - ▪ Noted injury to mother or infant
  - ▪ Consultations requested during birth
  - ▪ Request for pediatric care for birth
- Seek opportunity for peer support
  - o   Peer review (non-discoverable)
  - o   Case presentation or discussion
  - o   Informal support

Collaborative Practice:

Criteria to Consider for Consultation or Referral

- When shoulder dystocia is anticipated
- As soon as shoulder dystocia is evident
- In anticipation of neonatal resuscitation
- For newborn evaluation after difficult birth
- For case discussion & support

Care of the Woman Undergoing Vacuum Assisted Birth

Key Clinical Information:

Vacuum-assisted birth carries with it significant risks to mother and baby. The benefits of using the vacuum extractor to aid in the birth of the baby should clearly outweigh the potential risks associated with this procedure. Midwives who assist birth with a vacuum device should be educated and trained in evaluation its' use.

Client History:

Components of the History to Consider

- Verify LMP, EDC and term gestation
- Relevant prenatal and OB history
  - o   Progress of labor, including second stage
  - o   Fetal and maternal response to labor
  - o   Presence of any contraindications to vacuum assisted birth
- Indications for vacuum-assisted birth
  - o   2nd stage arrest of labor
  - o   Fetal distress
  - o   Uterine inertia
  - o   Maternal exhaustion
- Contraindications to vacuum-assisted birth
  - o   CPD
  - o   Unengaged fetal head
  - o   Premature infant (<37 weeks)
  - o   Suspected macrosomia
  - o   Non-vertex presentation

Physical Examination:

Components of the Physical Exam to Consider

- Abdominal exam
  - o   Fetal lie, presentation, position
  - o   Estimated fetal weight (EFW)
  - o   Presence of adequate, effective regular contractions
- Pelvic exam
  - o   Dilation – must be complete
  - o   Station

- ▪ +2 station = mid-forceps delivery (physician management recommended)
- ▪ Vertex visible at introitus = outlet delivery (CNM or physician management)
  - o   Presence of caput or marked molding – increases risk of fetal trauma
  - o   Evaluate pelvimetry
  - o   Assess fetal presentation and position

Clinical Impression:

Differential Diagnoses to Consider

- Vacuum assisted birth for
  - o   Maternal fatigue
  - o   2nd stage arrest of labor
  - o   Fetal distress
  - o   Uterine inertia
  - o   Uterine inertia
- Obstructed labor
- Potential for
  - o   Shoulder dystocia
  - o   Postpartum hemorrhage
  - o   3° or 4° laceration
  - o   Newborn injury

Diagnostic Testing:

Diagnostic Tests and Procedures to Consider

- Pre-op labs
- Evaluate effectiveness of uterine contractions
  - o   Palpation
  - o   Electronic fetal monitoring
- Evaluate fetal response via FHT

o   Auscultation
o   Electronic fetal monitoring

Providing Treatment:

Therapeutic Measures to Consider

- Oxytocin stimulation to improve contractions
- Vacuum assisted birth
  o   Empty bladder and rectum
  o   Consider local anesthesia
  o   Consider episiotomy,
    - May increase risk of 3° or 4° laceration
    - Mediolateral epis. may give more room
- Apply vacuum cup to posterior fontanel
  o   Verify that no maternal tissues are under cup rim
  o   Request suction
  o   4 in Hg or 100mm Hg between contractions
  o   15-23 in Hg or 500 mm Hg with contractions
- *Do not allow vacuum to remain at maximum levels for more than 10 accrued minutes*
- Apply gentle steady traction
  o   With contractions only
  o   Follow curve of Carus
- Discontinue attempts to assist birth with vacuum if
  o   Cup disengages 3 times
  o   Scalp trauma visible after cup disengages
  o   No progress following 3 attempts at traction
  o   15-30 minutes with no success
  o   Birth has not occurred within 10 *accrued* minutes of maximum suction

Providing Treatment:

Alternative Measures to Consider

- Allow rest period
  o   Provide for adequate hydration & nutrition
  o   Assess for maternal & fetal well-being
  o   Be patient
- Continue maternal pushing efforts
  o   Encourage voiding
  o   Push only with urge
- Vigilant assessment of maternal & fetal status
  o   Vital signs
  o   Fetal descent
- Position changes
  o   Side-lying
  o   McRoberts position
  o   Lithotomy with leg support
  o   Squatting
  o   Birthing stool
  o   Hand & knees
  o   Floating in birthing tub

Providing Support:

Education and Support Measures to Consider

- Discuss with client/family
  o   Concerns related to slow progress
  o   Options for care
  o   Recommendations and indications
  o   Vacuum assisted birth procedure
- Discuss risks and benefits with client
  o   Risks
  o   Fetal trauma
    - Cephalohematoma
    - Intracranial trauma
    - Shoulder dystocia, ecchymosis, abrasions
  o   Maternal trauma
    - 3rd or 4th degree laceration
    - Sulcus tears
    - Possible need for cesarean birth
  o   Benefits
    - Vaginal birth of infant
    - Faster than forceps or C-section
    - Less risk of fetal trauma than forceps
    - May decreased need for C-section

Follow-up Care:

Follow-up Measures to Consider

- Document
  o   Indications for vacuum assisted birth
  o   Physical findings
  o   Fetal position & presentation
  o   Station
  o   Clinical impression
  o   Discussion with client
  o   Client preferences
  o   Consultations
  o   Technique used
  o   Maternal and fetal
- Evaluate for maternal or neonatal injury
- Examine vagina carefully for lacerations
- Examine infant carefully for injury
- Discuss birth with mother/family
- Allow exploration of feelings
- Review indications for assisted birth

Collaborative Practice:

Criteria to Consider for Consultation or Referral

- With indications for vacuum extraction
- Maternal indications – C-Section may be necessary
- Pediatric service
  o   Fetal distress
  o   Fetal injury
  o   For fetal observation of delayed signs of injury

Care of the Woman During Vaginal Birth after Cesarean

Key Clinical Information:

Vaginal birth after Cesarean, or VBAC, provides select women with an alternative to surgical delivery of the infant. A scarred uterus, however, is at greater risk of rupturing than an unscarred uterus. Many factors contribute to scar integrity, among them are the type of closure (i.e. 1 layer vs 2 layers[25]), adequate tissue nutrition and oxygenation to support wound healing, an intact and functioning immune system, and minimal stress on the wound during and immediately following wound healing.

Uterine ruptures can and do occur, at a documented rate of approximately 0.5-1%[26]. This rate is increased in women with a single-layer uterine closure, 2 or more previous Cesarean births, an interdelivery interval of 24 months or less, history of post-operative fever or infection, and women who have their labor augmented or induced with oxytocin. When uterine rupture does occur, outcomes are improved with the immediate availability of skilled surgical services.

---

[25] Bujold, E et al. The impact of single-layer or double-layer closure on uterine rupture. Am J Obstet Gynecol 2002;186:1326-30

[26] Shipp, TD et al. Intrapartum uterine rupture and dehiscence inpatients with prior lower uterine segment vertical and transverse incisions. Obstet Gynecol 1999;94:735-40.

Client History:

Components of the History to Consider

- Current pregnancy course
- Obtain operative records for previous C-section
  - Indication for primary C-section
  - Gestational age with prior C/S
  - Type of uterine incision
  - Type of uterine closure
  - Post-operative course
- Negative factors for the VBAC candidate
  - Classical uterine incision
  - Documented CPD
  - Non-vertex presentation of baby
  - 2 or more previous Cesareans
  - Single-layer uterine closure
  - Maternal age >30
  - Less than 18 mo. since previous C/S
  - Non-progressive labor
- Positive factors for the VBAC candidate
  - Non-repeating cause
  - Client motivated for vaginal birth
  - Previous vaginal birth
  - Vertex presentation
  - 2-layer uterine closure
  - No hx post-op fever
  - Maternal age <30
  - 24+ months since previous C/S
  - Spontaneous onset of labor
  - Progressive labor

Physical Examination:

Components of the Physical Exam to Consider

- Comprehensive labor evaluation
  - Clinical pelvimetry with history CPD or FTP
  - EFW
  - Presentation, position, engagement
- Maternal and fetal vital signs
  - Fetal bradycardia
  - Maternal tachycardia
- Re-evaluate progress at frequent intervals
  - Maternal and fetal response to labor
  - Contraction pattern
  - Cervical change
  - Fetal decent

Clinical Impression:

Differential Diagnoses to Consider

- VBAC candidate
  - Non-repeating condition
  - Appropriate candidate per practice
  - Client preference for labor and vaginal birth
  - Access to surgical support
  - Informed choice and consent
- Repeat C/S candidate
  - Repeating cause for C/S
  - Client preference
  - Non-progressive labor
  - Informed choice and consent
- Uterine scar dehiscence or rupture
  - May result in fetal &/or maternal death
  - Access surgical services STAT

Diagnostic Testing:

Diagnostic Tests and Procedures to Consider

- Continuous evaluation of maternal and fetal status
  - 1:1 nurse or midwife care with auscultation *or*
  - External fetal monitor *or*
  - Internal fetal monitor
- Pre-op labs
  - CBC
  - Type and screen

Providing Treatment:

Therapeutic Measures to Consider

- Evaluate for onset of progressive labor
- Provide a supportive labor and birthing environment
- Limit invasive exams or procedures
- Oral intake
  - NPO
  - Ice chips
  - Clear liquids
  - As desired and tolerated
- IV access
  - Saline lock
  - IV
- Maternal and fetal evaluation of well-being
- Cytotec contraindicated for use with scarred uterus
- Oxytocin, as indicated
  - May facilitate vaginal birth due to uterine inertia
  - Overstimulation may increase risk of rupture
- Pain relief as needed

Providing Treatment:

Alternative Measures to Consider

- Facilitate physiologic labor
  - Ambulation
  - Hydrotherapy
  - Positioning
  - Doula support
  - Adequate hydration & nutrition
- Foster maternal autonomy
- Provide a supportive labor environment

Providing Support:

Education and Support Measures to Consider

- Comprehensive discussion and informed choice and consent during early pregnancy
  - Risks of catastrophic uterine rupture 1:5000 +/-
  - Risks of maternal or fetal death with catastrophic rupture
  - Risks, benefits and alternatives to VBAC
- Discussion regarding facility/practice parameters for VBAC
  - Anticipated care of VBAC women in labor
  - Labor procedures, i.e., IV, labs, etc.
  - Average length of time for urgent C/S
    - At facility
    - If transport required

Follow-up Care:

Follow-up Measures to Consider

- Discuss options with client and family
  - VBAC vs. repeat C-section
  - Surgical coverage
  - Locations for birth
  - Options for labor care & support
- Consult OB/GYN (and Pediatrics where applicable) of client choice when applicable
- Document
  - Review of previous C/S operative notes
  - Discussions with client/family
    - Client preference
    - Informed choice and consent

- o   Consultation, if obtained
- o   Midwifery plan of care
  - ▪   Parameters for
    - •   Evaluation
    - •   Consultation
    - •   Referral
    - •   Transport
- o   Update notes frequently, especially in labor

Collaborative Practice:

Criteria to Consider for Consultation or Referral

- •   Client for
  - o   Previous incision that is not low transverse
  - o   Planned repeat C-section
  - o   Planned VBAC
- •   STAT for client in labor with
  - o   Symptoms of uterine rupture
  - o   Evidence of developing dystocia/obstruction
  - o   Demand for repeat C/S

References

1. ACNM Clinical Bulletin No. 2. (Jan. 1997). Early-onset group B strep infection in newborns; prevention and prophylaxis. The Journal of Nurse-Midwifery, 42, 403-408.

2. ACOG (1990). Diagnosis and Management of Postpartum Hemorrhage. ACOG Technical Bulletin #143. Author.

3. American Academy of Pediatrics/American Heart Association. (1995). Textbook of Neonatal Resuscitation: Author.

4. Barger, M. K. Ed. (1988). Protocols for Gynecologic and Obstetric Health Care. Philadelphia, PA: W. B. Saunders.

5. Briggs, G.G., Freeman, R. K., Yaffe, S. J. (1994) Drugs in Pregnancy and Lactation (4th Ed.). Philadelphia, PA: Williams & Wilkins.

6. Enkin, M., Keirce M., Renfrew, M., Neilson, J. (1995). A Guide to Effective Care in Pregnancy and Childbirth (2nd Ed.). New York, NY: Oxford University Press.

7. Fennell, E. (1994). Urinary tract infections during pregnancy. The Female Patient, 19 (11), 27-35.

8. Frye, Anne. (1998). Holistic Midwifery. Portland, OR. Labrys Press

9. Gordon, J. D., Rydfors, J. T., et al. (1995) Obstetrics, Gynecology & Infertility (4th Ed.) Glen Cove, N.Y., Scrub Hill Press.

10. Graves, B.W. (1992). Newborn Resuscitation revisited. Journal of Nurse-Midwifery, 37, (supplement) 36s-42s.

11. Hunter, L. P., & Chern-Hughes, B. (1996) Management of prolonged latent phase labor. The Journal of Nurse-Midwifery, 41, 383-388.

12. Mandsager, N. (1997). Cervical Ripening: An update on prostaglandins. The Female Patient (OB/GYN Edition), 22 (5), 33-37.

13. Murray, M. (1997) Advanced Fetal Monitoring; Antepartal & intrapartal assessment and intervention. Program presented Milwaukee, WI 6/98.

14. Nolan, T. E., (1994) Chronic hypertension in pregnancy, The Female Patient, 19 (12), 27-42.

15. Paszkowski, T. (1994). Amnioinfusion; a review. The Journal of Reproductive Medicine, 39, 588-594.

16. Pearlman, M. D. (1995). Management of group B streptococcus during pregnancy. The Female Patient, 20 (1), 25-27.

17. Phelan, J. P. (1997, October). <u>Intrauterine Fetal Resuscitation; Betamimetics & Amnioinfusion.</u> Presented at Issues & Controversies in Perinatal Practice, Bangor, ME.

18. Piper, D.M., & McDonald, P. (1994). Management of anticipated and actual shoulder dystocia. <u>Journal of Nurse-Midwifery, 39,</u> 91s-103s.

19. Roberts, J. (1994). Current perspectives on preeclampsia. <u>The Journal of Nurse-Midwifery, 39,</u> 70-90.

20. Rothrock, J. C. (1993). The RN First Assistant (2nd Ed.). Philadelphia: J.B. Lippincott.

21. Scott, J. R., Diasaia, P.J., et al. (1996). <u>Danforth's Handbook of Obstetrics and Gynecology.</u> Philadelphia, PA, Lippincott - Raven.

22. Sheikh, A. & Ernest, J., (1994). Preterm rupture of membranes: The enigma remains. <u>The Female Patient, 19</u> (2), 13-24.

23. Soule, D. (1996). <u>The Roots of Healing.</u> Secaucus, NJ: Citadel Press.

24. Summers, L. (1997). Methods of cervical ripening and labor induction, <u>The Journal of Nurse-Midwifery, 42,</u> 71-83.

25. Varney, H., (1997). <u>Varney's Midwifery</u> (3rd ed.). Boston, MA: Jones and Bartlett.

26. Weed, S. (1985). <u>Wise Woman Herbal for the Childbearing Year.</u> Woodstock, NY: Ashtree Publishing.

27. Wood, C. L., (1994). Meconium-stained amniotic fluid. <u>Journal of Nurse-Midwifery, 39,</u> 106s-109s.

Chapter
6

Care of the Mother and Baby after Birth

Midwifery includes the care and support of the mother and her baby after birth. During this time of transition both mother and infant are particularly vulnerable to disruption.

Fostering mother/baby bonding is an essential component of midwifery practice. Continuation of the supportive care that was offered during pregnancy allows the mother and her infant time to focus on each other, and adapt to their respective changes under the watchful surveillance of the skilled midwife. Evaluation for post-partum depression, effective infant feeding, and individual variations from the expected norm offers an opportunity for early intervention in potential complications that may result in harm to mother or baby.

Care of the Post-Partum Mother: 1-4 Weeks

Key Clinical Information

The postpartum mother undergoes vast changes as her body returns to the non-pregnant state, and she adapts emotionally to the change in her family with the birth of her child. While the physiologic process is much the same in each individual, every woman responds differently to the birth of a child, and will have specific and distinct personal needs to be met..

Client History:
Components of the History to Consider
- Age, G, P
- Review prenatal course
- Review labor and birth information
  - Length of labor
  - Complicating factors for labor and/or birth
  - Manner of birth
    - Vaginal vs C/S
    - Lacerations or episiotomy
      - Hemorrhoids
  - Infant well-being since birth
- Inquire as to general well-being
- Return to non-pregnant status
- Ambulation
  - Voiding
  - Bowel function
  - Appetite
- Pain
  - Location
  - Severity

- o   Relief measures used & results
- Adaptation to postpartum status
- Maternal emotional response to
  - o Labor and birth
  - o Changes post-partum
  - o Changes in family dynamics
- Infant interactions
  - o Feeding
  - o Bonding
  - o Caretaking

Physical Examination:

Components of the Physical Exam to Consider

- Vital signs: BP, T, P
- Exam specific to medical or obstetrical conditions
- Chest
  - o Heart and lungs
  - o CVA tenderness
- Breasts & nipples
  - o Cracks or fissures
  - o Engorgement
  - o Colostrum or milk
- Abdomen
  - o Fundus; location, consistency, tenderness
  - o Incision: dressing, redness erythema, exudate
  - o Bladder: distention, tenderness
  - o Bowel sounds
  - o Muscle tone: diastasis, hernia
- Lochia
  - o Type, amount, odor
- Perineum & rectum
  - o Approximation of tissues
  - o Bruising, inflammation, hematoma
  - o Edema
  - o Hemorrhoids
- Extremities
  - o Edema
  - o Homan's sign
  - o Redness, heat or pain
  - o Varicosities

Clinical Impression:

Differential Diagnoses to Consider

- Postpartum, Vaginal birth
  - o With or without episiotomy or laceration
  - o Spontaneous vaginal birth
  - o Assisted vaginal birth
- Postpartum Cesarean birth
- Post-op tubal ligation
- Post-partum or post-operative course with complicating factors
  - o Post-partum hemorrhage
  - o Retained placental parts
  - o Cervical laceration
  - o Puerpural infection

Diagnostic Testing:

Diagnostic Tests and Procedures to Consider

- H&H on 1st or 2nd pp day
- Rh studies
- As indicated for complications of
  - o Pregnancy
  - o Postpartum
  - o Medical conditions

Providing Treatment:

Therapeutic Measures to Consider

- Bowel care
  - o Colace
  - o Senokot
  - o Milk of magnesia
- Urinary care
  - o Encourage frequent voiding
  - o Catheterize prn for urinary retention
  - o Insert Foley catheter if unable to void x 2
- Uterine care
  - o Heavy lochia &/or uterine atony
    - ▪ Methergine 0.2 mg po q 4 h x 6 doses
- Afterpains
  - o Darvocet- N 100: 1 po q 4 hr prn pain
  - o Empirin #3: 1-2 tabs q 4 hr prn
  - o Tylenol # 3: 1-2 tabs q 4 hr prn
- Sleep
  - o Encourage frequent rest periods
  - o Ambien 5-10 mg at HS
  - o Dalmane 30 mg at HS
  - o Nembutal Sodium 50-100 mg at HS
- Immune status
  - o Rh immune Globulin IM
  - o Rubella vaccine SC

Providing Treatment:

Alternative Measures to Consider

- Bowel care
  - o Encourage fiber & fluids
  - o Psyllium seed
  - o Prune juice
  - o Dried fruits
- Perineal care
  - o Comfrey compresses
  - o Homeopathic Arnica montana
  - o Sitz baths
- Urinary care
  - o Encourage frequent voiding
  - o Comfrey compress to vulva
- Urinary retention
  - o Oil of peppermint drops in toilet
- Uterine care
  - o Heavy lochia &/or uterine atony
    - ▪ Blue cohosh
    - ▪ Shepherd's purse
  - o Afterpains
    - ▪ Hot pack to abdomen
    - ▪ Nurse frequently
    - ▪ Void frequently
- Sleep
  - o Encourage frequent rest periods
  - o Chamomile tea to promote rest

Providing Support:

Education and Support Measures to Consider

- Active listening about
  - o Birth experience
  - o Maternal/family response to baby
  - o Feeding
  - o Feelings
- Provide information about
  - o Contraception options
  - o Infant care and feeding
  - o Medication instructions
  - o Prenatal vitamins
  - o FeSo4
  - o Other medications as indicated
  - o Postpartum return visit
  - o Signs & symptoms of post-partum complications

Follow-up Care:

Follow-up Measures to Consider

- Document

- o   Relevant history
- o   Physical findings
- o   Maternal responses
- o   Clinical impression
- o   Midwifery plan of care
- 2 week office check
  - o   New mothers
  - o   Complicated prenatal or postpartum course
  - o   Wound check post Cesarean
  - o   Initiate oral contraceptives
  - o   Screen for post-partum depression
- 4-6 week office check
  - o   Post-partum exam
    - ▪   Involution
    - ▪   Lactation
    - ▪   Perineum
  - o   Bowel & bladder function

- o   Sleep patterns
- o   Family adaptation
- o   Concerns and questions
- 8 weeks for
  - o   IUD insertion
  - o   Diaphragm or cap fitting

Collaborative Practice:
Criteria to Consider for Consultation or Referral

- Evidence of maternal complications post-partum
- Infection
- Acute urinary retention
- Sub-involution of the uterus
- Thrombophlebitis
- Hematoma
- Pulmonary embolism

Post-Partum Care, 4-6 Weeks

Key Clinical Information

By 4-6 weeks after the birth most women are returning to usual functioning, and adapting to the changes that the baby has brought to her, and the family's life. Maternal evaluation at this time is directed toward determining the presence of any complications or concerns, and addressing any need for birth control information or supplies. Support for the woman's new role, especially with first-time mothers, fosters a positive self-image and feelings of competency as she cares for her infant.

Women who have difficulty with the transition to mother may benefit from referrals to local resources such as parenting groups or classes, breastfeeding groups, play groups and other support services. Isolation during this time is not uncommon, and many women need to be actively directed (given permission) toward participation in activities other than newborn care.

Client History:
Components of the History to Consider

- Labor and birth events and outcomes
- Post-partum course
  - o   Physical return to non-pregnant status
  - o   Amount, color and consistency of lochia
  - o   Breasts, status of lactation
  - o   Perineal or abdominal discomfort
  - o   Voiding & stooling
  - o   Sexual activity
  - o   Adjustment to parenting
  - o   Signs or symptoms of depression
  - o   Sleep patterns
- Interactions with infant
  - o   Infant feeding
  - o   Satisfaction with parenting
  - o   Interactions & support of family/significant others
- Preference for contraception as indicated
  - o   Review of gyn history
  - o   General medical/surgical history
- Social history

Physical Examination:
Components of the Physical Exam to Consider

- Vital signs including temp
- Thyroid
- Breast exam
  - o   Lactation
  - o   Nipple integrity
- Abdominal exam
  - o   C-Section incision
  - o   Diastasis
  - o   Muscle tone
- Pelvic exam
  - o   External genitalia for status of perineum/lacerations
  - o   Speculum exam for appearance of cervix
- Bimanual exam
  - o   Uterine involution
  - o   Vaginal muscle tone
  - o   Presence of cystocele or rectocele
- Rectal exam
- Extremities
  - o   Varicosities
  - o   Phlebitis

Clinical Impression:

Differential Diagnoses to Consider

- Normal post-partum course
- Undesired fertility
- Post-partum complications, i.e.
  - Sub-involution of the uterus
  - Endometritis
  - Breastfeeding difficulties
  - Mastitis
  - Post-partum depression
  - Maternal adaptation problems

Diagnostic Testing:

Diagnostic Tests and Procedures to Consider

- Pap smear
- STI screen as indicated by history
- Labs
  - H&/CBC
  - Fasting blood sugar for gestational diabetics
  - TSH
  - Other labs as indicated by history

Providing Treatment:

Therapeutic Measures to Consider

- Initiation of birth control, as desired
  - Natural family planning
  - Non-prescription methods
  - Prescription methods
- Vitamin & mineral supplementation
  - FeSo4 replacement
  - Calcium
  - Multi-vitamin

Providing Treatment:

Alternative Measures to Consider

- Nutritional support
  - Increased fiber to stimulate regular bowel function
  - Whole foods diet
  - Adequate fluid intake
  - Increased nutritional needs to promote healing and foster general well-being

Providing Support:

Education and Support Measures to Consider

- Provide emotional support

- Assistance and caring from family & friends
- Midwife or nurse home visit
- Provide information about
  - Recommended diet
  - Anticipated weight changes post-partum
  - Potential decrease in libido post-partum & with breastfeeding
  - Initiation of physical activity
  - Birth control options
- Play or support groups for new mothers
- Resources in the area for specific needs
  - Mothers of twins
  - La Leche League
  - Parenting skills classes
  - Teen parent groups

Follow-up Care:

Follow-up Measures to Consider

- Document
  - Relevant history
  - Maternal adaptation
  - Infant well-being
  - Physical findings
  - Diagnostic findings
  - Discussions with mother
  - Preferences for family planning
  - Clinical impressions
  - Midwifery plan of care
- Return for continued care
  - Return visit in 12 months or as indicated by visit, i.e.
  - Post-partum depression screening
  - Birth control
  - STIs
  - Sub-involution
- Call with questions or concerns

Collaborative Practice:

Criteria to Consider for Consultation or Referral

- For significant postpartum depression
- For poor wound healing or infection
- For diagnosis not within the midwife's scope of practice

Post-partum Depression

Key Clinical Information:

Postpartum depression may range from 'the blues' to significant depression or postpartum psychosis. Depression may occur within 3-6 months after giving birth Anticipatory screening of every postpartum woman allows early identification of those women who may require more than simple support to cope with their emotional changes during the postpartum period.

Many women may feel reluctant to divulge negative feelings about themselves or their baby. A support, non-judgmental environment, where active listening is consistently demonstrated fosters the trust many women need to talk about their feelings. Postpartum depression affects up to 12% of women who give birth, with as many as 50% of women experiencing postpartum blues. Postpartum depression occurs in 26-32% of adolescent women who give birth, and is more common in women with history of mood disorder.

Client History:

- Risk factors for postpartum depression
  o Adolescent women
  o History of mood disorder
  o Postpartum for 3-6 months
- Components of the History to Consider
  o Age
  o Baby's age
  o Sleep patterns
  o Method of infant feeding
  o Hormone intake
  o Risk factors for postpartum depression
  o History of mood disorder
  o Family history of mood disorder
  o Expression of feeling unloved, esp. by infant or father of child
  o Unplanned and/or unwanted pregnancy
  o Single or separated with minimal support
- Indicators of postpartum depression
  o Onset and type of symptoms (present x 2 weeks)
  o Presence of sleep disorder
  o Thoughts of harming infant
  o Feelings of inadequacy
  o Extreme fatigue
  o Crying
  o Anxiety
  o Appetite changes
  o Irritability/mood changes
- Identify
  o Stressors
  o Sleep/wake patterns
  o Social support
    ▪ Housing
    ▪ Financial issues
    ▪ Living situation
    ▪ Support systems
  o Potential for harming self or infant

Physical Examination:

Components of the Physical Exam to Consider

- Vital signs, including temp
- Signs or symptoms of
  o Postpartum thyroidosis
  o Anemia
  o Infection
- Evaluate for
  o Sleep deprivation
  o Changes in personal appearance
  o Lethargy
  o Apathy
- Attitude toward
  o Self
  o Partner
  o Child(ren)

Clinical Impression:

Differential Diagnoses to Consider

- Postpartum depression
  o Mild/Moderate
  o Severe/risk of suicide or infanticide
- Depression exacerbated by birth
- Other mood disorder
- Thyroid dysfunction

Diagnostic Testing:

Diagnostic Tests and Procedures to Consider

- Thyroid profile
- Urinalysis
- CBC with diff.

Providing Treatment:

Therapeutic Measures to Consider

- Consider trial of anti-depressant
  o SSRI if bottle feeding
  o Tricyclic if breast feeding
- May consider trial of estrogen
  o Mild symptoms with early onset
  o Estrogen patch 0.05 or 0.1 mg for 3-6 months
  o Oral contraceptives
  o May improve or exacerbate depression

Providing Treatment:

Alternative Measures to Consider

- Herbal remedies
  o St. John's Wort, 300 mg tid
  o Lemon balm tea, 2 cups daily
  o Blessed thistle
    ▪ Infusion 1 cup daily
    ▪ Tincture 10-20 drops 3-4 times daily
- Adequate nutrition
  o Whole foods
  o Adequate fluids
  o Avoid caffeine, alcohol, cigarettes
- Support or women's groups
- Light therapy
- Daily walking or activity
- Time away from baby
- Time scheduled for
  o Personal time
  o Sleep
  o Personal care
  o Favorite activities
  o Intimate time with partner

☛ Alternative therapies should not be a substitute for supervised psychiatric care for the women who threatens, or appears at risk, to harm her self or her family

Providing Support:

Education and Support Measures to Consider

- Prenatal education
  o Signs and symptoms of postpartum depression
  o Normalcy of feelings associated with postpartum depression
  o Local resources
    ▪ Support groups
    ▪ La Leche league
    ▪ Parenting organizations
    ▪ Crisis hotline number
    ▪ Mental health professionals
- After birth
  o Review resources
  o Encourage
    ▪ Family support
    ▪ Rest with baby
    ▪ Avoid isolation
    ▪ Maintain nutrition

- Signs & symptoms of pp depression
- How to access help & support

Follow-up Care:

Follow-up Measures to Consider

- Telephone contact 24-48 hours
- Weekly visits (home or office) while acute
- As needed for titration of medication
- Document midwifery plan of care
  - o Relevant history
  - o Physical findings
  - o Diagnostic findings
  - o Discussions with client/family
    - Support systems
    - Danger signals
    - Medication use
    - Potential for harm to self or family
  - o Clinical impression with recommendations
  - o Client preferences for care
  - o Referrals & consultations

- o Plan for follow-up
- o Update plan as condition changes

Collaborative Practice:

Criteria to Consider for Consultation or Referral

- For psychotherapy, counseling, education with a mental health professional
- For medication, as indicated by client need and midwife scope of practice
- Patients who do not respond to therapy within 7-14 days
- For any woman or her infant who may be at risk
- Presence of psychotic symptoms
- For any patient who is suicidal or homicidal
- Rejection of, or physical aggression (threatened or actual) against, infant
- Social services

Endometritis

Key Clinical Informarion:

Endometritis is an infection of the lining of the uterus. Infection can extend into the fallopian tubes and pelvic peritoneum. Endometritis is more common following Cesarean birth, however, it can occur in any postpartum woman. Other common sites of postpartum infection include episiotomy or laceration sites and areas of bruising or hematoma formation. Prompt recognition and treatment is required to prevent onset of systemic infection, or localized tissue necrosis.

Two temperature elevations to 38°C/100.4°F more than 24 hours after birth, or temperature of 38.7°C/101.5°F at any time are indicative of postpartum infection. Evlauation should be made to determine the location of the infection. Postpartum endometritis usually presents on second to seventh postpartum day.

Client History:

Components of the History to Consider

- Length of time since birth
- General well being
  - o Appetite
  - o Urinary function
  - o Respiratory function
- Prenatal risk factors
  - o GBS +
  - o Bacterial vaginitis
  - o STD diagnosis or treatment
- Complications of birth
  - o Prolonged labor
  - o Prolonged rupture of membranes
  - o More than 4-6 internal exams
  - o Breaks in aseptic technique
  - o Excessive blood loss
  - o Uterine or cervical manipulation
  - o Cesarean section
  - o Retained placental fragments
- Onset, duration and severity of symptoms

  - o Fever and chills
  - o Malaise
  - o Presence and location of pain
  - o Odor to lochia
  - o Wound exudate
  - o Redness & inflammation at wound site
  - o Other associated symptoms

Physical Examination:

Components of the Physical Exam to Consider

- Vital signs, BP, T, P, R
- Physical exam including
- Cardiopulmonary system
  - o Color
  - o Breath sounds
  - o Rales
  - o Respiratory effort
- Breast exam
  - o Redness
  - o Mass
- Abdominal exam
  - o Uterine size

- o   Location of pain
- o   Tenderness with uterine motion
- Wound or laceration exam
  - o   Exudate
  - o   Redness
  - o   Swelling
  - o   Evaluate for hematoma
- Pelvic
  - o   Evaluation of lochia
    - ▪   Odor
    - ▪   Amount
- Extremities
  - o   Edema
  - o   Homan's sign
  - o   Pulses

Clinical Impression:

Differential Diagnoses to Consider

- Uterine infection
- Urinary tract infection
- Respiratory infection
- Deep vein thrombosis/pulmonary embolus
- Wound infection
  - o   Surgical incision
  - o   Incisional hematoma
  - o   Vaginal hematoma
  - o   Episiotomy
  - o   Laceration
- Breast infection
  - o   Mastitis
  - o   Abscess
- Drug reaction

Diagnostic Testing:

Diagnostic Tests and Procedures to Consider

- CBC w/ diff.
- Urinalysis
- O2 saturation
- Cultures as indicated
  - o   Urine
  - o   Blood
  - o   Wound
- Radiology studies as indicated
  - o   Chest x-ray
- Ultrasound
  - o   Pelvic
  - o   Abdominal
  - o   Extermities

Providing Treatment:

Therapeutic Measures to Consider

- Hydration
  - o   PO fluids
  - o   IV therapy
- Prevention of DVT
  - o   Anti-embolitic stockings
  - o   Isometric exercises

- Antimicrobial therapy
  - o   Cefotetan 1-2 G IV q 12 h
  - o   Mezlocillin 4 G IV q 4-6 h
  - o   Ticarcillin/clavaniculate 3.1 G IV q 6 h
  - o   Ampicillin/sulbactam 3 G IV q 4-6 h
  - o   Gentamycin 1.5 mg/kg load, then 1 mg/kg q 8 h, *plus* Clindamycin 900 mg I V q 6 h

Providing Treatment:

Alternative Measures to Consider

- Rescue remedy to pulse points
- Hot pack to abdomen
- Echinacea tea or tincture
- Homeopathic arnica for soft tissue injury

Providing Support:

Education and Support Measures to Consider

- Supportive measures
  - o   Rest
  - o   Adequate nutrition
  - o   Emotional support
  - o   Provision for infant care
- Discuss with client/family
  - o   Working diagnosis
  - o   Urgency of condition
  - o   Need for diagnostic testing
  - o   Potential need for
    - ▪   Medical evaluation
    - ▪   Hospitalization
    - ▪   Treatment
  - o   Compatibility of medications with breastfeeding, prn
- Provide emotional support
- Listen
- Provide information as situation demands

Follow-up Care:

Follow-up Measures to Consider

- Anticipate response to medication within 48 hours
- Consider abscess or hematoma if minimal or no response
- Document
  - o   Relevant history
  - o   Presenting complaint
  - o   Physical findings
  - o   Diagnostic findings
  - o   Discussion with patient/family
  - o   Midwifery plan of care
  - o   Consultation/referral
- Update notes frequently and with any changes

Collaborative Practice:

Criteria to Consider for Consultation or Referral

- When evaluation or treatment of postpartum infection is outside the scope of practice of the midwife
- For transfer of care from home or birth center for women requiring hospitalization
- For other medical complications of the postpartum period that require medical evaluation and care

Hemorrhoids

Key Clinical Information:

Hemorrhoids are varicosities of the veins that line the anal canal. They are a common finding in the postpartum period. Hemorrhoids may be swollen and painful, or they may become thrombosed, and require incision and drainage. Prompt treatment of hemorrhoids post partum may prevent thrombosis of external hemorrhoids that have become trapped by the anal sphincter.

Client History:
Components of the History to Consider
- Length and positions used during second stage labor
- Prior history of hemorrhoids
- Relief measures used and their effects
- Usual bowel function
- Presence of rectal bleeding

Physical Examination:
Components of the Physical Exam to Consider
- Determine presence of hemorrhoids
  - Size
  - Location
  - Edema
- Rectal examination
  - Thrombosis
  - Abscess
  - Anal fissure
  - Hematoma
  - Undiagnosed third or fourth degree laceration

Clinical Impression:
Differential Diagnoses to Consider
- Hemorrhoids
- Thrombosed hemorrhoids
- Anal abscess
- Anal fissure
- Recto-vaginal hematoma
- Undiagnosed third or fourth degree laceration

Diagnostic Testing:
Diagnostic Tests and Procedures to Consider
- Palpation to verify presence of thrombosed hemorrhoid
  - Firm clot felt within vein
  - Exquisitely painful to touch

Providing Treatment:
Therapeutic Measures to Consider
- Manually reduce hemorrhoids as necessary
- Incise & drain thrombosed hemorrhoids
- Topical analgesics
  - Americaine spray
  - Nupercainal ointment or suppositories
- Hemorrhoidal preparations
  - Steroid preparations indicated for
    - Bleeding
    - Severe inflammation
  - Anusol cream
  - Anusol-HC suppositories
  - Preparation H
  - Proctocort
  - Proctofoam
  - Proctofoam-HC
- Relieve and/or prevent constipation
  - Stool softeners
    - Colace – 50-200 mg daily
    - Surfac – 240mg po daily until normal
  - Laxatives
    - Peri-colace (softener + stimulant)
    - 1-2 capsules hs
  - Perdiem (fiber + stimulant)
    - 1-2 tsp in 8 oz water hs or in am
  - Senocot (senna stimulant)
    - 2 tabs q hs
- Fiber supplements
  - Citrucel – 1 TBS in 8 oz water 1-3 x daily
  - Metamucil – 1 packet or 1 tsp in 8 oz water 1-3 x daily
- Gylcerine suppositories
- Enemas
  - Fleet enema
  - Soapsuds enema
- Severe hemorrhoids
  - Rectal packing
  - Lubricate with hemorrhoid cream

Providing Treatment:
Alternative Measures to Consider
- Sitz baths
  - Warm water
  - Herbal infusions
    - Comfrey
    - Red clover
    - Nettle
- Ice packs
- Adequate dietary fiber & fluids
- Knee chest position to drain hemorrhoids
  - Hands & knees
  - Head on pillow
  - Bottom elevated
- Witch hazel compresses
- Measures to speed soft tissue healing
  - Aloe vera gel
  - Comfrey compresses used tid
  - Homeopathics
    - Arnica 30x 2 tabs qid
    - Hamamelis 30C

Providing Support:
Education and Support Measures to Consider
- Provide information regarding
  - Diet adequate in fluids & fiber
    - Dried fruit
    - Psyllium seed
    - Prune juice
    - Rhubarb
    - Blueberries
  - Treatment options & instructions
  - Avoidance of
    - Straining
    - Prolonged sitting on toilet
    - Holding stool
  - When to call

- ▪ Bleeding
- ▪ Increasing pain

Follow-up Care:

Follow-up Measures to Consider

- Reevaluate hemorrhoids
  - o 12-24 hours after treatment
  - o 1 week
  - o Persistent rectal bleeding
- Document
  - o Relevant history
  - o Physical findings
  - o Clinical impression

- o Midwifery plan of care
- o Consultations

Collaborative Practice:

Criteria to Consider for Consultation or Referral

- Thrombosed hemorrhoids for I&D
- Suspected third or fourth degree laceration
- Rectal
  - o Abscess
  - o Anal fissure
  - o Hematoma
  - o Bleeding

Mastitis

Key Clinical Information:

Mastitis may present itself in the early or late postpartum period. Prompt treatment at the first signs may prevent the need for antibiotic treatment. Delay in treatment may result in abscess formation, or systemic infection. All breastfeeding women should be aware of the presenting signs and symptoms of mastitis, preventive measures, when and how to contact their midwife for evaluation and possible treatment.

Client History:

Components of the History to Consider

- Breastfeeding history
  - o Duration of breastfeeding
  - o Infant feeding style
  - o Recent changes to nursing patterns
  - o Usual breast care
- Previous history of breast problems
  - o Mastitis
  - o Abscess
  - o Breast biopsies
  - o Breast reduction or implants
- Onset, duration & severity of symptoms
  - o Painful breast(s), worse when nursing
  - o Redness of breast
  - o Induration of breast
  - o Fever and/or chills
  - o Malaise or flu-like symptoms
  - o Headache
- Self-help measures used & effectiveness

Physical Examination:

Components of the Physical Exam to Consider

- Vital signs, esp. temp and pulse
- General well-being
- Breast exam
  - o Engorgement
  - o Tenderness, redness, swelling
  - o Induration
  - o Warmth; generalized or local
  - o Cracks or fissures in nipples
  - o Masses
    - ▪ Firm or soft
    - ▪ Fixed or mobile
    - ▪ Tender or non-tender
- Axillary exam
  - o Engorgement

- o Lymph nodes

Clinical Impression:

Differential Diagnoses to Consider

- Simple mastitis
- Breast abscess
- Severe mastitis with systemic involvement

Diagnostic Testing:

Diagnostic Tests and Procedures to Consider

- Breast ultrasound if abscess suspected
- Culture of breast milk for pathogen
- Mammograms are not recommended during lactation for evaluation of breast mass

Providing Treatment:

Therapeutic Measures to Consider

- Fever
  - o Acetominophen
  - o Ibuprofen
  - o Aspirin
- Antibiotic therapy for infection
  - o Dicloxacillin 250 mg qid x 10 days
  - o Keflex 500 mg po bid x 10 d
  - o Erythromycin
  - o Eryc 250 mg po q 6 h x 10 d
  - o Ery-tab 400 mg q 6 h x 10 d, or 333mg q 8 h, or 500 mg q 12 h
  - o EES 1.6 G/d in 2,3, or 4 evenly divided doses
  - o Nafcillin 250-500 mg po q 4-6 h x 10 d (or other penicillinase-resistant penicillin)

Providing Treatment:

Alternative Measures to Consider

- Adequate hydration & nutrition
- Rest with baby at breast
- For rest
  - o Hops infusion

- o   Skullcap tincture
- For fever, infusion of
  - o   Echinacea
  - o   Yarrow
  - o   Peppermint
- Echinacea tea or tincture
- Comfrey compresses to affected area
- Homeopathics[27]
  - o   Arnica 30C
  - o   Bryonia 30C
  - o   Phytolacca 30C
  - o   Belladonna 30 C

Providing Support:

Education and Support Measures to Consider
- Careful hand washing and breast care
- Warm compresses to affected area
- *Gentle* massage toward nipple
- Frequent nursing and/or pumping

- Change infant's suckling positions
  - o   Cradle
  - o   Side-lying
  - o   Football
  - o   Belly to belly
- Increase fluid intake
- Rest
- Request family assistance with
  - o   Housekeeping
  - o   Childcare
  - o   Promoting rest
- Provide medication instructions
- Instructions for when & how to contact
  - o   Fever (100.4 or >)
  - o   Chills
  - o   Malaise
  - o   Worsening symptoms

Follow-up Care:

Follow-up Measures to Consider
- Follow-up within 24 hours
  - o   To confirm effectiveness of therapy
  - o   For evaluation if no improvement
- Document
- Relevant history
- Physical findings
- Clinical impression
- Discussion with client
- Midwifery plan for on-going care and follow-up evaluation

Collaborative Practice:

Criteria to Consider for Consultation or Referral
- For Rx medications as indicated by midwife scope of practice
- For mastitis unresponsive to therapy
- For breast abscess

---

[27] Davis, E. (1997). Hearts and Hands. P172.

Newborn Resuscitation

Key Clinical Information:

Most babies make the transition at birth without needing anything more than gentle supportive care. Occasionally, however, some babies do not begin to breathe as anticipated, and may need intervention to assist them. Maintaining an intact cord may foster a gentle transition for the baby, and as long as the cord is pulsing, provides a secondary source of oxygen to the baby during the transition period.

Client History:

Components of the History to Consider

- Presence of risk factors for fetal asphyxia:
  - Cord factors:
    - Cord prolapse
    - Cord compression
  - Placental factors
    - Placental abruption
    - Placental insufficiency
    - Placenta previa
  - Maternal factors
    - Maternal vascular disease
    - Maternal hypotension
    - Uterine hyperstimulation
  - Fetal factors
    - Prematurity
    - Fetal isoimmunization
    - Meconium stained amniotic fluid
- Causes of respiratory distress include:
  - Sepsis
  - Meconium aspiration
  - Choanal atresia
  - Diaphragmatic hernia

Physical Examination:

Components of the Physical Exam to Consider

- Evaluate for presence of meconium
- Basic steps:
  - Prevent heat loss
  - Place on warm surface (i.e. radiant warmer)
  - Dry
  - Remove wet linen
  - Position
  - Suction
  - Tactile stimulation
- Evaluate respirations
  - Normal rate 40-60/min
  - May be irregular
  - No abdominal retractions
  - No grunting, gasping, or wheezing
- Evaluate heart rate
  - Normal rate 120-160 bpm
  - Regular rate & rhythm
- Evaluate color
  - Should pink easily with respirations
  - Cyanosis of hands & feet is common
  - Pallor or central cyanosis is worrysome

Clinical Impression:

Differential Diagnoses to Consider

- Primary apnea
- Secondary apnea
- Meconium aspiration
- Choanal atresia
- Diaphragmatic hernia
- Sepsis
- Assisted ventilation < 30 min
- Assisted ventilation > 30 min
- Hyaline membrane disease or RDS

Diagnostic Testing:

Diagnostic Tests and Procedures to Consider

- Endotracheal intubation
  - Non-vigorous infant, with meconium
  - Evaluate for meconium below cords
- Chest x-ray
  - Placement of ET tube
  - Pneumothorax
  - Pneumonia
  - Meconium aspiration
  - Respiratory distress

Providing Treatment:

Therapeutic Measures to Consider

(Per 2000 AAP/AHA Guidelines)

- Non-vigorous infant with meconium
  - Use meconium aspirator on perineum to suction:
    - Mouth
    - Nares
    - Pharynx
  - Endotracheal intubation to suction meconium
- 100 % O2 via bag and mask or ET tube
  - Infants with absent or weak respiratory efforts:
  - Heart rate less than 100
- Chest compressions
  - After 30 seconds positive pressure ventilation
  - Infants with heart rate under 60
- Medications as indicated by respiratory effort and heart rate
- Free flow O2 as indicated by
  - Respiratory effort
  - Color

Providing Treatment:

Alternative Measures to Consider

- Maintain cord intact to provide additional oxygenation
  - If cord is pulsing baby is getting oxygen
  - Cord pulses with baby's heart rate

o   Do not put traction or pressure on cord
o   May resuscitate baby with cord intact
- Application of homeopathic remedies (i.e. Rescue Remedy®) to pulse points is considered safe
  o   *Oral administration of any medication, homeopathic or herbal remedy may cause aspirations pneumonia and further compromise the infant and should be done with caution.*
- Prayer, talking to baby, physical touch

Providing Support:
Education and Support Measures to Consider
- Discuss care of infant when time allows
- Provide information about ongoing infant care and support when indicated
- Listen to parents concerns and fears
- Provide information about support groups or services as indicated

Follow-up Care:
Follow-up Measures to Consider
- Document resuscitation events
  o   Evaluation
  o   Treatments

o   Infant response
o   Consultation/referral/transport
- Notify appropriate personnel that infant required resuscitation
  o   Infant should be evaluated promptly as indicated by condition following resuscitation
  o   Provide for close follow-up of any baby who has required more then minimal support
    ▪   Vital signs every 1-4 hrs x 24 hrs

Collaborative Practice:
Criteria to Consider for Consultation or Referral
- For anticipated need of neonatal resuscitation
- For any infant who does not have improvement with initial 30 seconds O2 therapy
- Infant with signs or symptoms of
  o   Respiratory distress
  o   Meconium aspiration syndrome
  o   Difficulty with temperature regulation
  o   Cyanosis or pallor
  o   Vital signs outside of normal range

Initial Examination and Evaluation of the Newborn Baby

Key Clinical Information:

Every midwife should be skilled in examination of the newly born baby. The initial examination serves to determine if the baby is making a successful transition to the outside world from the total support provided within the womb. Babies vary tremendously, and the midwife must evaluation which variations require additional expertise in newborn care.

Client History:
Components of the History to Consider
- Birth information
  o   Age
  o   Gestational age
  o   Significant events or findings since birth
- Condition since birth
  o   General well-being
  o   Vital signs
  o   Feeding
  o   Voiding/stooling
- Family history of genetic disorders
- Maternal medical factors
  o   Chronic illness
    ▪   Hepatitis B
    ▪   HIV
    ▪   GC/CT
    ▪   Thyroid on replacement
    ▪   Diabetes
    ▪   Other
  o   Contributing obstetrical history
- Prenatal factors
  o   Onset of prenatal care
  o   Use of drugs, tobacco, alcohol
  o   Pregnancy complications
- Labor and birth factors
  o   Duration of pregnancy
  o   Duration of labor

o   Use of medications in labor
o   Complications of labor and/or birth
  ▪   Cesarean birth
  ▪   Vacuum extractor
  ▪   Fetal distress
  ▪   Meconium-stained fluid
  ▪   Other

Physical Examination:
Components of the Physical Exam to Consider
- Newborn resuscitation as indicated (see Newborn Resuscitation)
- Apgar scores at 1 and 5 minutes
- Vital signs
- Vital statistics
  o   Weight
  o   Head circumference
  o   Length
  o   Chest circumference
- Evaluation of gestational age
- General physical exam
- Skin
  o   Color
  o   Vernix
  o   Cracking
  o   Presence of lesions
  o   Evidence of birth trauma
- Head
  o   Molding

- o   Caput
- o   Cephaphematoma
- o   Fontanels
- Eyes
  - o   Red reflex
  - o   Position, size, shape of orbits
  - o   Color of iris and sclera
  - o   Subconjunctival hemorrhage
  - o   Conjunctivitis
- Ears
  - o   Position and shape
  - o   Presence of periauricular sinus or skin tags
  - o   Hearing testing
- Nose
  - o   Patency
  - o   Flaring
- Mouth
  - o   Lips
  - o   Gums
  - o   Palates
  - o   Tongue
  - o   Suck
- Back and spine
  - o   Breath sounds
  - o   Presence of anomalies
  - o   Curvature of spine
  - o   Pilonidal sinus
  - o   Spinal bifida
  - o   Patency of anus
- Chest
  - o   Respiratory effort and breath sounds
  - o   Heart rate and rhythm
  - o   Shape
- Abdomen
  - o   Number of cord vessels
  - o   Presence of bowel sounds (>1 hr after birth)
  - o   Palpation of kidneys, liver margin, presence of masses
  - o   Femoral pulses
- Genitalia
  - o   Male
    - ▪ Position of urinary meatus
    - ▪ Descent of testes in scrotum
  - o   Female
    - ▪ Configuration
    - ▪ Edema
    - ▪ Discharge
- Extremities
  - o   Range of motion
  - o   Congenital hip dislocation
  - o   Extra digits
- Reflexes
  - o   Rooting
  - o   Moro

Clinical Impression:

Differential Diagnoses to Consider

- Normal newborn
- Newborn course complicated by
  - o   Pregnancy factors
  - o   Labor and/or birth factors
  - o   Congenital factors
  - o   Other conditions

Diagnostic Testing:

Diagnostic Tests and Procedures to Consider

- Glucose (heelstick normal value >45 mg/dl)
- Cord blood studies
- Metabolic screening tests

- Consider additional testing for:
  - o   Cord blood gases
  - o   Anemia (HCT normal value 45-65%)
  - o   Hyper-bilirubinemia (normal value <13 mg/dl)
  - o   Syphilis
  - o   HIV
  - o   Sickle cell anemia
  - o   Hepatitis B
  - o   Gram stain of eye exudate
  - o   Culture of eye exudate for GC/CT

Providing Treatment:

Therapeutic Measures to Consider

- Vitamin K
  - o   Injection: AquaMEPHYTON (Phytonadione)
    - ▪ 0.5-1 mg IM within 1 hour of birth
  - o   Oral: Konakion MM (Mixed micellular preparation)[28]
    - ▪ 2 mg po within 1 hour of birth followed by
    - ▪ Additional doses at 7 and 30 days of age
- Prophylactic opthalmic treatment
  - o   Erythromycin ophthalmic ointment
    - ▪ 0.5 % x 1 dose
  - o   Tetracycline ophthalmic ointment
    - ▪ 1% x 1 dose
  - o   Silver nitrate, aqueous solution
    - ▪ 1% as single application
- Neonatal conjunctivitis
  - o   Ceftriaxone 25-50 mg/kg IV or IM
    - ▪ Single dose
    - ▪ Max dose 125 mg
- Hepatitis B vaccine
- Hepatitis B immune globulin if hepatitis B positive mother
- Photo-therapy for hyperbilirubenemia

Providing Treatment:

Alternative Measures to Consider

- Defer vitamin K
  - o   Incidence of hemorrhagic disease of the newborn without vitamin K ranges from 0.25-0.50 %
  - o   Greatest incidence in breastfed infants who did not receive vitamin K
  - o   Vitamin K is concentrated in colostrum and hind milk
  - o   Formula fed infants get significant vitamin K from cow's milk formula
- Defer erythromycin ophthalmic ointment
  - o   Negative GC/CT results
  - o   Culture and treat if conjunctivitis occurs
  - o   Use plain water wash, prn

Providing Support:

Education and Support Measures to Consider

- Discuss physical findings
  - o   Range of normal
  - o   Potential or actual concerns
  - o   Signs and symptoms to watch for
- Discuss purpose of testing and/or medications
  - o   Encourage questions
  - o   Engage parents in decision-making
  - o   Discuss
    - ▪ Potential options for care
    - ▪ Anticipated results/benefits
    - ▪ Risks/side effects
    - ▪ Alternatives
- Anticipatory guidance for parenting of newborn:

- [28] Clark, F.I., James, E.J., (1995). Twenty-seven years of experience with oral vitamin K1 therapy in neonates. J. Pediatrics 127(2): 301-304.

o   Expected feeding and activity levels
o   Evaluation of adequate hydration
o   Common patterns of voiding and stooling
o   Warning signs
- Poor feeding
- Lethargy
- Irritability
- Jaundice
- Dehydration
- Fever
- Poor color
- Vomiting
- Follow-up plans for newborn care
o   When to contact
o   How to contact

Follow-up Care:

Follow-up Measures to Consider

- Daily evaluation in first two to three days of life

- Weight check at one-two weeks
- Observation of feeding
o   Determine suck/swallow
o   Note latch if breastfeeding
o   Maternal/infant interaction
- Document examination & findings
- Note recommendations for continued care

Collaborative Practice:

Criteria to Consider for Consultation or Referral

- If newborn evaluation is not within scope of midwife's practice
- Presence of anomalies
- Evidence of infection
- Hyperbilirubenemia
- Lactation referral for breast feeding difficulties
- Other conditions not within the range of normal or expected findings

Care of the Infant Undergoing Circumcision

Key Clinical Information:

Circumcision is the surgical removal of part, or all, of the foreskin of the penis. It may be performed for social or religious reasons. Discussion with parents before birth provides an opportunity for questions. In the event that the baby is a boy, parents will have had time for reflection about whether circumcision is right for their family. There is no medical reason for newborn circumcision. Parents whose son is intact may need education regarding genital hygiene, especially if circumcision has previously been the norm for children in the family.

The midwife who plans to include circumcision in her or his practice should learn the skills needed from an experienced midwife, physician or Mohel until skilled at the procedure. Some form of local anesthesia is recommended in order to minimize the stress to the baby from the procedure.[29]

---

[29] ACOG (2001). Committee Opinion # 260, Circumcision. In 2002 Compendium of Selected Publications. ACOG.

Client History:

Components of the History to Consider

- Neonatal course since birth
  - Vitamin K
    - Oral vitamin K requires up to three doses before full effectiveness
  - Demonstrated voiding since birth
  - Review infant record
    - Physical exam
    - Lab tests
    - Temperature stability
    - Feeding & voiding since birth
- Contraindications to circumcision
  - Hypospadias
  - Medically unstable infant
  - Parents decline procedure

Physical Examination:

Components of the Physical Exam to Consider

- Vital signs including temp
- Examination of the penis
  - Evaluate for hypospadias prior to procedure
  - Identify landmarks for penile block if used

Clinical Impression:

Differential Diagnoses to Consider

- Normal male neonatal genitalia
- Elective circumsision
- Congenital phimosis

Diagnostic Testing:

Diagnostic Tests and Procedures to Consider

- As indicated to ensure infant's stability prior to procedure

Providing Treatment:

Therapeutic Measures to Consider

- Prepare equipment
  - Gomco clamp
  - Plastibell clamp
  - Mogen clamp
- Provide for pain relief
  - EMLA cream
  - Dorsal penile block
  - Subcutanous ring block
  - Parental presence
  - Swaddling
  - Anagesics

Procedure using Gomco Clamp:

- Use strict aseptic technique
  - Sterile gloves
  - Mask
  - Antimicrobial prep
  - Sterile drape for genital area
- Create dorsal slit
  - Identify preputial ring, and lift clear of the glans
  - Apply curved hemostats to edge of preputial ring (grasp 2-3 mm of tissue)
  - Insert straight hemostat or probe dorsally under foreskin to level of corona
  - Spread hemostat and free foreskin off dorsal side of the glans
  - Insert one blade of open straight hemostat along dorsal foreskin
  - Lift foreskin away from glans and meatus
  - Clamp 1 cm of foreskin in the midline
  - Inset blunt tipped scissors and carefully cut the crush-line
- Application of the clamp
  - Free inner preputial tissue from glans to expose glans and coronal sulcus

- Using gentle traction on curved hemostats pull the foreskin over the glans
- Insert the bell dorsally to completely cover the glans
- Place straight hemostat through hole on base plate and grasp edges of foreskin to close margins of dorsal slit before fitting hole over glans
- Carefully maneuver tip of cone to work it through bevel hole, working the base plate down over the secured foreskin until the bell is seated
- Swing the top plate over and lift the arms onto the yoke
- Note: The apex of the dorsal slit should be completely visible
- Excision of the tissue
  - Ensure top plate is aligned in notch
  - Tighten the nut to crimp foreskin between base plate and bell
  - Carefully excise foreskin with scalpel at the junction of the base plate and bell
- Loosen the nut and gently loosen tissue from bell
- Retract remaining foreskin to below the glans
- Observe for active bleeding
- Apply Vaseline gauze and pressure if necessary for hemostasis

Providing Treatment:

Alternative Measures to Consider

- Maintain intact foreskin
- Remove only very tip of foreskin
- Circumcise later in life when and if indicated

Providing Support:

Education and Support Measures to Consider

- Provide information regarding risks, benefits and alternatives to parents
- Potential benefits of circumcision include prevention of:
  - Phimosis
  - Paraphimosis
  - Balanoposthitis
  - Urinary tract infections
- Obtain informed consent
- Provide education to parents who opt for circumcision regarding post-procedure care of the penis
- Crying is common with first voids post-circumcision
- Appearance
  - Head of penis may be quite red
  - Swelling just under the glans is normal
  - A blood clot may form at incision site
  - Pink or yellow serous drainage may occur
- Care of circumcised penis
  - Keep area clean
  - Wash hands before diaper change
  - Change diaper frequently
  - Apply petroleum jelly on gauze with each diaper change until healing occurs
  - If gauze sticks, soak with warm water to loosen
- Call with signs or symptoms of complications
  - Active bleeding. Apply direct pressure to area
  - Pus, foul odor, or increased redness or swelling at incision site
  - Fever
  - Lack of urination within 12-24 hours after circumcision
- Provide education regarding the care of the uncircumcised penis to parents who opt not for circumcision

Follow-up Care:

Follow-up Measures to Consider

- Document procedure
  - Technique used
  - Infant response

o   EBL
o   Complications, if any
- Delay discharge from care until bleeding minimal and infant voiding
- Observe for potential complications:
  o   Removal of excessive foreskin
  o   Bleeding
  o   Infection
  o   Amputation of distal glans

o   Sepsis

Collaborative Practice:
Criteria to Consider for Consultation or Referral
- For any infant with congenital defects of the genitals
- For physician or Mohel performed circumcision at midwife's or parents' preference or as indicated by midwife's scope of practice

Newborn Deviations from Normal

Key Clinical Information:

Every baby is unique, and the midwife must be able to assess whether variations from the expected simply represent the wide range of normal, or indicate the presence of a condition that requires additional assessment and possibly treatment. While the vast majority of babies born to healthy mothers are themselves healthy, the hallmark of midwifery is improving the heath and well-being of mothers and babies. This includes being observant for subtle signs and symptoms that may indicate a need for skilled medical care.

Client History:

Components of the History to Consider
- Family history
  o   Genetic history
  o   Congentital anomalies
  o   Pregnancy losses
  o   Social factors
- Pregnancy history
  o   Complications of pregnancy
  o   Maternal disease or illness
    - GBS
    - Herpes
    - Diabetes
    - Epilepsy
    - HIV
  o   Drug, alcohol, or tobacco use
- Labor and birth events
  o   Abnormal fetal heart rate patterns
  o   Resuscitation
  o   Complications at birth, such as
    - Presence of meconium
    - Endotracheal intubation or suctioning
    - Instrument or surgical birth
    - Shoulder dystocia
  o   Evidence of birth trauma
- Review initial assessment
  o   Gestational age
  o   Congenital anomalies
  o   Lab tests
  o   Unusual findings
- Presence of symptoms since birth
  o   Type of symptom(s)
  o   Onset
  o   Duration
  o   Severity
  o   Treatments tried and infant response

Physical Examination:

Components of the Physical Exam to Consider
- Vital Signs
  o   Temperature
  o   Respiratory rate, volume and effort
  o   Presence of apnea
  o   Heart rate & rhythm
- Reflexes
- Observe for signs and symptoms suggesting need for further evaluation
- Color
  o   Pallor
  o   Cyanosis
  o   Rubor
  o   Jaundice
    - Before 24 hours – most likely pathologic
    - After 24 hours – most likely physiologic
- Muscle tone
  o   Flacid
  o   Hypotonia
- Activity level
  o   Convulsions
  o   Lethargy
  o   Irritability
  o   Hyperactivity
- Failure to feed well
- Failure to move an extremity
- GI adaptation
  o   Vomiting
  o   Diarrhea
  o   Abdominal distention
- Presence of congenital anomalies
- Presence of birth related injuries
  o   Cephalohematoma
  o   Brachial plexus injury
  o   Pneumothorax
  o   Fractured ribs
  o   Subgaleal hemorrhage post vacuum

Clinical Impression:
Differential Diagnoses to Consider
- Term or preterm infant with
  o   Respiratory distress
  o   Birth trauma or injury
  o   Congenital malformations

- o Physiologic jaundice
- o Hyperbilirubenemia
- o Genetic disorders
- o Group B strep
- o Congenital anomalies
- o Drug withdrawal
- o Other conditions or illnesses

Diagnostic Testing:

Diagnostic Tests and Procedures to Consider
- Total bilirubin
- Blood cultures
- Other tests
  - o As indicated by infant presentation, and
  - o Within midwife's scope of practice

Providing Treatment:

Therapeutic Measures to Consider
- Provide neutral thermal environment
  - o Skin to skin on mother
  - o On warmed resuscitation unit
  - o With hot water bottle for transport
- Provide O2 for cyanosis
  - o Blow-by
  - o Mask
  - o Positive pressure ventilation
- As indicated by diagnosis, i.e.
  - o Phototherapy
  - o Antibiotics

Providing Treatment:

Alternative Measures to Consider
- Home phototherapy, lights or sunlight
- Homeopathic Rescue Remedy to pulse points
- Prayer and acceptance of baby as perfect being
- Other remedies as indicated by baby's condition or presentation

Providing Support:

Education and Support Measures to Consider
- At discharge, or following home birth, provide information regarding:
  - o Signs and symptoms of illness or injury
  - o Who to contact if symptoms develop
  - o How to contact infant's health care professional
- For ill infant
  - o Provide information about
  - o Diagnosis, if known
  - o Evaluation plan if diagnosis unknown
  - o Provide support to parents during
  - o Newborn work-up
  - o Diagnosis
  - o Treatment

Follow-up Care:

Follow-up Measures to Consider
- Reevaluate infant in relation to problem if uncertain re: normalcy of behavior
- Document
  - o Findings
  - o Concerns
  - o Parent teaching
  - o Consultations
  - o Follow-up plan
    - Plan for reevaluation
    - Appointments scheduled
    - Referrals made
  - o Parent response to condition

Collaborative Practice:

Criteria to Consider for Consultation or Referral
- Arrange for, or perform comprehensive newborn evaluation within 24 hour of age
- Consider consultation for any out of the ordinary behavior or findings
- Transport infant or transfer care of infant as indicated by problem

Ongoing Care of the Infant

Key Clinical Information:

The newborn infant may be cared for by a wide variety of health professionals, including midwives. The midwife who includes care of the infant after the immediate newborn period must develop working relationships with other infant care professionals who may provide care during times of illness, injury or other deviations from the norm Working with parents by providing information, education and support is essential.

Client History:

Components of the History to Consider
- Significant maternal history
- Course of labor and delivery and baby's response
  - o Apgar scores
  - o Resuscitative efforts and infant response
- Significant findings or events since birth
  - o Voiding and stooling patterns
  - o Feeding method and efforts
  - o Weight loss or gain
  - o Variations from expected newborn course
- Indication for present evaluation
  - o Routine care
  - o Problem-oriented care
  - o Signs and symptoms of
    - Infection
    - Injury
    - Neurologic disease
    - Birth defects
    - Drug addiction

Physical Examination:

Components of the Physical Exam to Consider

- Vital signs
- Skin color and turgor
  - o Pallor
  - o Cyanosis
  - o Ruddiness
  - o Jaundice
- General physical exam for signs of illness
  - o Tachycardia (HR > 170 bpm)
  - o Tachypnea (RR > 60 rpm)
  - o Jitteriness or irritability
  - o Poor muscle tone
  - o Bulging or sunken fontanels
  - o Hip clicks or laxity
  - o Absence of voiding or stooling
  - o Unusual sounding cry
  - o Feeding difficulties

Clinical Impression:

Differential Diagnoses to Consider

- Normal healthy newborn
- Newborn with signs or symptoms of
  - ▪ Infection
  - ▪ Injury
  - ▪ Neurologic disease
  - ▪ Birth defects
  - ▪ Drug addiction
  - ▪ Weight loss
  - ▪ Hearing or visual deficits
  - ▪ Failure to thrive

Diagnostic Testing:

Diagnostic Tests and Procedures to Consider

- Glucose
- Bilirubin
- Cord blood studies for Rh/ABO
- Other labs or tests as indicated by the infant's condition and within the scope of practice of the midwife

Providing Treatment:

Therapeutic Measures to Consider

- Nutritional supplements as needed
- Photo-therapy for hyperbilirubenemia
- Hepatitis B immunization
- Childhood immunizations

- o Diptheria, Pertussis, Tetanus (DPT)
- o Oral Polio/Inactivated Polio Vaccine (OPV/IPV)
- o Measles, Mumps, Rubella (MMR)
- o Hepatitis B
- o Varicella
- Treatment for underlying disease or illness
  - o Antibiotics
  - o Antiretroviral medications
  - o Hepatitis B immune globulin
  - o Other treatments as indicated

Providing Treatment:

Alternative Measures to Consider

- Supplement with Lact-aid® if breastfeeding
- Delay in onset of immunizations
- No immunizations

Providing Support:

Education and Support Measures to Consider

- Provide information on:
  - o Normal newborn behavior and findings
  - o Signs and symptoms of concern
  - o Warning signs
  - o When to call with concerns
  - o How to call in off-hours
  - o Routine for well infant care
  - o Immunization practices
- Encourage parental participation in decision-making
- Provide access to additional resources as needed

Follow-up Care:

Follow-up Measures to Consider

- Document all findings, especially any variations from normal
- Weight check at 1-2 wks of age
- Follow-up oral vitamin K at 1 and 4 week visits
- Monthly exams until 6 months

Collaborative Practice:

Criteria to Consider for Consultation or Referral

- For routine care when outside the scope of the midwife's practice
- In the presence of
  - o Variations from normal
  - o Illness
  - o Injury

References

1. American Academy of Pediatrics/American Heart Association. (2000). Textbook of Neonatal Resuscitation: Author.

2. Bachmann, G. A. (1993). Estrogen-androgen therapy for sexual and emotional well-being. The Female Patient. 18, 15-24.

3. Behrman, R.E., Kleigman, R.M., Arvin, A.M., (1996). Nelson Textbook of Pediatrics (15th Ed.). Philadelphia, PA: W.B. Saunders Co.

4. Barger, M. K. Ed. (1988). Protocols for Gynecologic and Obstetric Health Care. Philadelphia, PA: W. B. Saunders.

5. Briggs, G.G., Freeman, R. K., Yaffe, S. J. (1994) Drugs in Pregnancy and Lactation (4th Ed.). Philadelphia, PA: Williams & Wilkins.

6. Clark, C., Paine, L.L. (1996). Psychopharmacologic management of women with common mental health problems. Journal of Nurse-Midwifery 42, 254-274.

7. Davis, E. (1997). Hearts and Hands; A midwife's guide to pregnancy and birth. Berkely, CA: Celestial Arts.

8. Enkin, M., Keirce M., Renfrew, M., Neilson, J. (1995). A Guide to Effective Care in Pregnancy and Childbirth (2nd Ed.). New York, NY: Oxford University Press.

9. Foster, S. (1996). Herbs for Your Health. Loveland, CO: Interweave Press.

10. Frye, Anne. (1998). Holistic Midwifery. Portland, OR. Labrys Press

11. Gelbaum, I. (1993) Circumcision: Refining a traditional surgical technique. Journal of Nurse-Midwifery, 38 (Supplement), 18S-30S.

12. Gordon, J. D., Rydfors, J. T., et al. (1995) Obstetrics, Gynecology & Infertility (4th Ed.) Glen Cove, N.Y., Scrub Hill Press.

13. Graves, B.W. (1992). Newborn Resuscitation revisited. Journal of Nurse-Midwifery, 37, (supplement) 36s-42s.

14. Leopold, K. & Zoschnick, L., (1997). Postpartum depression. The Female Patient, (OB/GYN Edition), 22 (8), 40-49.

15. Miller, L., (1996), Beyond "The Blues": postpartum reactivity and the biology of attachment. Primary Psychiatry, April 1996, 35-38.

16. Scoggin, J., Morgan, G., (1997). <u>Practice Guidelines for Obstetrics and Gynecology.</u> Philadelphia, PA, Lippincott.

17. Scott, J. R., Diasaia, P.J., et al. (1996). <u>Danforth's Handbook of Obstetrics and Gynecology.</u> Philadelphia, PA, Lippincott - Raven.

18. Speroff, L., Glass, R. H., Kase, N. G. (1994) <u>Clinical Gynecologic Endocrinology and Infertility</u> (5th Ed.) Philadelphia, PA, Williams & Wilkins.

19. Swartz, M. H. (1994) <u>Textbook of Physical Diagnosis</u>: History and examination. (2nd Ed.) Philadelphia, PA, W. B. Saunders Co.

20. Varney, H., (2004). <u>Varney's Midwifery</u> (4th ed.). Boston, MA: Jones and Bartlett.

21. Weed, S. (1985). <u>Wise Woman Herbal for the Childbearing Year.</u> Woodstock, NY: Ashtree Publishing.

Care of the Woman with Reproductive Health Needs: Care of the Well Woman

Midwives are specialists in the care of the well woman. Providing women's health care in an environment of support and understanding fosters women's ability to care for themselves.

Women have a history of meeting others needs before attending to their own in almost every culture. This may be due to social constraints, lack of education about their health needs, communication barriers, transportation issues, or a lack of funds with which to pay for services. In our fragmented American society, many women may not know how to access services, or may be unable to navigate the complex health care system in a manner that meets their most basic needs.

Midwives are needed to reach out to the women of the communities in which they live and practice to bridge this chasm. Community midwifery may range from home-based care, to a local clinic, to a complex service that functions within the confines of a tertiary care hospital. No matter what the setting, each individual midwife can make a difference.

Listening to women is an essential component of midwifery care that includes validating women's experiences, offering non-judgmental support, and considering how the information reveal affects this woman, as a person, within her family, and her community.

Opportunities for midwifery include providing grass-roots encouragement for women to develop support networks within their own neighborhood, cultural enclave, or ethnic group. Midwives may offer women's health education programs, or informal counseling services even if there is no opportunity for the midwife to provide birth care. A commitment to women and an inquiring mind are all that is necessary to begin the adventure of improving the health of women using the midwifery model of care.

The Well Woman Exam

Key Clinical Information

The well woman exam is an opportunity for women to learn about their bodies while at the same time caring for themselves. The Pap smear is performed as a screening test for pre-malignant conditions of the cervix. Sexually transmitted infections (STI) may be screened for, as well breast disease or other health problems. The visit also offers both the woman and the midwife to work in partnership to address the unique concerns that that may affect each individual's life.

For an initial visit and exam the client history required will be quite comprehensive, while on repeat visits, especially in a community where the midwife provides ongoing care to the same women, a brief update of the history may be all that is required.

Client History:
Components of the History to Consider
- Reason for visit
- Last menstrual period (LMP)
- Obstetrical history
  - Gravity, parity
  - Infertility or losses
  - Problems/concerns
  - Plans for future pregnancies
- Menstrual patterns
  - Length of flow
  - Amount of flow
  - Pain/clots etc.
- Sexual history
  - Sexual orientation
  - New or change in partners
  - Method of birth control if applicable
  - Concerns
- Medical/Surgical history
  - Allergies
  - Medications & remedies
    - Over the counter
    - Prescription
    - Herbal/homeopathic remedies
  - Current immunization status
  - Diseases, conditions, or problems
  - Surgeries
  - Current health care
    - Primary care provider
    - Specialist care
    - Diagnostic testing
    - Treatments
- Health philosophy & care
  - Survival
  - Medically oriented
  - Alternative
- Social history
  - Use of alcohol, tobacco, drugs
  - Family community support systems
  - Domestic violence screen
  - Emotional well-being screen
  - Diet and physical activity
- Family history

- Medical conditions
- Hereditary conditions
- Review of systems (ROS)
  - Client impression of her health
    - Physical
    - Emotional
  - Changes in weight/appetite
  - Bowel and bladder function
  - Weakness/fatigue/malaise
  - Shortness of breath/palpitations
  - Other symptoms by body system
    - HEENT
    - Cardiopulmonary
    - Gastrointestinal
    - Neurologic
    - Reproductive
    - Musculoskeletal
    - Endocrine
    - Integumentary

Physical Examination:
Components of the Physical Exam to Consider
- Vital signs
  - Height/weight
  - Blood pressure/pulse/respirations
- Skin
  - Lesions
  - Scars
  - Bruises
- Head, eyes ears, nose & throat
  - Vision
  - Hearing
  - Condition of teeth & gums
  - Thyroid
  - Lymph nodes
- Back/Chest
  - Configuration/symmetry
  - CVA tenderness
  - Scoliosis/kyphosis
- Lungs
  - Rate, rhythm & depth of respirations
  - Breath sounds
- Heart
  - Rate and rhythm
  - Extra or unusual sounds

- Breasts
  - Symmetry
  - Masses
  - Discharge
- Abdomen
  - Configuration
  - Masses/pain
  - Diastasis recti
- Extremities
  - Range of motion
  - Symmetry
  - Strength
- Pelvic exam
  - External genitalia & rectum
    - Bartholin's, urethra Skene's
    - Configuration
    - Lesions/discharge
    - Hemorrhoids
  - Speculum exam
    - Vagina
      - Discharge
      - Odor
    - Cervix
      - Discharge
      - Lesions
      - Configuration
    - Specimen collection
  - Bimanual exam
    - Uterine position
    - Size & shape
    - Pain on cervical motion
    - Adnexa
      - Masses
      - Pain
      - Mobility
    - Rectal exam
      - Hemorrhoids
      - Masses
      - Bleeding
      - Specimen collection

Clinical Impression:

Differential Diagnoses to Consider

- Well women preventive health exam NOS
- Well woman exam with significant findings, i.e.,
  - Undesired fertility
  - Sexually transmitted infection
  - Other infection
  - Infertility
  - Pregnancy
  - Rectal bleeding

Diagnostic Testing:

Diagnostic Tests and Procedures to Consider

- Specimens collected during exam/visit
  - Dip urinalysis
  - Pregnancy testing
  - Finger-stick Hct or Hgb
  - Pap smear
  - STI testing
  - Wet prep for BV or Trich
  - Stool for occult blood
- Lab testing
  - CBC or H&H

- Hepatitis profile
- HIV
- Q-β HCG
- Sickle cell prep
- Fasting blood sugar
- Urinalysis &/or culture
- Radiology
  - Ultrasound
  - Mammogram

Providing Treatment:

Therapeutic Measures to Consider

- Provide immunizations prn
  - Tetanus/diptheria
  - Hepatitis B
  - Measles, Mumps, Rubella
  - Varicella
  - Influenza (over 50)
  - Pneumococcal vaccine (over 65)
- Treatment based on diagnosis

Providing Treatment:

Alternative Measures to Consider

- Treatment based on diagnosis

Providing Support:

Education and Support Measures to Consider

- Discuss
  - Reason for visit
  - Significant findings
  - Options for care
  - When to follow-up
  - Notification process for results
- Address client concern

Follow-up Care:

Follow-up Measures to Consider

- Document visit
  - History & ROS
  - Significant findings
  - Clinical impression
  - Plan of continued care
- Notify clients of testing results
- Report adverse reactions to vaccines
  - Vaccine Adverse Reporting System
  - www.vaers.org
  - 1-800-822-7967

Collaborative Practice:

Criteria to Consider for Consultation or Referral

- Based on midwife scope of practice & client needs
- Abnormal pap smears
- Abnormal breast exam
- Confirmed occult blood in stool
- Initial HIV diagnosis
- Other diagnoses as indicated by client preference and need for medical care
- As needed for
  - Social service
  - Transportation services
  - Mental health services
  - Drug & alcohol rehab services
  - Homeless shelters
  - Abused women's services

Pre-conception Counseling

Key Clinical Information

Preconception counseling provides an opportunity to address health needs that may affect pregnancy before the pregnancy occurs. Midwife initiated discussions may spark awareness and interest in modifying health behaviors as a prelude to a planned pregnancy, or foster correct use of birth control for pregnancy prevention.

Client History:
Components of the History to Consider

- Age
- Previous OB/GYN history
  - G, P
  - Result of previous pregnancies
  - STDs/HIV status
  - Abnormal pap smears/cervical treatment
- Medical and surgical history
  - Current medical problems
  - Previous surgery
  - Medications
- Social history
  - Mental well-being
  - Nutrition
  - Eating disorders
  - Over/under-weight
  - Pica
  - Substance abuse
  - Physical abuse
  - Partner/family support
- Family reproductive history
  - Birth defects
  - Genetic disorders
  - Multiple births
  - Losses
- Personal concerns
  - Readiness (self and partner)
  - Financial concerns
  - Spouse and/or family concerns

Physical Examination:
Components of the Physical Exam to Consider

- Complete physical exam as indicated by
  - History
  - Interval since last physical
  - Primary focus on
    - Thyroid
    - Breast exam
    - Pelvic exam

Clinical Impression:
Differential Diagnoses to Consider

- Preconception reproductive health care
- Screening for health risks related to pregnancy
- Preconception counseling related to risk factors, i.e.,
  - Diabetes
  - Hypertension
  - Genetic disorders
  - Neural tube defects

- Advanced maternal age
- HIV
- Substance abuse

Diagnostic Testing:
Diagnostic Tests and Procedures to Consider

- PPD
- Cervico-vaginal screening
  - Pap smear
  - BV
  - GBS
  - Chlamydia
  - Gonorrhea
- Blood tests
  - Rubella & Hepatitis B titers
  - Blood type & Rh
  - H & H
  - TSH
  - Toxoplasmosis screen
  - HIV testing
  - Other as indicated by history

Providing Treatment:
Therapeutic Measures to Consider

- Treat medical conditions
  - Adjust medications according to drug pregnancy category
- Vitamin and mineral supplement
  - Folic acid 0.4 mg/400mcg po daily
  - Begin at least 4 weeks prior planned conception
  - Continue through at least 13 weeks gestation
  - Consider multivitamin with or without iron
- Update immunization status
  - Rubella
    - Avoid pregnancy for 3 months following Rubella immunization [30]
  - Hepatitis B
  - Tetanus/diphtheria

Providing Treatment:
Alternative Measures to Consider

- Whole foods diet
- Iron and folic acid food sources
- Natural family planning methods for determining ovulation

---

[30] Sweet BR Ed. (1999) Mayes Midwifery (12th ed.) London: Balliere Tindall. P 175

Providing Support:

Education and Support Measures to Consider

- Health Promotion
    - Counsel regarding pertinent issues as determined by history
    - Encourage dental work prior to conception
    - Encourage regular physical exercise
    - Provide nutrition information
    - Avoidance of cigarettes alcohol, recreational drugs
    - Environmental concerns
    - Workplace hazards
    - Toxic chemicals
    - Radiation contamination
- Provide pregnancy information/resources for your community
- Address birth options/locations & services

Follow-up Care:

Follow-up Measures to Consider

- With onset of amenorrhea for HCG testing
- If no pregnancy within 12 months
- With questions or concerns

Collaborative Practice:

Criteria to Consider for Consultation or Referral

- As indicated for care that is outside the scope of the midwife's practice
    - Genetic counseling
    - Infertility evaluation or treatment
- Abnormal pre-conception labs
- Substance abuse centers
- Nutritional risk assessment by dietician
- Physical abuse
- Psychosocial issues

Smoking Cessation

Key Clinical Information

Smoking is an addiction that is both physical as well as psychological. In order to successfully stop smoking there must be desire to quit, a method to address the physical symptoms of nicotine withdrawal, and exploration and cultivation of more positive coping skills and habits.

Client History:

Components of the History to Consider

- Age
- Medical and surgical history
    - Current medical problems
    - Heart disease
    - Diabetes
    - Elevated cholesterol
    - Hypertension
- Mental health disorders
    - Eating disorders
    - Depression
    - Bi-polar disease
    - Psychosis
- Medications
    - Estrogen products
    - Oral contraceptives
    - ERT
    - Antidepressants
    - Wellbutrin (same as Zyban)
    - MAOIs
- Social history
    - Duration of smoking history
    - Attempts at quitting
    - Current ppd habit
    - Partner/family support
- Personal concerns
    - Readiness/motivation
    - Previous attempts to stop smoking
    - Coping skills
    - Weight gain
- Family medical history
    - Heart disease

- Diabetes
- Elevated cholesterol
- Hypertension
- Stroke

Physical Examination:

Components of the Physical Exam to Consider

- BP, WT
- Physical exam
    - As indicated by history and interval since last exam
    - Focus on cardio pulmonary system

Clinical Impression:

Differential Diagnoses to Consider

- Smoking cessation

Diagnostic Testing:

Diagnostic Tests and Procedures to Consider

- Lipid profile
- ECG

Providing Treatment:

Therapeutic Measures to Consider

- Nicotine containing medications are pregnancy category D
- Nicoderm CQ (transdermal)
    - 7 mg/24 hr, 14 mg/24 hr, or 21 mg/24hr
    - Begin with 21 or 14 mg patch
    - Use 2-6 weeks then decrease dose
- Nicotrol step-down patch (transdermal)
    - 5-15 mg/16 hr patch, or
    - Use during waking hours
- Nicorette gum
    - 2 mg, 4 mg strength
    - Use 2 mg if < 1 ppd smoker
    - Max 24 pieces/day

- Nicotrol NS/Inhaler
  - o   0.5 mg/spray, 10 mg/cartridge inhaler
  - o   1-2 doses/hr
- **Non-nicotine medication**
- Bupropion HCL (Zyban)
  - o   150 mg po x 3 days
  - o   150 BID with 8 hrs between doses
  - o   Stop smoking within 1-2 weeks of use
  - o   May use with nicotine medications
  - o   Pregnancy category B
  - o   Not for use in those with
    - ▪   Eating disorders
    - ▪   Seizures
    - ▪   Wellbutrin or MAOIs

Providing Treatment:
Alternative Measures to Consider

- Decrease cigarette use by 1-2 cig/week
- Learn new coping skills
- Avoid situations that increase desire to smoke
- Keep gum or healthy finger food available for oral satisfaction
- Increase physical activity

Providing Support:
Education and Support Measures to Consider

- Provide advise & support for smoking cessations
- Provide clear medication instructions
- Nicotine containing medications
  - o   Stop smoking with prior to or with onset of use
  - o   Use lower dose with + cardiac history
- Bupropion HCL

- o   Take as instructed
- o   May decrease appetite
- o   May cause medication interactions
- Counsel as determined by history
  - o   Encourage regular physical exercise
  - o   Provide nutrition information
  - o   Provide information regarding
    - ▪   Local resources for developing healthy coping mechanisms
    - ▪   Smoking support groups

Follow-up Care:
Follow-up Measures to Consider

- 2 weeks after beginning smoking cessation
  - o   Client support
  - o   Evaluation of
  - o   Current smoking habit (Bupropion HCL)
  - o   BP, WT
  - o   Symptoms or side effects since use of medication
- Refer for counseling/support for addictions prn
- Register pregnant clients by calling (800) 336-2176

Collaborative Practice:
Criteria to Consider for Consultation or Referral

- For prescription of medications if not within midwife's scope of practice
- For clients with
  - o   Cardiac history
  - o   Adverse medication reaction
  - o   Onset of cardiac symptoms with use of nicotine containing medications

Barrier Methods

Key Clinical Information

Barrier methods provide not only contraception, but also some protection from sexually transmitted infections. Use of barrier methods requires that couples take the time to learn and use their method consistently. Barrier methods may be an adjunct to other methods, or used alone. More information on latest products is available at www.birthcontrol.com.

Client History:
Components of the History to Consider

- Allergies
- Medications
- OB/GYN history
  - o   LMP – normal menstrual pattern
  - o   G,P
  - o   Last exam, pap, and STD testing, as applicable
  - o   History of STDs – diagnosis and treatment
  - o   History of abnormal pap smears - diagnosis and treatment
- Past and current medical and surgical history
- Social history
  - o   Cigarette smoking, drug and/or alcohol use
  - o   Living situation and resources
  - o   Sexual partner support for method of birth control
- Method related considerations
  - o   Assess ability to learn and use method reliably
  - o   Assess impact of unplanned pregnancy

Physical Examination:
Components of the Physical Exam to Consider

- Complete physical exam, with focus on
  - o   Reproductive system
  - o   Vaginal/cervical anatomy & position
  - o   Fit of diaphragm or cap
  - o   Woman's ability to insert/remove device

Clinical Impression:
Differential Diagnoses to Consider

- Contraceptive management
  - o   Diaphragm fitting
  - o   Cervical cap fitting
  - o   Contraceptive education, condoms

Diagnostic Testing:
Diagnostic Tests and Procedures to Consider

- Pap smear
- Urinalysis

- STD screening as indicated
- Other screening tests according to age and health history

Providing Treatment:

Therapeutic Measures to Consider

- Diaphragm
  - o Not recommended for patients with history of UTIs
  - o Female superior position decreases effectiveness
  - o Must be used with spermicide
- Cervical cap
  - o May cause increased rate of cervical erosion
  - o Recommended to be used with spermicide
  - o Prentif cavity rim cervical cap
    - ▪ 4 sizes
  - o Lea's cap
    - ▪ 1 size
    - ▪ Available from Canada
  - o Oves cap
    - ▪ Medical grade silicone
    - ▪ 3 sizes
    - ▪ Available from Canada
- Male condom
  - o Provides some measure of protection against STIs
  - o May contribute to latex allergy
  - o Requires male cooperation to use effectively
- Contraceptive sponge
  - o Today sponge
    - ▪ Nonoxyl-9
    - ▪ 89-91% effective
  - o Protectaid
    - ▪ Available in Canada
    - ▪ F5 gel
    - ▪ 90% effective
  - o Pharmatex sponge
    - ▪ Available in Canada
    - ▪ Benzalkonium chloride
    - ▪ 83% effective
- Reality® female condom
  - o Allows female control for STI protection & contraception
  - o Greater protection than male condom

Providing Treatment:

Alternative Measures to Consider

- Fertility awareness
- Abstinence

- Withdrawal
- Natural spermicide
- Spermicidal solution for use with cervical cap or diaphragm (Use instead of nonoxyl-9)
  - o 1 cup water
  - o 1 teaspoon fresh lemon juice
  - o 5 teaspoons table salt
  - o 10 teaspoons cornstarch
  - o 10 teaspoons glycerine
  - o Mix solids, add liquids while stirring, cook over low heat until thick. Store in sealed containers. Discard unused portions after 30 days.

Providing Support:

Education and Support Measures to Consider

- Instruct in proper use, cleaning and care of reusable devices
- Have client perform a return demonstration of insertion and removal of diaphragm or cervical cap
- Review effectiveness of chosen method
- Review other birth control methods and their effectiveness
- Condoms are recommended to protect against STIs
- Call or return for care if amenorrhea or positive pregnancy test occurs

Follow-up Care:

Follow-up Measures to Consider

- Document discussions regarding
  - o All methods of birth control
  - o Client preferences for birth control
  - o Fitting for cap or diaphragm
  - o Client instructions for use
  - o Planned follow-up
- Follow-up
  - o 2 week visit for evaluation of fit of diaphragm or cervical cap
  - o 3-4 month return visit for repeat pap smear in cervical cap users
  - o Annual return for pap smear screening
  - o PRN with problems

Collaborative Practice:

Criteria to Consider for Consultation or Referral

- For pelvic anatomy that does not allow for fitting of diaphragm or cervical cap
- For prescription birth control if not offered through midwife

Injectable Contraceptiive Hormones

Key Clinical Information

Depo provera and Lunelle contraceptive injections offer a hormonal method of birth control for women who cannot reliably use other hormonal methods. While there may be a prompt return to fertility after the injection, there may also be a significant delay in return to fertility. Some women report PMS-like symptoms while on Depo, which is a progestin-only medication.

Client History:

Components of the History to Consider

- Allergies
- Medications

- OB/GYN history
  - o LMP + normal menstrual pattern
  - o G,P
  - o Last exam, pap and STD testing if applicable

- o   History of
- o   STIs – diagnosis and treatment
- o   Abnormal pap smears - diagnosis and treatment
- Breast/mammogram abnormalities – diagnosis and treatment
- Risk factors for osteoporosis
  - o   Low Ca+ diet
  - o   Sedentary
  - o   Small frame
  - o   Family history
- Past and current medical and surgical history
  - o   Thrombophlebitis, current or past
  - o   Liver dysfunction or disease
  - o   Hyperlipemia
  - o   Hypertension
- Social history
  - o   Smoking
  - o   Risk factors for STIs
- Contraindications to injectable contraceptive use
  - o   Pregnancy
  - o   History of breast cancer
  - o   Undiagnosed genital bleeding
- Assessment of reliability to return for injections as scheduled

Physical Examination:

Components of the Physical Exam to Consider

- Complete physical exam with focus on
- Breasts
- Reproductive tract
- Thyroid

Clinical Impression:

Differential Diagnoses to Consider

- Contraceptive management
  - o   Contraceptive injection
    - ▪   Depo provera
    - ▪   Lunelle

Diagnostic Testing:

Diagnostic Tests and Procedures to Consider

- Pap smear
- Urinalysis
- STI testing
- Pregnancy test

Providing Treatment:

Therapeutic Measures to Consider

- Initial injection must be given *only*
  - o   Within first 5 days of normal menses
  - o   Within first 5 days postpartum if not breastfeeding
  - o   At 4-6 weeks postpartum if breastfeeding
- Depo-Provera
  - o   150 mg IM
  - o   Repeat q 12-13 weeks
- Lunelle
  - o   0.5 mg IM
  - o   Repeat q 28-30 days

Providing Treatment:

Alternative Measures to Consider

- Fertility awareness
- Abstinence
- Withdrawal
- Natural spermicides

Providing Support:

Education and Support Measures to Consider

- Counsel regarding all birth control options
- Review common side effects
- Depo-Provera, side effects
  - o   Spotting or amenorrhea
  - o   PMS-type symptoms
  - o   Weight gain
  - o   Pregnancy may be delayed
  - o   10-18 months following last injection
  - o   Pregnancy may occur within 14 weeks of last injection
  - o   Condoms recommended to protect against STDs
  - o   Bone density changes
  - o   Encourage weight-bearing activity
  - o   Calcium & Vit D intake
  - o   Review signs and symptoms of potential risks (see patient labeling)
  - o   Thrombophlebitis
  - o   Ocular disorders
  - o   Ectopic pregnancy
- Lunelle, side effects
  - o   Weight gain
  - o   Menorrhagia
  - o   Amenorrhea
  - o   Moodiness
  - o   Breast pain
  - o   Increased risk of gallbladder disease
  - o   Increased risk of blood clots and associated complications, i.e., stroke

Follow-up Care:

Follow-up Measures to Consider

- Document
  - o   Discussions about birth control methods
  - o   LMP, or if no menses last injection date
  - o   Side effects & client response
  - o   Route & location of injection
  - o   Dosage & name of medication
  - o   Plan for continued care
- Schedule return visit to allow grace period in case of illness, rescheduling, etc.
- ☛ Don't miss pap screening due to frequent visits
- For persistent bleeding on Depo
  - o   Oral contraceptives x 1-3 months
  - o   Conjugated estrogens 0.625 mg daily x 21 days

Collaborative Practice:

Criteria to Consider for Consultation or Referral

- As indicated by history or physical exam
- For side effects/complications of medication use such as gallbladder disease or thrombus formation

Emergency Contraception (ECP)

Key Clinical Information

Emergency contraception is most effective as soon as possible after unprotected intercourse, but must be used within 72 hours after unprotected sexual exposure. It is not recommended for regular use as contraception. When prescribed as *Preven*, the emergency contraceptive kit includes a pregnancy test and both *Preven* and *Plan B* include detailed client instructions. Side effects include nausea & vomiting, and an antiemetic may be prescribed in addition. To access the Emergency Contraceptive Hotline call 1-888-NOT-2-Late.

Client History:

Components of the History to Consider

- Allergies
- Medications
- Number of hours since unprotected intercourse
- OB/GYN history
  o LMP – normal menstrual pattern
  o G,P
  o Current or recent use of contraception
  o Last exam, pap and STD testing if applicable
  o History of STDs
  o History of abnormal pap smears
- Contraindications to ECP use
  o Pregnancy
  o Undiagnosed genital bleeding
- Assess feelings about
  o Potential unplanned pregnancy
  o Reasons for unprotected sexual exposure
- Determine client plans for birth control

Physical Examination:

Components of the Physical Exam to Consider

- Complete physical exam within past 12 months
- Focus on reproductive system
- Not required for Rx, but may be useful when
  o History is unclear
  o STD testing indicated
  o Other symptoms are present

Clinical Impression:

Differential Diagnoses to Consider

- **Contraceptive management following unprotected sexual exposure**

Diagnostic Testing:

Diagnostic Tests and Procedures to Consider

- Pregnancy testing
  o If menstrual history is uncertain or unclear
- STD screening as indicated
- Other screening tests
  o According to age and health history

Providing Treatment:

Therapeutic Measures to Consider

- Provide antiemetic one hour before first dose[31]
- Compazine
  o 5-10 mg tablet
    ▪ Repeat q 6-8 hrs prn

o   15 mg spansule
  ▪ Repeat in 24 hours prn
- Phenergan
  o 25 mg tablet or suppository
  o Repeat q 8-12 hours prn
- Benadryl
  o 25-50 mg PO
  o Repeat prn q 4-6 hour
- Emergency Contraceptive Pills
- First dose ASAP but at least within 72 hours
- Second dose 12 hrs after 1st dose
- Plan B
  o Progestin only
  o May cause less nausea
  o 0.75 mg levonorgestrel per dose
  o 1 tab per dose, 2 doses
- Preven (ECP Kit)
  o Estogen/Progesin
  o 0.05 mg ethinyl estradiol/0.25 mg levonorgestel
  o 2 tabs, 2 doses
- Lo/Ovral
  o 0.03 mg ethinyl estradiol/0.30 mg levonorgestrel
  o 4 tabs, 2 doses
- Levelen/Nordette (light orange pills)
  o 0.03 mg ethinyl estradiol/0.15 mg levonorgestrel
  o 4 tabs, 2 doses
- Tri-Levelen/Triphasil (yellow pills)
  o 0.03 mg ethinyl estradiol/0.125 mg levonorgestrel
  o 4 tabs, 2 doses

Providing Treatment:

Alternative Measures to Consider

- Nausea
  o Seabands
  o Ginger tea
- Herbs that foster onset of menstruation
  o Blue cohosh
  o Angelica root
  o Dong-quai
  o Vitex or Chasteberry
  o Black cohosh
  o Evening primrose oil
- Homeopathic remedies that foster onset of menstruation[32]
  o Pulsatilla
  o Sepia
  o Caulophyllum
  o Calcarea carb.
- For additional information about herbal remedies to prevent or avoid pregnancy See

[31] ACOG (2001). ACOG Practice Bulletin: Energency Oral Contraception. In 2002 Compendium of Selected Publications. Washington, DC: ACOG.

[32] Smith, T (1984). A Woemn's Guide to Homeopathic Medicine. New York: Thorson Publishers.

- o   *A Difficult Decision: A Compassionate Book About Abortion*
      by Joy Gardner
- o   *The Roots of Healing* by Deb Soule

Providing Support:

Education and Support Measures to Consider

- Make certain patient does not want to become pregnant
- Explain how to use ECPs correctly
- Emphasize that ECPs are for emergency use only
- Counseling regarding common side effects
  - o   Nausea and vomiting
    - Menses
    - May be earlier or later than usual
    - Within 21 days of ECP
    - Return for care if no menses within 21 days
  - o   Breast tenderness
- Discuss
  - o   Safe sexual practices
  - o   Pregnancy and STD prevention
  - o   Other contraceptive options
- Options if ECP is not effective
  - o   Not teratogenic
- ECP is more likely to be used when women obtain information and a prescription with a routine visit

Follow-up Care:

Follow-up Measures to Consider

- Document client education for ECP
  - o   Medication instructions
  - o   When to return for care
  - o   Findings from exam or testing, if done
- Have client return for care with
  - o   Symptoms suggesting complications
  - o   Amenorrhea that continues over 21 days after ECP
  - o   For initiation of regular contraception
  - o   Client requires further information or counseling regarding STDs or pregnancy prevention

Collaborative Practice:

Criteria to Consider for Consultation or Referral

- For prescription of ECP if not within midwifery scope of practice
- For emergency IUD insertion (effective within 5 days of unprotected intercourse)
- If ECP not effective for termination of pregnancy per client choice
- For complications of medication requiring medical care

The Intrauterine Device

Key Clinical Information

The IUD is a highly effective method of birth control that may be hormonal or non-hormonal. The Mirena IUD releases levonorgestrel, while the Para-Guard IUD releases copper. Like any method of birth control, careful selection of the client who is an appropriate candidate for this method is essential. Benefits include the IUD's effectiveness (99+%), and ease of use. The common side effect of heavy bleeding has been minimized by the Mirena; the progestin thins the lining of the uterus, and menses tend to be light. Perforation, infection, and expulsion remain potential problems associated with the IUD, and must be considered when counseling the woman considering this method of birth control.

Client History:

Components of the History to Consider

- Age
- G, P
- Allergies
- Medications
- Medical/surgical history
- Verify
  - o   LMP or date of delivery
  - o   Contraceptive history & current use
  - o   Last pap/gyn exam
    - Pap results
    - STI test results
  - o   No history of fibroids or unusual configuration of uterus
- Prior to removal determine
  - o   Indication for removal
  - o   Birth control method desired, if any
- The ideal history for IUD insertions includes
  - o   No history PID
  - o   Mutually monogamous long-term relationship
  - o   One or more full term pregnancies
  - o   Negative history of heavy menses
  - o   Negative history of severe dysmenorrhea
  - o   Comfortable with the thought of an IUD in her uterus
  - o   Does not want a pregnancy for 3-10 years
  - o   Is able to check for the IUD string
- Contraindications to IUD insertion
  - o   Pregnancy
  - o   Abnormalities of the uterus
  - o   PID past or present
  - o   Uterine or cervical malignancy
  - o   Copper allergy or Wilson's disease (copper IUD)
  - o   Previous ectopic pregnancy
  - o   Immuno-compromised state
  - o   Valvular heart disease
  - o   Unresolved abnormal pap or cervical cancer
  - o   Decreased immune response
  - o   Acute liver disease (hormonal IUD)
  - o   Current DVT (hormonal IUD)

Physical Examination:

Components of the Physical Exam to Consider

- Physical exam as indicated by client history
- Prior to insertion
  - o Obtain pap smear and STI testing prn
    - ▪ Obtain results prior to IUD insertion
  - o Bimanual exam to determine
    - ▪ Uterine size & contour
    - ▪ Uterine position
    - ▪ Involution if postpartum
  - o Speculum exam
    - ▪ Sound uterus (6-9 cms is recommended)
- Prior to removal
  - o Speculum exam for visualization of strings
  - o Based on indication for removal

Clinical Impression:

Differential Diagnoses to Consider

- Contraceptive management:
  - o IUD insertion
  - o IUD removal
  - o Complications of IUD insertion/use
    - ▪ Vasovagal syncope
    - ▪ Perforation of the uterus
    - ▪ Expelled IUD
    - ▪ Lost IUD
    - ▪ Intermenstual bleeding
    - ▪ Pregnancy with IUD in situ

Diagnostic Testing:

Diagnostic Tests and Procedures to Consider

- Pap smear
- Chlamydia and gonorrhea testing
- Hepatitis profile
- HIV testing
- Other labs as indicated by health status

Providing Treatment:

Therapeutic Measures to Consider

- Ibuprofen or naproxen 1 hr before procedure
- Have atropine sulfate available for vagal response
- Antibiotic prophylaxis not recommended
- Procedure for insertion:
  - o Read manufacturer's instructions
  - o Obtain informed consent (see client education)
- Timing of insertion
  - o 4-8 weeks postpartum
  - o During menses
  - o Any time, as long as pregnancy is ruled out
- Use sterile technique
- Swab cervix with antiseptic solution (i.e. betadine prep)
- Position tenaculum gently
  - o Close slowly to decrease cramping
  - o Position on anterior lip for anteverted cervix
  - o Position on posterior lip for retroverted uterus
  - o Avoid vessels at 3 & 9 o'clock positions
- Sound uterus prior to insertion
  - o Apply traction to tenaculum
  - o Gently insert sterile sound until slight resistance is felt
  - o Do not use force
  - o Note depth of sound
  - o Use sound to prepare IUD insertion device for correct uterine size
- Load IUD into insertion device using sterile technique
- Gently insert IUD according to manufacturer's instructions
- Use traction on tenaculum to straighten uterine curvature
- Remove insertion device

- Remove tenaculum
- Obtain hemostasis
  - o Apply pressure to bleeding sites
  - o Apply silver nitrate to bleeding sites (may cause cramping)
- Trim strings to approximately 1.5 – 2 inches in length
- Observe for vagal response prior to discharge
  - o Trendellenber's position
  - o Smelling salts
  - o Atropine sulfate 0.4-0.5 mg IM for severe vagal response with bradycardia
- Procedure for removal
  - o Grasp strings and pull gently but firmly
- If strings not visible at os:
  - o Palpate cervical canal with sterile forceps
  - o Grasp string or IUD if felt and pull gently
- If unable to palpate evaluate for presence of IUD with ultrasound

Providing Treatment:

Alternative Measures to Consider

- Fertility awareness
- Abstinence
- Withdrawal
- Natural spermicides

Providing Support:

Education and Support Measures to Consider

- Review history with client, and spouse if needed
- Review all birth control options appropriate for this woman
- Discuss risks, benefits, effectiveness of IUD
- Provide information about the
  - o Pre-procedure preparation
  - o IUD cost
  - o Details of insertion procedure
  - o Potential side effects
    - ▪ Signs and symptoms
    - ▪ When to call
    - ▪ How to call in off hours
  - o Return visit post-procedure
- Teach client to feel strings after insertion

Follow-up Care:

Follow-up Measures to Consider

- Document
  - o Review of history
  - o Informed consent
  - o Findings on exam
  - o Details of procedure
  - o Complications or untoward events
    - ▪ Treatment
    - ▪ Client response
  - o Plan for continued care
- Return for care
  - o 2 weeks post-insertion or post next menses
  - o With onset of fever, pain or heavy bleeding
  - o For planned return to fertility
  - o For schedule replacement
    - ▪ 5 years for Mirena
    - ▪ 10 years for Para-Guard

Collaborative Practice:

Criteria to Consider for Consultation or Referral

- For IUD insertion if not within the scope of the midwife's practice
- For complications of IUD insertion
  - o Difficulty sounding uterus
  - o Perforation of uterus

- Uterine anomalies
- History of postpartum endometritis in past 3 months
- Client desire for paracervical block for insertion

- IUD string not visible or palpated and removal is desired
  o May need removal under anesthesia and direct visualization with hysteroscopy

Natural Family Planning

Key Clinical Information

Natural family planning, or fertility awareness can be an effective method of birth control for the couple who are attentive to the nuances of the female cycle and are committed to this form of birth control. Every woman can benefit from an increase awareness and understanding of her menstrual cycle, and the process of reproduction. This information can be used to prevent pregnancy alone or in conjunction with other non-hormonal methods of birth control.

Client History:
Components of the History to Consider
- Menstrual history
  o LMP
  o Frequency of menses
  o Duration of menses
  o Midcycle pain/discharge
- Current method of birth control
- Effect an unplanned pregnancy would have
- OB/GYN history
- Medical/Surgical history

Physical Examination:
Components of the Physical Exam to Consider
- Vital signs
- Weight/height
- Complete physical exam with focus on
  o Thyroid
  o Breasts
  o Pelvic exam

Clinical Impression:
Differential Diagnoses to Consider
- Contraceptive care
  o Education & counseling

Diagnostic Testing:
Diagnostic Tests and Procedures to Consider
- Pap
- STI testing
- Thyroid

Providing Treatment:
Therapeutic Measures to Consider
- Ovulation predictor tests
- www.birthcontrol.com

Providing Treatment:
Alternative Measures to Consider
- Fertility awareness
  o Menstrual calendar
  o Basal body temperature charting

  o Cervical mucous
- Abstinence
  o Periodic abstinence (rhythm method)
  o Avoid intercourse during fertile times
  o Abstinence
- Withdrawal
  o May work for some couples
  o There may/may not be sperm in pre-ejaculatory fluid
  o May or may not interrupt sexual satsifaction
- Natural spermicides (see Barrier Methods)
- Outercourse
  o Hugging & kissing
  o Holding and fondling
  o Sexual activity that does not include penis in vagina

Providing Support:
Education and Support Measures to Consider
- Discussion to determine if this is a realistic method for this couple
- Provide information & resources about
  o Changes throughout the menstrual cycle
  o Basal body temperature/thermometer
  o Option to add barrier methods or spermicide at midcycle
- Engage partner in discussions

Follow-up Care:
Follow-up Measures to Consider
- Document
  o Discussions with client regarding natural family planning
  o Exam & findings
  o Plan for continued care
- Return for care
  o On an as needed basis
  o As recommended by age & sexual activity
  o For Pap and STI testing

Collaborative Practice:
Criteria to Consider for Consultation or Referral
- For problems outside the scope of midwife's practice

Norplant Contraceptive Implant

Key Clinical Information

The Norplant System is a subdermal contraceptive implant that consists of Silastic capsules filled with a time-release form of levonorgestrel. The Norplant is not currently being marketed in the U.S., due to difficulty with consistency in hormonal release. However, there still may be numerous women with the system in place, and the system is still approved by the FDA. Another implant, Jadelle, is also available in other countries.

Client History:

Components of the History to Consider

- Allergies
- Medications
- G, P, LMP or days/weeks postpartum
- History of hormonal contraceptive use
- Presence or indications of contraindications to Norplant use
- Contraindications for Norplant use
  o Active thrombophlebitis or thromboembolitic disease
  o Undiagnosed genital bleeding
  o Acute liver disease
  o Benign or malignant liver tumors
  o Known or suspected breast cancer

Physical Examination:

Components of the Physical Exam to Consider

- Complete physical exam prior to insertion with focus on
  o Bimanual and speculum exam
  o Breast exam
  o Palpation for liver margins

Clinical Impression:

Differential Diagnoses to Consider

- Contraceptive management
  o Contraceptive implant insertion
  o Contraceptive implant removal
  o Complications of contraceptive implants
    ▪ Unplanned pregnancy
    ▪ Infection at insertion site
    ▪ Intermenstrual bleeding
    ▪ Headaches
    ▪ Unacceptable weight gain
    ▪ Difficult removal

Diagnostic Testing:

Diagnostic Tests and Procedures to Consider

- Pap smear
- STI screen
  o Chlamydia & gonorrhea
  o Hepatitis profile
  o HIV
- Mammogram

Providing Treatment:

Therapeutic Measures to Consider

- Consider trial of Nordette x 1 month to evaluate client response prior to insertion of implants
- Ibuprofen or acetaminophen prior to procedure
- Have atropine sulfate available for vagal response

- Procedure for insertion
  o Obtain informed consent
  o Insert within 7 days of start of LMP
  o Insert prior to discharge postpartum or at 6 weeks if breastfeeding
- Using sterile technique follow manufacturer's insertion instructions
  o Use template to mark site of insertion
  o Sterile prep and drape
  o Local anesthesia using 1-2% lidocaine with epinephrine
  o Consider buffering lidocaine with sodium bicarbonate to reduce stinging
    ▪ 10:1 lidocaine:bicarb
    ▪ Mix well before injecting
  o Close incision with steri-strips
- Removal techniques vary
  o May need larger incision
  o Capsules will be covered by fibrous sheath
  o Allow 30+ minutes for removal
  o Use sterile technique
  o One removal technique
    ▪ Palpate capsules and using digital pressure push capsule into wound
    ▪ Grasp implant with fine tipped clamp
    ▪ Pull end of capsule into wound
    ▪ Abrade fibrous sheath from capsule end
    ▪ Grasp capsule with second clamp
    ▪ Release first clamp
    ▪ Pull capsule from wound
    ▪ Repeat for additional capsules
  o May need return visit for removal of all capsules
  o Close incision with steri strips or suture
- Post insertion/removal
  o Apply sterile dressing
  o Wrap insertion/removal site with pressure dressing
  o Ice and elevate x 2 hours to decrease bruising
- For irregular vaginal bleeding post-insertion consider
  o Ibuprofen 800 mg tid x 5 days, *may combine with*
    ▪ Conjugated estrogens 0.625 - 1.25 mg po daily x 10-21 days, or
    ▪ Low dose birth control pills x 1 pack
  o Consider other contraceptive method

Providing Treatment:

Alternative Measures to Consider

- Fertility awareness
- Abstinence
- Withdrawal

- Natural spermicides

Providing Support:

Education and Support Measures to Consider

- Counseling regarding insertion and/or removal
- Provide manufacturer's written information to client
- Counsel regarding potential side effects
  - o Bruising and tenderness at site
  - o Irregular bleeding
  - o Headaches
  - o Weight gain
  - o Breast tenderness
  - o 0.2 –1.1 % risk of pregnancy
- More complex procedure for removal
- Encourage condom use as indicated by history
- Decreased effectiveness while on TB and seizure medications

Follow-up Care:

Follow-up Measures to Consider

- Document

- o Informed consent
- o Details of procedure
- o Client response
- o Complications of procedure
  - ▪ Treatment
  - ▪ Response
- o Plan for continued care
- Return to office
  - o 2 weeks for insertion/removal site check
  - o With persistent vaginal bleeding
  - o With amenorrhea for evaluation for pregnancy
  - o For signs and symptoms of infection
  - o For planned return to fertility

Collaborative Practice:

Criteria to Consider for Consultation or Referral

- For removal if not within the scope of the midwife's practice
- For difficult insertion or removal
- For + pregnancy test

Hormonal Contraceptives; Pills, Patches, & Rings

Key Clinical Information

Birth control pills offer a well-established woman-controlled method of hormonal birth control. They may result in a decrease in ovarian cancer risk, a decrease in the rate of endometrial cancer, allow woman to suffer less dysmenorrhea, and result in a lighter menstrual flow. As with all medications, they are not without risks and side effects.

Client History:

Components of the History to Consider

- Allergies
- Medications
- OB/GYN history
  - o LMP – normal menstrual pattern
  - o G,P – date of most recent birth if postpartum
  - o Last exam, pap and STD testing if applicable
  - o History of STDs – diagnosis and treatment
  - o History of abnormal pap smears - diagnosis and treatment
- Past and current medical and surgical history
  - o Depression
  - o Gallbladder disease
  - o Hypertension
  - o Thrombophlebitis
- Social history
  - o Cigarette smoking, drug and/or alcohol use
  - o Living situation and resources
  - o Sexual partner support for method of birth control
- Family history
  - o Gallbladder disease
  - o Coronary artery disease before age 50
  - o Stroke before age 50
- Contraindications to oral contraceptive use
  - o Pregnancy
  - o Liver disease
  - o Undiagnosed abnormal genital bleeding
  - o Thrombophlebitis or thromboembolitic disease
  - o Coronary heart disease or cerebrovascular disease
  - o Cancer of the reproductive organs

- Relative contraindications
  - o Women who smoke and are > 35 years old
  - o BP 140/90 or greater
  - o Diabetes
  - o Asthma
  - o Kidney disease
  - o Gallbladder disease
  - o Lupus
  - o Depression
- Assess the woman's ability & motivation to use client regulated hormonal contraception
  - o Daily routine for pill taking
  - o Weekly routine for patch
  - o 3-week cycle for ring
  - o Ability to cope with side effects while adjusting to hormones
  - o Motivation to prevent pregnancy

Physical Examination:

Components of the Physical Exam to Consider

- BP
- Height/weight - BMI
- Complete physical exam
- Focus on reproductive system
- Thyroid
- Breasts
- Pelvic
  - o Speculum exam
  - o Bimanual exam

Clinical Impression:

Differential Diagnoses to Consider

- Contraceptive management
  - o   Oral contraceptive use
  - o   Oral contraceptive use complicated by
    - ▪   Hypertension
    - ▪   Hyperlipidemia
    - ▪   Non-compliance
    - ▪   Intermenstrual bleeding
    - ▪   Mood changes
    - ▪   Depression
    - ▪   Pregnancy

Diagnostic Testing:

Diagnostic Tests and Procedures to Consider

- Pap smear
- Urinalysis
- STD screening as indicated by history
- Other screening tests according to age and health history
  - o   Lipid profile for + family history of CAD
  - o   Fasting blood sugar
  - o   TSH
- Pregnancy testing

Providing Treatment:

Therapeutic Measures to Consider

- Progestin only birth control pills, i.e.,
  - ▪   Micronor
  - ▪   Nor-QD
  - ▪   Ovrette
  - o   Must take same time each day
  - o   Breakthrough bleeding common
  - o   Reduced effectiveness with
    - ▪   TB medications
    - ▪   Anticonvulsants
    - ▪   Barbituates
- Combination OCs
- Very low dose birth control pills, i.e.,
  - ▪   Alesse
  - ▪   Levlite
  - ▪   Nordette
  - o   Contain both estrogen and progestin
  - o   May have improved side effect profile than regular dose OC
  - o   Lo-Estrin 1/20
- Low dose birth control pills, i.e.,
  - ▪   Tri-Levelen
  - ▪   Demulen
  - ▪   Jenest
  - ▪   Necon
  - o   Slightly higher dose
  - o   Often less menstrual irregularity
  - o   May have increased side effects
- Recommended effective lowest dose
- Higher doses available for specific indications
- Transdermal patch: Ortho Evra
  - o   Combination patch
    - ▪   Effectiveness approx 99%
    - ▪   ↓ Effectiveness in women > 198 lbs.
- NuvaRing Contraceptive Vaginal Ring
  - o   Combination ring
    - ▪   Lower dose of medication is needed
    - ▪   Effectiveness approx 98-99%

Providing Treatment:

Alternative Measures to Consider

- Fertility awareness
- Abstinence

- Withdrawal
- Natural spermicides

Providing Support:

Education and Support Measures to Consider

- Instruct in starting and daily use of hormonal contraceptives
- Pills
  - o   Barrier or alternate method recommended x 2-3 weeks of first cycle
  - o   Condoms recommended to protect against STDs
  - o   Breakthrough bleeding is common in first cycles
  - o   Take pill daily at same time
  - o   Take pills ASAP if forgotten
  - o   Use backup method if 2+ pills are missed
- Patches
  - o   Applied every 7 days x 3 weeks
  - o   Apply to clean, dry skin of the
    - ▪   Buttocks
    - ▪   Upper outer arm
    - ▪   Lower abdomen
    - ▪   Upper torso
  - o   1 week off patch
  - o   Use additional method or abstinence during 1st week of use
  - o   Replace if full or partial detachment occurs
  - o   Side effects same as with OC
- Ring
  - o   Inserted into vagina and left for 3 weeks
  - o   No ring for 1 week
  - o   Side effects same as OC
- All methods: Call if the following occur
  - o   Amenorrhea
  - o   Persistent Intermenstrual bleeding
  - o   Chest pain or shortness of breath
  - o   Numbness or tingling of arms or legs
  - o   Severe headaches
  - o   Depression
  - o   Visual disturbances
- Review health benefits
  - o   Regulation of menses
  - o   Decreased cramping and flow
  - o   Protection against uterine & ovarian cancer
  - o   Decreased risk of bone loss
  - o   Potential decrease in risk of pelvic infections

Follow-up Care:

Follow-up Measures to Consider

- Document
  - o   Exam findings
  - o   Evaluation for contraindications to hormone use
  - o   Client preference for hormonal birth control
  - o   Client education for use of medication
  - o   Plan for continued care
- Return for care
  - o   3 months for evaluation of oral contraceptive use
  - o   BP & weight
  - o   Review of correct hormone use
    - ▪   Satisfaction with method
    - ▪   Questions or concerns
    - ▪   Side effects

Collaborative Practice:

Criteria to Consider for Consultation or Referral

- For prescription of hormonal contraceptives if not within the midwife's scope of practice
- Clients with relative contraindications to hormonal contraceptives who wish to trial this method
- Development of complication(s) of hormonal contraceptive use

Voluntary Interruption of Pregnancy

Key Clinical Information

It is the hope of most midwives that every baby that is conceived represents a wanted pregnancy. However, the reality is that this is not always the case. Unplanned or unwanted pregnancies can result from sexual assault, birth control failures, or poor judgment stemming from a multitude of factors. Our job as midwives, is to provide women with sound information and supportive, non-judgmental care so that they may make an informed personal decision when confronted with this difficult situation.

Medical or surgical termination of pregnancy offer one alternative to women with an unplanned and/or unwanted pregnancy. They are successful approximately 95-99% of the time when initiated *before* 8 weeks gestation. In pregnancies 8 weeks gestation or greater, surgical abortion is recommended.

Client History:
Components of the History to Consider
- Age
- Obstetric history
  - G, P
  - Current pregnancy
    - LMP, cycle history
    - Date of conception, if known
    - Current or prior method of birth control
    - Date of pregnancy test
    - Signs and symptoms of pregnancy
    - Dating ultrasound results
    - Alpha fetal protein or triple screen results
    - Amniocentesis or level II ultrasound results
    - Blood type & Rh factor if known
- GYN History
  - Last pap & exam
  - STI screening & results
- Medical/surgical history
  - Allergies
  - History of genetic disorders
  - Medical conditions
  - Prior surgery
- Social issues
  - Feelings about pregnancy
  - Personal support systems
  - Financial concerns regarding pregnancy options
  - ⊕Cultural considerations affecting decision
  - Other social issues
    - Drug, alcohol & tobacco use
    - Domestic violence
    - Mental health concerns
- Contraindications to medical abortion[33]
  - Abnormal pelvic exam, potential for ectopic pregnancy
  - IUD in situ
  - Potential for non-compliance with required follow-up
  - Presence of significant medical problems
    - Cardiopulmonary
    - Endocrine
    - Hepatic
    - Hematologic
  - Refusal to follow-up with definitive surgical treatment if medical treatment fails

Physical Examination:
Components of the Physical Exam to Consider
- Vital signs
- Pelvic exam for sizing of pregnancy
- General well-being

Clinical Impression:
Differential Diagnoses to Consider
- Pregnancy
  - For medical abortion
  - For surgical abortion, 1st trimester
  - For surgical abortion, 2nd trimester
- Pregnancy, complicated by
  - Fetal anomalies
  - Abnormal genetic testing

Diagnostic Testing:
Diagnostic Tests and Procedures to Consider
- Blood type, Rh and antibody screen
- Serum or urine HCG
- CBC, or H&H
- Pelvic ultrasound
  - Rule out ectopic pregnancy
  - Estimate gestational age

Providing Treatment:
Therapeutic Measures to Consider
- Verify surgical coverage for client in case does not pass products of conception spontaneously
- Obtain informed consent
- Mifepristone (Mifeprex)

[33] Varney, H. (2004). Varney's Midwifery. Boston: Jones & Bartlett.. pp. 576.

o   Dose: 600 mg PO in presence of provider
o   Observation x 30 minutes
- Provide for pain relief
  o   Acetaminophen
  o   Acetaminophen with codeine
  o   NSAIDS
     ▪ Do not interfere with mifepristone
     ▪ Provide significant pain relief
- Return visit scheduled for 36-48 hours
  o   40 μg misoprostol PO
  o   Observe for +/- 4 hours (expulsion of products of conception occurs during this time in 60% of patients)
- Rh immune globulin 1 dose (full or mini) for Rh negative women post-abortion
- Return visit in 7-10 days
  o   History for sign or symptoms of
     ▪ Complications
     ▪ Incomplete abortion
  o   Pelvic exam to verify complete abortion
  o   Post-abortion counseling
  o   Contraceptive management
- Surgical interruption scheduled if full POC not passed by 2 weeks after initial dose

Providing Treatment:

Alternative Measures to Consider

- Herbal remedied to foster interruption of pregnancy (see Natural Family Planning)
- Remedies to support the reproductive system during medical or surgical abortion
  o   Herbals
     ▪ Red raspberry leaf
     ▪ Dong-quai
     ▪ Vitex
     ▪ Lemon balm
     ▪ Alfalfa leaf
     ▪ Nettle leaf
  o   Homeopathic
     ▪ Arnica
     ▪ Sabina
     ▪ Pulsatilla

Providing Support:

Education and Support Measures to Consider

- Provide factual, unbiased information during options counseling
- Available options may be based upon
  o   Age of client
  o   Availability of services
  o   Philosophy of care
  o   Gestational age of pregnancy
  o   Maternal medical factors
  o   Financial considerations
- Potential options
  o   Adoption outside the family
  o   Adoption within the family
  o   Keeping and caring for the baby
  o   Voluntary termination of pregnancy
     ▪ Medical
     ▪ Surgical
- Clear information should be provided regarding
  o   All available services
  o   The termination procedure(s)
     ▪ Medical

- Avoids invasive procedure
- No anesthesia
- High success rate (⊇95%)
- Requires careful follow-up
- May take up to 14 days to complete
- Requires client participation
  ▪ Surgical
    - Invasive procedure
    - Sedation or anesthesia
    - One visit
    - High success rate (99%)
    - May not require follow-up
  ▪ Coverage options should surgical services be required or desired
o   Potential side effects of medical abortion
  ▪ Nausea & vomiting
  ▪ Diarrhea
  ▪ Malaise
o   Necessary follow-up for medical abortion
  ▪ 36-48 hours, and
  ▪ 7-10 days
o   Warning signs and symptoms post-procedure
  ▪ Saturating sanitary pads in 30 minutes x 4
  ▪ Heavy flow x 24 hrs
  ▪ Severe pain
  ▪ Fever & chills lasting > 24 hours
o   Resources for emotional support

Follow-up Care:

Follow-up Measures to Consider

- ASAP for scheduling following verification of dates
- For prenatal care at patient preference post options counseling
- For medical abortion
  o   36-48 hours
     ▪ Provide misoprostol
     ▪ Observe for passage of products of conception
     ▪ Send to pathology for verification of tissue
     ▪ Provide RhIG if indicated
  o   7-10 days
     ▪ Check β-HCG levels
       - Should be 50% of previous levels
       - Should drop continuously
       - May take up to 90 days to return to non-pregnant range
     ▪ Follow-up ultrasound prn
       - If no FHR may wait up to 36 days post-mifepristone before surgical intervention is necessary
- For post-termination exam 1-4 weeks

Collaborative Practice:

Criteria to Consider for Consultation or Referral

- If midwife cannot provide objective care based on client preference for termination
- For genetic counseling if genetic disorder noted in fetus
- For adoption resources
- For voluntary termination of pregnancy when not within the midwife's scope of practice
- To obtain surgical coverage for clients undergoing medical abortion when service is provided by the midwife

Care of the Women with Care of the Woman with Reproductive Health Needs: Women Undergoing the Challenges of Aging

The changes that occur as women age cannot be quantified simply by where she is on the chart of reproductive-life stages, but must include a broad view of how she sees herself and how the challenges of aging affect her.

The population is aging, and so is the clientele of midwives who provide comprehensive woman-centered care across the lifespan. Caring for women as they age requires a broad knowledge-base of the changes that occur, and the ability to listen to women as they explore the many possibilities available to them in traditional and alternative health care.

During this time of transition women may have families that range from small children to adult children, grandchildren, and may include aging parents. The dream of retirement or financial security may be receding with the demands of providing care for aged parents, or a diminished ability to work. Health problems may become more prevalent, and use up a significant proportion of energy that was previously directed to home, family, or livelihood.

The hormonal changes that occur with aging may impact a woman's emotional responses to her life situation, her ability to rest well or sleep, her strength and stamina, and her self-image. Compassionate midwifery care offers women an opportunity to create a new view of themselves and the aging process, and provide a gateway to necessary services when problems develop.

Evaluation of the Menopausal Woman

Key Clinical Information

Evaluation the woman who is stands on the threshold of menopause offers an opportunity to assess health attitudes and practices, while screening for common health problems that may occur following the change of life. This time of transition may last one day, the day when it has been 12 months since the last menstrual period, or it may last several years during which there are multiple sighs and symptoms signaling the impending change. Each woman responds differently to the precursors of menopause, some may sign with relief that their time of bleedings is nearly done, while others may rage against the passing of their fertility, and mourn their lost youth. The midwife may smooth the transition with a listening ear, and carefully selected treatments for the problems that present.

Client History:

Components of the History to Consider

- Age
- Reproductive history
  - o LMP, G, P
  - o Presence or absence of cervix, uterus, ovaries
  - o GYN condition
  - o Menstrual status
    - ▪ Frequency, duration and flow
    - ▪ Associated vasomotor symptoms
      - • Hot flashes
      - • Night sweats
      - • Flushing
- Uro-genital symptoms
  - o Vaginal dryness
  - o Urinary symptoms
  - o Decreased libido
- Other symptoms
  - o Insomnia
  - o Emotional changes
    - ▪ Lability
    - ▪ Depression
    - ▪ Diminished coping ability
- Medical/Surgical history
  - o Chronic illnesses
  - o Surgeries
  - o Allergies
  - o Medications
- Family History
  - o Osteoporosis
  - o Female reproductive cancers
  - o Colon or GI malignancy
  - o Heart disease
- Social history
  - o Drug/ETOC & tobacco use
  - o Family support systems
  - o Social activities
  - o Ability to care for self
    - ▪ Food/shelter
    - ▪ Activities of daily living
    - ▪ Ability to seek assistance prn
  - o Physical activity
  - o Nutritional assessment
- Review of Systems
  - o Integumentary
    - ▪ Skin changes
    - ▪ Lesions
  - o HEENT
    - ▪ Hearing loss
    - ▪ Visual changes
  - o Cardiopulmonary
    - ▪ SOB
    - ▪ Palpitations
    - ▪ Edema
  - o Gastrointestinal
    - ▪ Bowel changes
    - ▪ Rectal bleeding
  - o Genitourinary
    - ▪ Urinary frequency
    - ▪ Dysparunia
  - o Endocrine

- ▪ Fatigue
- ▪ Intolerance to cold/heat
  - o Neurologic
    - ▪ Confusion
    - ▪ Headaches
  - o Musculoskeletal
    - ▪ Pain
    - ▪ Range of motion

Physical Examination:

Components of the Physical Exam to Consider

- Vital signs, including BP
- Height/weight
  - o BMI
  - o Changes
- HEENT
  - o Skin turgor
  - o Hearing
  - o Vision
  - o Thyroid
- Back
  - o CVA tenderness
  - o Evaluate for kyphosis
  - o Respiratory exam
- Cardiac exam
  - o Rate & rhythm
  - o Murmurs
  - o Pulses
  - o Peripheral edema
- Breast exam
  - o Masses
  - o Discharge
  - o Axilla
- Abdomen
  - o Bowel sounds
  - o Liver margins
- Extremities
- Genital exam
  - o Genital atrophy
  - o Lesions
  - o Pap
  - o Bi-manual exam
    - ▪ Uterine
      - • Size
      - • Consistency
      - • Contour
      - • Mobility
    - ▪ Adnexa
      - • Size
      - • Consistency
      - • Mobility
- Rectal exam
  - o Palpate for lesions/masses
  - o Stool for occult bleeding

Clinical Impression:

Differential Diagnoses to Consider

- Peri-menopausal woman
- Menopausal woman
- Endocrine disorder
- Mood disorder
- Woman at risk for

o   Osteoporosis
o   Heart disease
o   Diabetes
o   Colon cancer, etc.

Diagnostic Testing:

Diagnostic Tests and Procedures to Consider

- Pap smear
- Endometrial biopsy
- Mammogram
- Thyroid testing
- Liver function tests
- Fasting blood sugar
- Bone density testing
- Lipid profile
- ECG
- Stool for occult blood
- Colonoscopy
- TB testing

Providing Treatment:

Therapeutic Measures to Consider

- Hormone therapy (See HRT)
  - o   Estrogen Replacement Therapy
  - o   Combination Hormone Replacement Therapy
  - o   Estrogen/Androgen Therapy
- Treatment of medical conditions (i.e. hypertension)

Providing Treatment:

Alternative Measures to Consider

- Dietary changes
  - o   Decrease fat, caffeine, sugar, alcohol
  - o   Increase soy, whole grains
  - o   Vitamin E, vitamin D, calcium & magnesium
- Wise Woman Tea (The Roots of Healing p. 236)
- Maintain regular weight-bearing exercise
  - o   Walking
  - o   Weight training
- Non-weight bearing exercise for joint mobility
  - o   Swimming
- Utilize creative outlets
  - o   Journal writing
  - o   Dance, meditation, or singing
  - o   Prayer
- Community involvement/groups
  - o   Schools/childcare
  - o   Church
  - o   Libraries
  - o   Nature preserves
  - o   Homeless shelters
  - o   Soup kitchens
  - o   Non-profit organizations
- Sexual comfort
  - o   Vaginal lubricants
  - o   Alternate sexual practices

Providing Support:

Education and Support Measures to Consider

- Common side effects of the peri-menopausal period

o   Headaches
o   Hot flashes/flushes
o   Night sweats
o   Insomnia
o   Menstrual changes

- Medical therapies available for symptoms
  - o   Risks
  - o   Benefits
  - o   Alternatives
- Benefits and drawbacks to testing
  - o   Prep for testing, prn
  - o   Interpretation of test results
- Alternative therapies for symptoms
  - o   Risks
    - ▪ May stimulate similar to estrogens
    - ▪ Difficult to quantify dose
  - o   Benefits
    - ▪ Natural
    - ▪ Client regulated
    - ▪ May relieve symptoms
  - o   Options
    - ▪ Soy
    - ▪ Plant estrogens
    - ▪ Regular physical activity
    - ▪ Sleep aids
      - Valarian root
      - Chamomile
      - Melatonin
- Warning signs of female reproductive cancers
  - o   Bleeding
    - ▪ Irregular
    - ▪ Post-menopausal
  - o   Pain
  - o   Masses
  - o   Lesions
- Local support groups or resources as indicated

Follow-up Care:

Follow-up Measures to Consider

- Document
- Results of history & ROS
- Physical findings
- Clinical assessment
- Diagnostic testing & results
- Plan for continued care
- Referral or consultations
- Return for continued care
  - o   As indicated by test results
  - o   Annually
  - o   With onset of problem/symptoms

Collaborative Practice:

Criteria to Consider for Consultation or Referral

- For abnormal physical findings or test results
- For testing or Rx not within the scope the midwife's practice
- For continued care of medical problems

Hormone Replacement Therapy

Key Clinical Information

Hormone Replacement Therapy (HRT), like many other treatments is a double-edged sword. It offers significant benefits to a carefully selected group of women, while for other women it holds significant risks. One major criticism of HRT is the way it was 'mandated' for every woman after menopause as if it was a panacea for all the ills of women as they age. Obviously, no therapy should be used globally without evaluation the risks and benefits for the individual, and offering information so that the client herself can be an active participant in her care. That being said, HRT offers profound relief of vaso-motor symptoms for women with severe effects of hormone depletion at menopause, or during the peri-menopausal period. The peri-menopause is a period of time, usually about 3-5 years preceding the menopause, during which multiple vaso-motor symptoms are commonly troublesome.

Unopposed estrogen (ERT) has been demonstrated to increase the risk of endometrial cancer over women who used it in combination therapy or women who declined ERT.. All women who have a uterus and use supplemental estrogen from *any* source should have it balanced with progesterone. Women who use long term HRT are at increased risk of heart disease and breast cancer over women who decline HRT. In women with severe symptoms planning short-term therapy (<5 yrs) to help them through menopause this risk is considered low when there is no significant risk of breast cancer or heart disease.

Client History:

Components of the History to Consider

- Age
- Reproductive history
  - LMP or age at menopause
  - Current pattern of menstruation
    - Frequency
    - Duration
    - Amount of flow
  - Presence or absence of vasomotor symptoms:
    - Hot flashes
    - Night sweats
    - Vaginal atrophy and dryness
    - Urinary problems
    - Mood disturbance
  - Facial hair increase
  - Reproductive cancers and disorders (i.e. leiomyomata)
  - Last exam
    - Pap
    - Mammogram
    - Bone density testing
- Medical/surgical history
  - Allergies
  - Medications
  - Hx of thromboembolus or thrombosis
  - Recent fractures
  - Anorexia nervosa
  - Long-term Depo-Provera use (especially immediately prior to menopause)
  - Gallbladder disease
  - Liver disease
- Family history:
  - Osteoporosis
  - Heart disease
  - Alzheimer's disease
  - Colon cancer
  - Breast cancer
- Social history
  - Tobacco & ETOH use
  - Physical activity patterns
  - Nutritional statush
- Contraindications for HRT
  - Estrogen sensitive tumors, especially history of breast or endometrial cancer
  - Undiagnosed post-menopausal bleeding
  - Impaired liver function
  - Hx of thromboembolus or thrombosis
  - Heart disease
- Review of Systems

Physical Examination:

Components of the Physical Exam to Consider

- Vital signs, BP, WT (BMI)
- Height, compare to previous
- General physical exam with focus on
  - Thyroid palpation
    - Size, contour
  - Breast exam
    - Presence of masses

- Documentation of contour
- o Pelvic exam
  - Atrophy, pallor
  - Presence of masses
- o Bony integrity
  - Range of motion
  - Arthritis
  - Kyphosis
- o Rectal exam

Clinical Impression:

Differential Diagnoses to Consider

- HRT for the following indication(s)
  - o Severe vaso-motor symptoms
  - o Osteoporosis (consider non-hormonal therapies first)
  - o ASC-US pap smear
  - o Mood disturbance related to hormone changes (consider other medications first)
- Medical contraindication to HRT in client with symptoms

Diagnostic Testing:

Diagnostic Tests and Procedures to Consider

- Pap smear
- Endometrial biopsy
- FSH/LH
- Blood lipid evaluation
- ECG
- Bone mineral density testing
- Mammogram
- Pelvic ultrasound
- Post-menopausal woman
  - o Prior to initiation of HRT consider
  - o Endometrial biopsy
  - o Progestin challenge
    - Provera 5-10 mg daily x 10 days
    - Anticipate withdrawal bleed within 10 days of completion of medication
    - If little or no bleed consider continuous HRT therapy
    - If vigorous bleed consider cyclic HRT

Providing Treatment:

Therapeutic Measures to Consider

- Peri-menopausal woman with moderate to severe vasomotor symptoms:
  - o Consider oral contraceptives
    - Do not use in smokers!!!
  - o Consider transdermal estrogen
  - o Progestin not required with regular monthly menses
  - o Add progestin when menses irregular
- Post-menopausal woman
- Continuous Hormone Replacement Therapy
- Combination therapy
  - o CombiPatch (estradiol/norethindrone acetate transdermal system)
    - Apply patch at twice weekly interval
    - For more info: 1-877-266-2448 or www.combipatch.com
  - o PremPro (oral conjugated estrogens/progestin)
    - 0.625/2.5 1 po daily
    - 0.625/5 1 po daily
  - o Estrogen – daily
    - Conjugated estrogen 0.625 mg
    - Estropipate 0.625 mg
    - Esterified estrogen 0.625 mg
    - Micronized estradiol 1 mg
  - o Transdermal estrogen 0.05 mg
  - o Progestin – daily

- Provera 2.5 mg
- Cyclic Hormone Replacement Therapy
  - o Estrogen - days 1-25 of month or continuously
  - o Dose range 0.3 mg-1.25 mg daily, varies with brand
  - o 0.625 mg is lowest dose recommended to treat osteoporosis
- Plant-based estrogens
  - o EstraTab
  - o Ogen
- Progestin use with cyclic estrogen
  - o Provera 5-10 mg x 5-10 days
  - o Prometrium 200mg qhs x 12 days
  - o Use estrogen days 1-25 of cycle month
  - o Use progestin days 11-25 to 16-25 of cycle month
- Estrogen-Androgen Therapy
  - o For decreased libido
  - o Given cyclically (i.e. three weeks on, 1 week off)
  - o Short term therapy
  - o Virilization may occur
  - o Must use progestin in client with intact uterus
  - o Products available
    - Esterified estrogen 0.625 mg/methyltesterone 1.25 mg
    - Esterified estrogen 1.25 mg/methyltesterone 2.5 mg
    - Conjugated estrogen 0.625 mg/methyltesterone 5 mg
    - Conjugated estrogen 1.25 mg/methyltesterone 10 mg

Providing Treatment:

Alternative Measures to Consider

- See "vaso-motor symptoms"
- Natural Hormones
  - o Custom compounding of natural hormones
  - o Professional compounding pharmacies
  - o Hormone creams, absorbed via skin
- Phytoestrogens may combat symptoms of menopause
  - o Peanuts
  - o Oats
  - o Corn
  - o Apples
  - o Soy
  - o Flaxseed
- Homeopathic Remedies
  - o Hot Flashes
    - Belladonna
    - Lachesis
  - o Vaginal dryness
    - Bryonia
    - Natrum mur.
- For additional herbal formulas see *The Roots of Healing* by Deb Soule
- Vitamin & mineral supplements
  - o Calcium and magnesium supplementation
  - o Vitamin E supplements 400 IU b.i.d. with meals

Providing Support:

Education and Support Measures to Consider

- Review method of HRT, dose, timing, side effects
- Reinforce need to return for evaluation if unscheduled vaginal bleeding or other symptoms occur while on HRT
- Osteoporosis prevention and evaluation
- Avoid caffeine, fat, white sugar, flour, cigarettes and alcohol
- Add to the diet: whole grains, dark leafy green vegetable, sea vegetables, protein from legumes, nuts and seeds
- Lifestyle changes to add regular exercise, rest and relaxation

- Encourage participation in activities that support acceptance of the life changes

Follow-up Care:

Follow-up Measures to Consider

- Document
  - Relevant history & ROS
  - Physical findings
  - Indication for HRT
  - Discussions with client
    - Risks/benefits
    - Indications
    - Anticipated response
    - Informed choice
    - Signs & symptoms requiring return for care
  - Medication
    - Dose
    - Regimen
    - Instructions
  - Plan for continued care
  - Consultations or referrals
- Return for continued care

- Evaluate in 3 months after initiating HRT
  - Reduction in symptoms
  - Bleeding patterns
  - Satisfaction with treatment
  - Concerns or unexpected side effects
- Annually for well woman exam
- Following any unanticipated or unscheduled vaginal bleeding for evaluation
- For breast changes

Collaborative Practice:

Criteria to Consider for Consultation or Referral

- For tests or Rx of HRT not within the midwife's scope of practice
- Symptoms that do not respond to standard HRT regimens
- Unexplained or persistent vaginal bleeding
- Breast mass or abnormal mammogram
- Osteoporosis
- Signs or symptoms of heart disease
- Complications of HRT

Screening for Osteoporosis

Key Clinical Information

Osteoporosis is defined as a disease that is characterized by a decrease in the level of bone mass itself, resulting in bones that are more porous. This leads to deterioration of the structural integrity of the remaining bone, and contributes to fragile bones that are more likely to fracture with minimal trauma. The diagnosis of osteoporosis and osteopenia (the onset of bone loss, but not yet to the degree that equals osteoporosis) are made using Bone Mineral Density (BMD) evaluation. Ostoeporosis is said to be present when the BMD is more than 2.5 standard deviations below the mean. Prevention measures include regular weight-bearing activities to both increase bone stress and maintain muscle mass to support the bone. Treatment is aimed at slowing the loss of bone and preferably building bone mass. Any woman with a history of a fracture after age 40 should consider BMD testing.

Client History:

Components of the History to Consider

- Age
- Reproductive history
  - LMP, G, P
  - Age at menarche
  - Age at menopause
  - Length of time post-menopause
  - Use of hormonal
    - Contraceptives
    - Hormone replacement therapy
    - Herbs or plant extracts
  - Breastfeeding history
- Assess for risk factors for osteoporosis:
  - Small or thin frame or body size
  - Positive family history of osteoporosis
  - Prior fracture after minor trauma after age 40
  - Current history of cigarette smoking
  - Early/surgical menopause without estrogen replacement

  - Sedentary lifestyle
  - Low calcium intake
  - Corticosteroid use
  - Excessive use of thyroid hormone
  - History of anorexia
  - Long-term depo-provera use
  - ETOH abuse
- Assess for symptoms of osteoporosis
  - Complaints of back pain
  - Changes in posture/height
  - Fractures after peri-menopausal period
- Current prevention measures
  - Vitamin D intake/sun exposure
  - Calcium intake
  - Mineral supplementation
  - Weight bearing exercise
- Health habits
  - Daily physical activity
  - Tobacco use
  - Alcohol use

Physical Examination:

Components of the Physical Exam to Consider

- Vital signs
- Height, compare to previous
- Weight
- Presence of kyphosis, 'dowager's hump'
- Palpation of vertebrae for pain
- Evidence of increased risk for falls
  o Physical limitations
  o Frailty
  o Balance and coordination
  o Eyesight
- Other exam components as indicated by history

Clinical Impression:

Differential Diagnoses to Consider

- Osteoporosis
- Osteopenia (decreased bone density)
- Calcium & Vit. D deficiency
- Risk factors for fracture
- Compression fracture
- Disc compression

Diagnostic Testing:

Diagnostic Tests and Procedures to Consider

- Bone density testing
  o Dual-energy x-ray absorptiometry (DXA)
- Osteomark® urine test for bone collagen breakdown
  o (1-800-99OSTEX)

Providing Treatment:

Therapeutic Measures to Consider

- For women with no contraindications to HRT
  o Single or combination hormone replacement therapy (see HRT)
    ▪ Short term therapy (<5 yrs)
    ▪ Weigh risks vs benefits
- For women whom estrogen is contraindicated due to its effects on the uterus and/or breast
  o Raloxofene (Evista)
    ▪ 60 mg po daily
  o Calcitonin-salmon (Miacalcin)
    ▪ 200 units intranasally daily
  o Alendronate (Fosamax)
    ▪ Must swallow whole
    ▪ Prevention – 5 mg po daily
    ▪ Treatment – 10 mg po daily

Providing Treatment:

Alternative Measures to Consider

- Nutritional support
  o Calcium foods
    ▪ Sea vegetables
    ▪ Deep green leafy vegetables
    ▪ Canned fish with bones
    ▪ Molasses
    ▪ Tofu, soy milk
    ▪ Corn tortillas
  o Herbs
    ▪ Red raspberry leaf

- Oatstraw
- Nettles
- Borage
- Dandelion greens
- Vitamin and mineral therapy
  o Vitamin D
  o Calcium
- Weight bearing exercise
- Sunlight exposure for vitamin D synthesis
  o Hands and face
  o 10 minutes daily

Providing Support:

Education and Support Measures to Consider

- Provide information regarding
  o Calcium sources & intake
  o Weight bearing exercise
    ▪ Walking
    ▪ Weight training
    ▪ Rowing
    ▪ Sweeping, vacuuming
  o Medication use
    ▪ Side effects
    ▪ Benefits
    ▪ Risks
- Community preventive health programs
  o Smoking cessation
  o Alcoholics anonymous
  o Exercise programs
- Encourage client to avoid or limit use of
  o Tobacco
  o Alcohol
  o Caffeine

Follow-up Care:

Follow-up Measures to Consider

- Document
  o Risk factors for osteoporosis
  o Bone density test results
  o Treatment, if indicated
  o Client education/discussions
  o Plan for continued care
  o Consultation or referral
- Offer bone density testing at 1-2 year intervals
- Evaluate behavioral modification for modifiable risk factors
  o Smoking
  o Alcohol use
  o Physical activity patterns
- Review risk status annually with well woman exam

Collaborative Practice:

Criteria to Consider for Consultation or Referral

- To order bone density testing if not within the midwife's scope of practice
- Physical therapy referral for strengthening program
  o Ability to maintain activities of daily living
  o Improve balance
  o Assess for risk of falls
- For initiation and management of treatment plan for diagnosis of osteoporosis

Care of the Woman with Vaso-Motor Symptoms

Key Clinical Information

Vaso-motor symptoms are a common occurrence during both the peri-menopausal period and early post-menopause. They can make women quite miserable, and significantly affect quality of life. Many women prefer not to use HRT for treatment of vaso-motor symptoms due to the inherent risks associated with hormone use. For centuries women coped without HRT, and did very well. Some women, however have severe vaso-motor symptoms and may benefit from treatment

Client History:

Components of the History to Consider

- Age
- Reproductive history
  - LMP or age at menopause
  - Current pattern of menstruation
    - Frequency
    - Duration
    - Amount of flow
- Presence and severity of vasomotor symptoms:
  - Hot flashes
  - Night sweats
  - Vaginal atrophy and dryness
  - Urinary problems
  - Facial hair
  - Insomnia
  - Decreased libido
  - Mood disturbance
- Medical/surgical history
  - Allergies
  - Medications
  - Conditions
    - Gallbladder disease
    - Heart disease
    - Blood clots
    - Liver disease
- Family history
  - Heart disease
  - Breast cancer
- Review of systems
- Social history
  - ETOH/tobacco use
  - Support systems
  - Significant life stressors

Physical Examination:

Components of the Physical Exam to Consider

- BP, WT, HT
- General physical exam with focus on
  - Thyroid palpation
  - Breast exam
  - Pelvic exam
  - Rectal exam
- Observe for atrophy of tissues
  - Pale
  - Thin
  - Fragile

Clinical Impression:

Differential Diagnoses to Consider

- Vasomotor symptoms related to menopause
- Medical conditions with similar symptoms
  - TB
  - Thyroid disorder
  - Adrenal disorder

  - Mood disorder

Diagnostic Testing:

Diagnostic Tests and Procedures to Consider

- Pap smear
- Endometrial biopsy
- FSH/LH
- Blood lipid evaluation
- Bone density testing
- Mammogram
- Pelvic ultrasound

Providing Treatment:

Therapeutic Measures to Consider

- Hormone Replacement Therapy (see HRT)
- Peri-menopausal woman
  - Moderate to severe vasomotor symptoms:
  - Consider oral contraceptives
  - Consider transdermal estrogen
- Menopausal woman
  - Consider HRT therapy
- Antidepressants (see Mental Health Problems)
- Sleep aids (short term therapy)
  - Use caution if
    - Depression suspected
    - ETOH use
    - Hepatic or renal disease
  - Revaluate 2-3 weeks
  - Ambien 10 mg po hs
  - Dalmane 15-30 mg hs
  - Halcion 0.125-0.25 mg hs
  - Sonata 10 mg hs

Providing Treatment:

Alternative Measures to Consider

- Nutritional support
- Phytoestrogens
  - Peanuts
  - Oats
  - Corn
  - Apples
  - Soy
  - Flaxseed
- Calcium and magnesium supplementation
- Vitamin E supplements 400 IU b.i.d. with meals
- Natural Hormones
- Custom compounding of natural hormones
  - Portland Professional Pharmacy, Portland, ME
- Homeopathic Remedies
  - Hot Flashes
    - Belladonna
    - Lachesis
  - Vaginal dryness
    - Bryonia
    - Natrum mur.

- For herbal formulas see *The Roots of Healing* by Deb Soule
- Physical activity to release endorphins
  - o Yoga
  - o Dance
  - o Aerobics, etc.

Providing Support:

Education and Support Measures to Consider

- Methods of treatment for vasomotor symptoms
- Informed choice regarding treatment
- Need to return for evaluation for
  - o Unscheduled vaginal bleeding
  - o Breast mass
  - o Osteoporosis prevention and evaluation
- Dietary recommendations
  - o Whole grains
  - o Dark leafy green vegetables
  - o Sea vegetables
  - o Protein from legumes, nuts and seeds
  - o Limited animal proteins & fats
- Lifestyle changes
  - o Add regular exercise, rest & relaxation
  - o Avoid
    - ▪ Caffeine
    - ▪ Fat
    - ▪ Refined sugar & flour
    - ▪ Cigarettes & alcohol
- Provide information about
  - o Menopause and vasomotor symptoms
  - o Local support or women's groups
  - o Signs & symptoms that indicate a need to seek care

Follow-up Care:

Follow-up Measures to Consider

- Document
  - o Vasomotor symptoms and perceived severity
  - o Relevant history
  - o Findings on physical exam
  - o Diagnostic test results
  - o Discussions with client regarding options for treatment and care
  - o Recommendations
  - o Consultations or referrals
  - o Plan for continued care
- Return for continued care
  - o As needed to provide ongoing support and information regarding changes with peri-menopause & menopause
  - o Following any unscheduled vaginal bleeding for evaluation
  - o For worsening symptoms of depression
  - o For evaluation of treatment side effects
  - o For annual evaluation

Collaborative Practice:

Criteria to Consider for Consultation or Referral

- For Rx not within the midwife's scope of practice
- Symptoms that do not respond, or worsen with
  - o Alternative therapy
  - o Standard HRT regimens
- Unexplained or persistent vaginal bleeding
- Breast mass
- Osteoporosis
- Abnormal liver or renal function test results
- Symptoms of heart disease

References

1. Bachmann, G. A. (1993). Estrogen-androgen therapy for sexual and emotional well-being. The Female Patient. 18, 15-24.

1. Barger, M. K. Ed. (1988). Protocols for Gynecologic and Obstetric Health Care. Philadelphia, PA: W. B. Saunders.

2. Barton, S. Ed. (2001). Clinical Evidence. London. BMJ Publishing Group.

3. CDC (2002). National Immunization Program. Accessed on-line at www.cdc.gov/nip/recs/adult-schedule.htm

4. Ferris, D, Brotzman, G., Mayeaux, E.J., (1998). Improving compliance with estrogen therapy for osteoporosis. The Female Patient. Vol. 23, No.4, 29-45.

5. Frye, Anne. (1998). Holistic Midwifery. Portland, OR. Labrys Press

6. Foster, S (1996). Herbs for Your Health. Loveland, CO: Interweave Press.

7. Gordon, J. D., Rydfors, J. T., et al. (1995) Obstetrics, Gynecology & Infertility (4th Ed.) Glen Cove, N.Y., Scrub Hill Press.

8. Mackenzie, S.J., Yeo, S. (1997), Pregnancy interruption using Mifepristone (RU-487); A new choice for women in the USA. The Journal of Nurse-Midwifery, 42, 86-98.

9. Murphy, J. L., Ed. (2003). Nurse Practitioner's Prescribing Reference. New York, NY. Prescribing Reference, Inc.

10. Program for Appropriate Technology in Health. (1997, May). Emergency contraception: A resource manual for providers. Seattle, WA: Author

11. Rieder, J., Coupey, S.M., (2000). Contraceptive compliance. The Female Patient, (supplement). March 2000, 12-19.

12. Ringel, M (1998). HRT: Is it for you? The Female Patient. 11(S), 13-17.

13. Scherger, J. E. (1993). *Preconception care: A neglected element of prenatal services.* The Female Patient. 18, 78-83.

14. Scott, J. R., Diasaia, P.J., et al. (1996). Danforth's Handbook of Obstetrics and Gynecology. Philadelphia, PA, Lippincott - Raven.

15. Siris, E. S., Schussheim, D. H. (1998). Osteoporosis: Assessing your patient's risk. <u>Women's Health in Primary Care. 1(1),</u> 99-106

16. Smith, Trevor. (1984). <u>A Woman's Guide to Homeopathic Medicine.</u> New York, NY, Thorsons Publishers Inc.

17. Soule, D. (1996). <u>The Roots of Healing.</u> Secaucus, NJ: Citadel Press.

18. Starr, D. S., (2000). *The Legal Advisor: Missing a smoking gun.* <u>The Clinical Advisor.</u> March 25, 2000, 105-106

19. Trapani, FJ (1984). <u>Contraception Naturally.</u> Coopersburg, PA: CJ Frompovich Publications

20. Varney, H., (2004). <u>Varney's Midwifery</u> (4th ed.). Boston, MA: Jones and Bartlett.

21. Weed, S. (1985). <u>Wise Woman Herbal for the Childbearing Year</u>. Woodstock, NY: Ashtree Publishing.

Care of the Woman with Reproductive Health Needs: Reproductive Health Problems

Midwifery care includes the care of select women's health problems and variations from normal.

The ability to discern the difference between which conditions or findings represent the wide spectrum of 'normal', and which may be subtle presentations of the abnormal is a skill that midwives must work to develop. Skill as a diagnostician is necessary if midwifery practice includes comprehensive care of women's reproductive health needs. Many women rely on their midwife to care for their women's health needs outside of pregnancy.

There are many resources available to the midwife to help her maintain and improve her competence in the diagnosis and treatment of commonly encountered women's health problems. A problem-oriented, directed history is essential to accurate diagnosis, and validation of the woman's concerns. The exam should focus on pertinent body systems and the organs that influence them. The resulting clinical impression, or list of potential differential diagnoses, should guide the midwife as to what diagnostic studies are appropriate, or whether prompt consultation or referral is indicated. The midwifery plan of care should clearly address diagnostic testing; treatments; anticipated results; client education about the problem, the treatment, and when to return for care; client preferences for care; and anticipated return for care, with and without resolution of symptoms.

Abnormal Mammogram

Key Clinical Information

Mammography is one method of identifying breast lesions that may be benign or malignant. An abnormal mammogram may indicate the presence of abnormality that requires biopsy to determine whether treatment is indicated or not. Women with an abnormal mammogram are understandably anxious. The prompt treatment of early breast cancer is a woman's best chance for long-term survival. Women who have negative lymph nodes at time of biopsy have a 70% chance for 5-year survival without recurrence.

Client History:

Components of the History to Consider

- OB/GYN history
  - Current menstrual status
  - G,P
  - Age at first birth
  - Infant feeding method(s)
  - Breast history
    - Mastitis
    - Prior breast masses
    - Previous breast surgery
    - Previous treatment for breast disease
- Current symptoms
  - Onset
  - Duration
  - Severity
- Family history
  - Breast cancer
  - Ovarian cancer
  - Benign breast disease
- Screening for risk factors for breast cancer
  - Most breast cancer is random, not risk associated
  - Older age
  - Early menarche
  - Alcohol use
  - Hormone replacement therapy
  - ⊕Eastern European Jewish heritage
  - Nulliparous status
  - Never having breast fed
  - Strong family history
  - Personal history of breast cancer

Physical Examination:

Components of the Physical Exam to Consider

- Complete breast exam
  - Positioning
    - Sitting
    - Supine
- Evaluate for
  - Mass
  - Dimpling
  - Nipple retraction
  - Nipple discharge
  - Redness
  - Induration
  - Axillary lymphadenopathy
  - Breast or axillary enderness

Clinical Impression:

Differential Diagnoses to Consider

- Breast cancer
  - In situ
  - Focal
  - Disseminated
- Benign breast mass
  - Fibroadenoma
  - Fibrocystic breast
  - Enlarged lymph nodes
  - Other benign lesions

Diagnostic Testing:

Diagnostic Tests and Procedures to Consider

- Ultrasound if benign process is suspected
- Follow-up mammogram
  - Based on radiologist recommendations
  - Magnification views
  - 3-6 months follow-up
- Biopsy
  - Fine needle aspirations
  - Core needle biopsy
  - Stereotactic biopsy
  - Excisional biopsy
- Genetic testing

Providing Treatment:

Therapeutic Measures to Consider

- Excisional biopsy
  - Definitive treatment for benign masses
  - May be sufficient for small malignancies when combined with chemo &/or radiation
- Cancer treatments
  - Surgery
    - Lumpectomy
    - Mastectomy
      - Partial
      - Simple
      - Radical
    - Axillary node evaluation
      - Sentinel node(s)
      - Axillary node dissection
  - Medical therapy
    - Radiation, &/or
    - Chemotherapy

Providing Treatment:

Alternative Measures to Consider

- Alternative therapies should not take the place of diagnostic measures
- Herbal and homeopathic remedies for
  - o Immune support:
    - Echinacea
  - o Emotional support:
    - Rescue remedy
    - Bach flower essences
    - Lemon balm
- Love & laughter have been shown to fight cancer
  - o Rent comedy videos
  - o Enjoy time with friends
  - o Enjoy each day as a gift

Providing Support:

Education and Support Measures to Consider

- Advise client of abnormal screening test results
- Provide information about options
  - o Tissue sample (biopsy) is diagnostic test
  - o Provide written information regarding
    - Abnormal mammograms
    - Options for diagnostic testing

- Options for treatments
- Allow time for client to express concerns
  - o Validate concerns/fears
- With cancer diagnosis, info on
  - o Community resources
  - o Reach to Recovery
  - o American Cancer Society
  - o Cancer support groups

Follow-up Care:

Follow-up Measures to Consider

- Document
  - o Mammogram results
  - o Discussion with clients
  - o Referrals
  - o Anticipated plan

Collaborative Practice:

Criteria to Consider for Consultation or Referral

- Community resources
  - o Social service
  - o Transportation
  - o Counseling
  - o Support groups
- Refer for evaluation of lesion

Abnormal Pap Smear

Key Clinical Information

Abnormal Pap smear results are a common occurrence. Triage of the woman with an abnormal smear can be confusing. The American Society for Colposcopy & Cervical Pathology (ASCCP) has developed algorithms for this process. The algorithms may be purchased from ASCCP, or viewed on line at www.asccp.org.

Pap smear slides remain the most effective & cost efficient means of screen a large population of women. However, liquid-based cytology offers the opportunity to perform 'reflex' HPV testing should an atypical result be returned. HPV testing is useful for determining which clients require more aggressive follow-up, but is of limited value with an abnormal result other than 'abnormal cells of unknown significance'.

AGUS, HSIL or cancer findings should prompt immediate evaluation by a skilled colposcopist. When in doubt about the interpretation of any Pap result, discussion with the cytology lab is recommended.

Client History:

Components of the History to Consider

- LMP, G, P
- History of prior
  - o Abnormal Pap smears
  - o Diagnostic testing
  - o Treatment
- Sexual history
  - o Age at onset of sexual activity
  - o Number of sexual partners
  - o Condom use
  - o History of STIs
    - HPV

- HIV
- Social history
  - o Smoking
  - o Drug & alcohol use
- Family history
  - o Cervical disease
  - o DES exposure in utero
- Medical history
- Risk factors for abnormal Pap
  - o More than 3 sexual partners
  - o History of STIs, esp. HPV & HIV
  - o Prior abnormal Paps
  - o Lack of self-care, no-show

- o   Cigarette smoking
- o   With CIN (cervical intraepithelial neoplasia)
  - ▪ Persistent CIN I
  - ▪ Progressive CIN
  - ▪ Any CIN II or greater lesion

Physical Examination:

Components of the Physical Exam to Consider
- Examination of the external genitalia for HPV lesions
- Visualization of the cervix and vaginal vault
- Colposcopic exam, if indicated
  - o   Squamo-columnar junction
  - o   Presence of gross lesions
  - o   Presence of aceto-white lesions
    - ▪ Punctation
    - ▪ Mosaicism
    - ▪ Abnormal vessels
    - ▪ Lesion borders
  - o   Abnormal Lugol's uptake

Clinical Impression:

Differential Diagnoses to Consider
- Genital infection
  - o   Cervicitis
  - o   Vaginitis
  - o   STI
- Trauma
- Abnormal cervical cytology
  - o   DES exposure
  - o   Atypical squamous cells of unknown significance
  - o   Atypical glandular cells of unknown significance
  - o   Atypical endometrial cells of unknown significance
  - o   Low grade squamous intraeptithelial lesion
  - o   High grade squamous intraeptithelial lesion
  - o   Suspicious for invasive cervical cancer
    - ▪ Adneocarcinoma
    - ▪ Squamous cell carcinoma

Diagnostic Testing:

Diagnostic Tests and Procedures to Consider
- ASCUS
  - o   Evaluation
    - ▪ HPV hybrid capture testing, or
    - ▪ Repeat pap smear in 3 months, or
    - ▪ Colposcopic evaluation
  - o   If evaluation is WNL repeat pap at next annual
  - o   Colposcopy for
    - ▪ Abnormal repeat pap
    - ▪ HPV + for high-risk types
- ASGUS
  - o   Colposcopic evaluation
  - o   Endocervical curettage
  - o   Endometrial biopsy
- LSIL
  - o   Colposcopic evaluation
  - o   Biopsy of lesions
  - o   Endocervical curettage
- HSIL
  - o   Colposcopic evaluation
  - o   Biopsy of lesions
  - o   Endocervical curettage
- High risk patient
- Inflammation
- Treat underlying condition
- Repeat pap smear
- Follow pap with acetic acid wash to look for gross lesions
- Arrange for biopsy if lesions present
- If repeat normal, repeat in 3 months

- If inflammation persists
- Evaluate cervix with acetic acid wash to look for gross lesions
- Arrange for biopsy if lesions present
- If repeat is abnormal, arrange for colposcopy
- Hyperkeratosis/parakeratosis (common post-LEEP)
- Repeat pap smear in 3 months
- Follow pap with acetic acid wash to look for gross lesions
- Arrange for biopsy if lesions present
- If repeat pap normal, follow up in 9 months when annual due
- If repeat pap shows persistent HK/PK
- Evaluate cervix with acetic acid wash to look for gross lesions
- Arrange for biopsy if lesions present
- If repeat pap abnormal, arrange for colposcopy
- ASCUS
- Based on number and type of risk factors
- Repeat pap smear in 3 months
- Arrange for colposcopy
- If repeat pap normal, follow up in 3-6 months
- If ASCUS persists, arrange for colposcopy
- If repeat pap abnormal, arrange for colposcopy
- AGCUS
- Arrange for
- Colposcopic evaluation
- Endocervical curettage
- Endometrial biopsy
- LGSIL
- Arrange for colposcopic evaluation
- Biopsy of lesions
- Endocervical curettage
- HGSIL
- Refer immediately for colposcopic evaluation
- Biopsy of lesions
- Endocervical curettage

Providing Treatment:

Therapeutic Measures to Consider
- Dietary support
  - o   Beta-carotene – 50,000 IU bid with meals
  - o   Vitamin C – 2000 mg tid
  - o   Vitamin E – 400 IU
  - o   Folic acid – 2 mg daily x 3 months then 0.4 mg daily
  - o   Selenium – 200 mg daily
  - o   Zinc – 30 mg daily
- Conservative management
  - o   Follow with Paps & colposcopy
  - o   Re-biopsy as indicated
  - o   Triage to treatment with progression
- Ablation therapies
  - o   Cryotherapy
  - o   Laser
- Excisional therapies
  - o   LEEP procedure
  - o   Cold knife cone

Providing Treatment:

Alternative Measures to Consider
- Alternative therapies are not a substitute for evaluation & treatment
- Herbs to support the immune & reproductive systems
  - o   Echinacea
  - o   Red raspberry leaf
  - o   Vitex
- Visualization of healing

Providing Support:

Education and Support Measures to Consider

- Provide information regarding cervical disease
  - o Meaning of abnormal Pap result
  - o Information about diagnostic testing options
  - o Potential treatment measures
  - o Importance of, and schedule for follow-up
- Information on smoking cessation, prn
- Information on supplements listed above

Follow-up Care:

Follow-up Measures to Consider

- CIN I
  - o Follow with pap smears (compliant clients)
    - q 4 months x 12 months then q 6 months x 12 months
    - Arrange for repeat biopsy for persistent lesion
    - Treat according to biopsy results
  - o Arrange for treatment (large lesion or non-compliant client)
    - Cryotherapy
    - LEEP
    - Laser
  - o Post-treatment

- Pap q 4 mo. x 12 mo. then q 6 mo. x 12 mo.
    - Arrange for repeat biopsy for persistent lesion
  - o Treat according to biopsy results
- CIN II or greater
  - o Arrange for treatment
    - LEEP
    - Laser
    - Cone biopsy
  - o Post-treatment
  - o Pap q 4 mo. x 12 mo. then q 6 mo. x 12 mo.
    - Arrange for repeat biopsy for persistent lesion
    - Treat according to biopsy results

Collaborative Practice:

Criteria to Consider for Consultation or Referral

- For colposcopy if not within the scope of the midwife's practice
- For unusual cervical configuration or appearance
  - o Visually
  - o By palpation
  - o By colposcopy
- Recommend referral for colposcopy for all HSIL lesions
- For treatment of CIN lesions

Amenorrhea

Key Clinical Information

Primary amenorrhea is no onset of menses by age 16 in a young woman who has developed secondary sex characteristics, or no menses by age 14 in the absence of secondary sex characteristics. Up to 10% of young women with primary amenorrhea will have a constitutional delay of menarche. Secondary amenorrhea is the absence of menses for 3-6 months in a woman who has previously menstruated, and is not pregnant. There is crossover between potential causes of primary and secondary amenorrhea, and all differential diagnoses should be considered when evaluating the woman with amenorrhea.

Client History:

Components of the History to Consider

- Age
- Development of secondary sex characteristics
- Age at menarche
- Previous menstrual pattern
- Onset and duration of amenorrhea
- Presence of other symptoms
  - o Galactorrhea
  - o Hirsutism
- Medical history
  - o Thyroid disorders
  - o Weight loss
  - o Systemic illness
  - o Medication & drug use history
- Sexual history
  - o Sexual activity
  - o Sexual abuse
  - o Contraceptive history
  - o Pregnancy and breastfeeding history, including pregnancy terminations
- Nutrition patterns, especially anorexia

- Physical activity level

Physical Examination:

Components of the Physical Exam to Consider

- Wt, vital signs
- Hair distribution
- Thyroid exam
  - o Enlargement
  - o Nodularity
  - o Physical findings consistent with thyroid disorders
- Breast exam
  - o Development
  - o Nipple discharge
- Bimanual exam
  - o Presence of secondary sex characteristics
  - o Examination for congenital anomalies
    - Presence or absence of vagina or uterus
    - Ambiguous genitalia

Clinical Impression:

Differential Diagnoses to Consider

- Amenorrhea, due to
  - o Pregnancy

- o Hormonal contraception use
- o Peri-menopause
- o Constitutional rate of maturation
- o Anorexia, causing hypothalamic dysfunction
- o Hormonal imbalance/insufficiency
  - Premature ovarian failure
  - Polycystic ovary syndrome
  - Androgen-producing tumors
  - Hyperprolactinemia
  - Hypothyroidism
  - Pituitary disease
- o Congenital anomalies
  - Congenital absence of uterus/ovaries
  - Congenital adrenal hyperplasia
- o Genetic factors

Diagnostic Testing:

Diagnostic Tests and Procedures to Consider

- Previous history of menstruation
  - o Serum HCG
  - o If HCG negative
    - TSH (elevated TSH = hypothyroidism)
    - Prolactin (<100ng/ml normal)
    - Consider progesterone trial
- Normal secondary sex characteristics
  - o Uterus present
    - Serum HCG
    - Serum T4, TSH
    - Prolactin level
      - ↑ Prolactin level get CT scan
      - Normal prolactin level evaluate for vaginal and cervical patency
  - o Uterus absent
    - Evaluate testosterone level, &/or
    - Karyotype
- No secondary sex characteristics
  - o FSH/LH levels
    - FSH 5-30 IU/L
    - LH 5-20 IU/L
    - ↑ FSH/LH ⇒ Karyotype
    - Normal or ↓ FSH/LH ⇒ refer for trial with gonadotropin releasing hormone

Providing Treatment:

Therapeutic Measures to Consider

- For progesterone trial
  - o Provera 10 mg x 10 days *or*
  - o Prometrium 400 mg qhs x 10 days or
  - o Crinone 4% Progesterone Gel 45 mg per vagina qod x 6 doses
  - o Expect withdrawal bleeding within 10 days following medication
- Based on differential diagnosis

Providing Treatment:

Alternative Measures to Consider

- Herbal remedies that support menstruation
  - o Red raspberry leaf tea
  - o Dong-quai tea (not to be used while pregnant or nursing)
  - o Wild yam root tea or tincture
  - o Blue cohosh root tea or tincture
  - o Use for three months, even after cycle resumes

Providing Support:

Education and Support Measures to Consider

- Reassure
- Provide age-level information regarding
  - o Testing and results
  - o Expectation for treatment
  - o Advise client, in age-related terms, of plan of care
- Provide information regarding appropriate support groups
- Provide information regarding exercise and amenorrhea as applicable
- Impact of condition on future childbearing

Follow-up Care:

Follow-up Measures to Consider

- Document
  - o Findings of H&P
  - o Testing & results
  - o Discussions
  - o Client response
  - o Ongoing plan of care
  - o Referrals
- Office follow-up
  - o As indicated by results and diagnosis
  - o Results of progestin challenge
    - + withdraw bleed with normal prolactin and TSH = anovulation
    - - withdraw bleed requires further work-up
  - o For support during additional work-up
  - o As indicated for routine care

Collaborative Practice:

Criteria to Consider for Consultation or Referral

- For primary amenorrhea
  - o In the presence of anomalies or abnormal lab results
  - o In the adolescent with eating disorder
  - o That does not resolve by age 18 in presence of normal exam and labs
- For abnormal hormone levels
- For amenorrhea that persists following progestin challenge
  - o If no withdrawal bleed
  - o Following a withdrawal bleed
- For malnutrition or eating disorder
- For progestin challenge or other evaluation not within the scope of the midwife's practice

Breast Mass

Key Clinical Information

Every breast mass must be considered suspicious for breast cancer until shown to be otherwise. Breast cancer is second only to lung cancer as a cause of mortality in women, and it is the leading cause of cancer-related deaths in women aged 35-54. Up to 80% of women who develop breast cancer have no risk factors for breast cancer. Pregnancy does not exclude breast cancer from the differential diagnosis; 2% of all breast cancers are diagnosed during pregnancy.

Client History:

Components of the History to Consider

- Characteristics of mass
  - When first noted
  - Pain
  - Associated breast changes
    - Nipple discharge
    - Relation to menstrual cycle
- Menstrual status
- Previous mammography
- Risk factors
  - Positive family history
  - Loss of ovarian function before age 35
  - Age at menopause (>40 menstrual years increases risk 2-5 times)
  - Obesity, diabetes, high fat diet
  - Nulliparous, or first child born after age 35
- Use & duration of HRT
- Previous or current breast conditions
  - Lactation
- Self breast exam habits

Physical Examination:

Components of the Physical Exam to Consider

- Complete breast exam, sitting and supine
  - Visual findings
    - Dimpling
    - Skin changes
    - Asymmetry
    - Nipple retraction
    - Redness
  - Palpable findings of mass(es)
    - Number
    - Location(s)
    - Contour
    - Size
    - Mobility
    - Consistency
    - Heat
  - Evaluation for spontaneous nipple discharge
  - Evaluation for palpable axillary nodes

Clinical Impression:

Differential Diagnoses to Consider

- Benign breast mass(es)
  - Fibroadenoma
  - Fibrocystic breasts
  - Traumatic hematoma
- Breast infection
  - Enlarged lymph node(s)
  - Breast abscess
  - Blocked duct
  - Mastitis
- Breast cancer

Diagnostic Testing:

Diagnostic Tests and Procedures to Consider

- Mammogram
  - Difficult to interpret with
    - Young women
    - During lactation
- Ultrasound
  - Cyst or abscess suspected
  - May support or oppose physical findings
  - Shows fluid-filled soft-tissue changes best
- Biopsy
  - Definitive diagnosis with tissue specimen
  - Each technique has limitations
    - Needle aspiration biopsy
    - Stereotactic biopsy
    - Excisional biopsy
- Genetic screening
  - Contoversial
  - Negative screen does not exclude risk

Providing Treatment:

Therapeutic Measures to Consider

- If cystic mass consider
  - Observation
  - Aspiration
  - Excision
- If abscess
  - Treat with oral antibiotics:
    - Keflex (or other cephalosporin) 500 mg q 12 hours or 250 mg qid for 7-14 days
    - Dicloxacillin
    - Erythromycin (if PCN allergic) 250 mg qid
  - May require incision & drainage
- If solid with sharp margins, uniform shape, no characteristics of malignancy consider
  - Close observation & re-evaluation
  - Needle or stereotactic biopsy
  - Excision of mass
- If characteristics of malignant or pre-malignant lesions
  - Needle or stereotactic biopsy
  - Excisional biopsy

Providing Treatment:

Alternative Measures to Consider

- Decrease/eliminate
    - o Caffeine
    - o Chocolate
    - o Alcohol
    - o Carbonated beverages
    - o Fat intake
- Increase vitamin intake
    - o Vitamin C
    - o Beta-carotene
    - o Vitamin E
    - o B-complex
- Amend diet to include lots of
    - o Deep green vegetables
    - o Grains
    - o Legumes
    - o Sea-vegetables
    - o Fruit
- Homeopathic treatment for fibrocystic breast discomfort:
    - o *Belladonna* for tenderness and sensitivity
    - o *Conium* for premenstrual tenderness
    - o *Lapis albis* for a painful nodule with burning
    - o Homeopathic remedies for cysts (after malignancy has been ruled out)
    - o *Calcarea* for single cyst without tenderness or pain
    - o *Conium* for right-sided, hard, mobile cyst
- Breast Cancer
    - o Healthy diet to promote healing
    - o Homeopathic arnica to promote healing
    - o Rescue remedy for emotional distress

Providing Support:

Education and Support Measures to Consider

- Teach self breast exam techniques
- Provide information about evaluation modalities to allow an informed choice
- Provide information and support measures related to diagnosis

Follow-up Care:

Follow-up Measures to Consider

- Cystic mass
    - o 1-3 months, immediately following menses if menstruating
    - o Immediately if enlargement occurs
- Solid masses, if not referred for biopsy (appears benign by mammogram &/or ultrasound)
    - o 1 month, following menses and frequently thereafter until demonstrated no growth or regression.
    - o Remember a benign breast mass can mask a malignancy making it more difficult to discover.

Collaborative Practice:

Criteria to Consider for Consultation or Referral

- For breast mass that is suspicious for cancer
- Following abnormal mammogram or ultrasound for diagnostic evaluation
- For excision if cyst recurs after aspiration
- To evaluate and order testing if not within the midwife's scope of practice
- Client preference for definitive therapy (i.e. excisional biopsy)

Bacterial Vaginosis

Key Clinical Information

Bacterial vaginosis is a commonly occurring problem. Controversy exists as to whether bacterial vaginosis (BV) contributes to the onset of preterm labaor. BV has been linked to background mycoplasma infection. BV may contribute to endometritis, and post-operative wound infections following gynecological procedures. Many women consider all vaginal infections 'yeast' and may self-treat with over-the-counter medications before coming for evaluation.

Client History:

Components of the History to Consider

- Age
- Symptoms
    - o Vulvovaginal irritation or burning
    - o Presence of thin gray/white discharge
        - ▪ Foul odor
        - ▪ Commonly described as "fishy"
    - o Onset, duration & severity of symptoms
    - o Treatments used & results
- Sexual history
    - o Change in sexual partner for self or partner
    - o Condom use
    - o Birth control method

Physical Examination:

Components of the Physical Exam to Consider

- Genital examination for
    - o Redness
    - o Erythema
    - o Lesions
    - o Discharge
    - o Retained tampon or foreign body
    - o Presence of odor
- STI testing as indicated by history

Clinical Impression:

Differential Diagnoses to Consider

- Bacterial vaginosis
- Monilial vaginosis
- Chronic cervicitis
- Foreign body

- Chlamydia
- Gonorrhea
- Mycoplasma

Diagnostic Testing:

Diagnostic Tests and Procedures to Consider

- Wet prep
  - o   Positive KOH whiff test
  - o   Positive clue cells
  - o   Negative mycelia or branching hyphae
  - o   Rare lactobacilli
  - o   Occasional WBCs
- Vaginal pH >4.5

Providing Treatment:

Therapeutic Measures to Consider

- MetroGel-Vaginal
  - o   1 applicator per vagina
  - o   Bid x 5 days or qhs x 7 days
- Flagyl ER (metronidazole)
  - o   750 mg po qd x 7 days
- Flagyl (metronidazole)
  - o   500 mg po bid x 7 days
- Flagyl (metronidazole)
  - o   250 po tid x 7 days
  - o   2nd or 3rd trimester pregnancy
- Flagyl (metronidazole)
  - o   2 gm po as single dose
  - o   2nd or 3rd trimester pregnancy
- Cleocin (clindamycin) vaginal cream
  - o   5 gm intravaginally QHS x 7 d
  - o   Not recommended in pregnancy
  - o   May use in 1st trimester of pregnancy
- Cleocin (clindamycin)
  - o   300 mg po bid x 7 days
- Ampicillin
  - o   500 mg po QID x 7 days
  - o   May use during pregnancy
- Amoxicillin
  - o   500 mg PO TID x 7 days
  - o   May use during pregnancy

Providing Treatment:

Alternative Measures to Consider

- Herbal douche
  - o   Calendula – 2 parts
  - o   Echinacea root – 2 parts
  - o   Myrrh – 2 parts
  - o   Make tincture
  - o   Place 50 gtts in 1-cup warm calendula tea.
  - o   Douche x 6 nights.
- Homeopathic remedies
  - o   Graphites – discharge is thin and watery and causes burning
  - o   Sepia - discharge is offensive and may be yellowish

Providing Support:

Education and Support Measures to Consider

- Provide information about diagnosis
- Encourage client to return if symptoms persist or return
- Advise patient that partner may need treatment for persistent infections
- Do not use condoms for 24 hours after insertion of vaginal medications

Follow-up Care:

Follow-up Measures to Consider

- Document
  - o   Symptoms and clinical findings
  - o   Clinical impression/diagnosis
  - o   Client education & response
  - o   Treatment & follow-up plan
- If symptoms recur or persist
  - o   Consider testing for chlamydia &/or mycoplasma
  - o   Treat partner and re-treat patient
- Re-evaluate at 28-35 weeks if positive diagnosis during pregnancy

Collaborative Practice:

Criteria to Consider for Consultation or Referral

- For persistent or unresponsive vaginitis
- For preterm labor
- For medication Rx if not within midwife's scope of practice

Chlamydia

Key Clinical Information

Chlamydia remains the most common sexually transmitted infection in the U.S. Women with chlamydial infection may present with symptoms that range from asymptomatic to fulminant PID. Chlamydia infection may cause or contribute to blocked tubes, infertility, persistent pelvic pain, ectopic pregnancy, preterm labor or rupture of membranes and neonatal conjunctivits and/or trachoma. Chlamydia and gonorrhea infection frequently co-exist

Client History:

Components of the History to Consider

- LMP
- Onset, duration, & type of symptoms
  - o   Pain
  - o   Discharge
  - o   Location
- Sexual history
  - o   Previous diagnosis of STIs
  - o   Change in sexual partner for self or partner
  - o   Current method of birth control, i.e. IUD
  - o   Consistency of condom use

Physical Examination:

Components of the Physical Exam to Consider

- Vital signs
- Abdominal palpation with focus on
  - Rebound tenderness
  - Guarding
- Pelvic exam with focus on
  - External genitalia
  - Vaginal discharge
  - Appearance of cervix
    - Presence of cervical discharge
    - Edema, erythema of cervix
  - Cervical motion tenderness
  - Uterine enlargement or tenderness
  - Palpation for adnexal mass

Clinical Impression:

Differential Diagnoses to Consider

- Vaginits
- Chlamydia
- Gonorrhea
- PID
- Cervicitis
- Cervical cancer
- Ectopic pregnancy
- Ovarian cyst

Diagnostic Testing:

Diagnostic Tests and Procedures to Consider

- Cervical swab for chlamydia and gonorrhea
- Vaginal wet mount
- Serum/urine pregnancy testing
- Serum testing for
  - HIV
  - Hepatitis B
  - Syphilis

Providing Treatment:

Therapeutic Measures to Consider

- Remove IUD if present
  - Provide alternate method of birth control
- Medications
  - Doxycycline 100 mg po bid x 7 days – pregnancy category D
  - Azithromycin 1 G po in a single dose – pregnancy category B
  - Ofloxacin 300 mg po bid x 7 days – pregnancy category C
  - Erythromycin base 500 mg po qid x 7 days – pregnancy category B
  - Erythromycin ethylsuccinate 800 mg po qid x 7 days – pregnancy category B

  - Sulfisoxazole (Gantrisin) 500 mg po qid x 10 days – pregnancy category C

Providing Treatment:

Alternative Measures to Consider

- Alternative measures are not a substitute for antibiotic therapy
- Supportive/comfort measures
  - Herbal/Homeopathic remedies to boost immune response
    - Echinacea
    - Homeopathic Merc. sol.
  - Dietary intake of acidophyllus to offset effects of antibiotics on gut
    - Capsules
    - Yogurt
    - Probiotics

Providing Support:

Education and Support Measures to Consider

- Provide information regarding
  - Infection cause and transmission
  - Effects on reproductive organs and future fertility
  - Treatment plan
  - Prevention measures
    - Risk behaviors
    - Safe sexual practices
  - Need to evaluate and/or treat partner(s)

Follow-up Care:

Follow-up Measures to Consider

- Document
  - Presenting symptoms
  - Physical & lab findings
  - Treatment plan
    - Medication
    - Education
    - Plan for continued care
- Return to office or clinic
  - 1-2weeks post-treatment for test of cure
  - For continued symptoms
  - For persistent pain
- Retest
  - With pregnancy
  - New partner for self or partner
- Consider early ultrasound with diagnosis of pregnancy and history of significant PID

Collaborative Practice:

Criteria to Consider for Consultation or Referral

- For Rx if not within midwife's scope of practice
- For persistent, severe, or unresponsive infection
- For + HIV or Hep B status
- For persistent pelvic pain following resolution of infection

Colposcopy

Key Clinical Information

Colposcopy is the 'gold standard' fro the evaluation of abnormal Pap smear results. It involves looking at the cervix under magnification, (using a colposcope) while applying one or more solutions that help delineate or highlight abnormal lesions. Biopsies are then taken from the most abnormal area(s).

Many midwives perform colposcopy on women who have low-grade lesion that usually do not require treatment. There is a significant education & training process that is required in order to become skilled as a colposcopist. For more information contact the American Society for Colposcopy & Cervical Pathology at 1-800-787-7227 or www.asccp.org.

Terms: **CIN:** Cervical Intraepithelial Lesion **VIN:** Vulvar Intraepithelial Lesion **VaIN:** Vaginal intraepithelial lesion

Client History:
Components of the History to Consider
- Indication for colposcopy
  - ASC-US
  - LGSIL
  - Genital lesions
- GYN History
  - History of STIs
  - Prior abnormal paps, diagnostic procedures, treatment
  - Inter-menstrual or post-coital bleeding
  - Maternal DES use
- Medical history
  - HIV infection
  - Decreased immune response
- Family history
  - Maternal or sibling history of abnormal pap smears or cervical cancer
- Social history
  - Smoking
  - Factors that contribute to risk

Physical Examination:
Components of the Physical Exam to Consider
- Vulvar examination
  - Apply 5% acetic acid soaked 4x4s
  - Examine for evidence of potential VIN
    - Pigmented or aceto-white lesions
    - Warts
    - Discharge
- Vaginal examination
  - Apply 5% acetic acid wash
  - Examine for evidence of VaIN
    - Aceto-white lesions
    - Warts or other signs of HPV
    - Punctation &/or mosaicism
  - Gentle biopsy if lesion present or refer for biopsy (vagina is very thin)
- Cervical examination
  - Obtain pap smear if necessary
  - Apply 5% acetic acid wash

  - Examine without magnification
  - Examine colposcopically
    - No filter
    - Green filter
    - Transformation zone
    - Squamo-columnar junction
    - Evaluate lesion(s)
      - Size
      - Location
      - Clarity of margins
      - Thickness of edge
      - Brightness of aceto-white tissue
      - Presence of punctation &/or mosaicism
      - Intercapillary distance
      - Fine vs coarse changes
      - Abnormal vessels
  - Apply Lugol's solution if needed to clarify presence of lesion or borders
- Following biopsies of lesion(s)
  - Ensure hemostasis
    - Pressure
    - Monsel's paste (ferric sub-sulfate solution allowed to thicken to a paste)
    - Silver nitrite application

Clinical Impression:
Differential Diagnoses to Consider
- Evaluation of abnormal pap smear
- Follow-up after diagnosis and/or treatment of CIN
- Persistent abnormal vaginal discharge in spite of negative testing
- Visible cervical lesion on gross exam
- Perinatal DES exposure

Diagnostic Testing:
Diagnostic Tests and Procedures to Consider
- Pap smear – if > 6 weeks since abnormal pap
- HPV testing

- Cervical biopsies as indicated by colposcopic exam
- Endocervical curettage
  - o If unsatisfactory exam *or*
  - o All patients

Providing Treatment:

Therapeutic Measures to Consider

- Client with consistent results
  - o No high risk HPV, no lesion, AS-US pap
    - ▪ Observation with close follow-up x 2 years
  - o High-risk HPV, AS-US/LSIL pap, lesion & biopsy consistent with CIN I
    - ▪ Treatment if lesion is persistent or progressive
    - ▪ Treatment if client is likely to be non-compliant with follow-up
  - o High-risk HPV, AS-US/LSIL pap, lesion & biopsy consistent with CIN II/III
    - ▪ Treatment
  - o Client with inconsistent results
    - ▪ Consult with pathologist, review
      - • Cytology
      - • HPV result
      - • Histology
      - • Clinical presentation
    - ▪ Close follow-up, or
    - ▪ Further evaluation w/ expert colposcopist
- Treatments
  - o Cryotherapy (ablative therapy)
  - o LEEP (excisional therapy)
  - o Laser (abalative teherapy)
  - o Cold knife cone (excisional therapy)

Providing Treatment:

Alternative Measures to Consider

- Increase folic acid intake
- Whole foods diet
- Support immune system
  - o Echinacea
  - o Visualization
  - o Herbal support formula see "The Roots of Healing" p 176-178

Providing Support:

Education and Support Measures to Consider

- Provide information about the colposcopic procedure
- Discuss post-colposcopy discharge, abstinence x 7 days, timing and contact for results
- Provide information about tentative diagnosis and anticipated treatment and/or follow-up
- Provide written information about abnormal paps, HPV, and anticipated 2 year follow-up

Follow-up Care:

Follow-up Measures to Consider

- Document
  - o Indication for colposcopy
  - o Findings, pictorial & desriptive
  - o Anticipated biopsy result(s)
  - o Actual biopsy result(s)
  - o Correlate results to formulate plan
    - ▪ Pap
    - ▪ HPV
    - ▪ Clinical picture
    - ▪ Biopsy results
- Close follow-up x 2 years
- Interval based on results & correlation
  - o Pap/colpo q 3-6 months
  - o Reevaluate with biopsy for
    - ▪ Persistent lesion on colposcopy
    - ▪ Progressive pap smear result

Collaborative Practice:

Criteria to Consider for Consultation or Referral

- Colposcopy is not within midwife's scope of practice
- High grade lesions
- Lesions CIN II or greater for treatment
- Clients with demonstrated progression
- Non-compliant clients for treatment
- For management plan for woman in whom results are not consistent

Dysfunctional Uterine Bleeding

Key Clinical Information

Dysfunctional uterine bleeding has many causes. Many of them may be a physiologic process that is age related, or it may be secondary to a pathologic processes. Differentiation of the reason for irregular or intermenstrual bleeding is essential to developing a plan of care that is acceptable to the woman and appropriate to treat the problem. A common cause of non-cyclic bleeding in adolescents and peri-menopausal women is anovulation. In the woman of childbearing age, other causes such as thyroid disease or pelvic infection are more common[34].

---

[34] ACOG (2000). ACOG Practice Bulletin #14. Management of Anovulatory Bleeding. In 2002 Compendium of Selected Publications. Washington, DC: ACOG

Client History:

Components of the History to Consider

- Age
- G, P, LMP, menarche
- Allergies
- Medications
  - Prescription
    - OCs
    - Depo Provera
    - HRT
    - Anticoagulants
  - Herbal or OTC remedies
    - Aspirin & NSAIDs
    - Blue or black cohosh
- GYN history
  - Current method of contraception
    - IUD
    - Hormonal methods
  - History of, and risk for STIs
  - Pap smears
    - Results of prior pap smears
    - Date of last pap & exam
  - Menses
    - Onset, frequency and duration of menses
    - Usual flow
    - Changes in menses
    - Onset, frequency and duration of bleeding
    - Association of bleeding with
      - Menstrual cycle
      - Intercourse
    - Pain associated with bleeding and or menses
- Other associated symptoms
  - Symptoms of hypotension, anemia
  - Changes in metabolism
  - Hirsutism
  - Eating disorder
  - Pain with intercourse
  - Urinary frequency
  - Abdominal bloating

Physical Examination:

Components of the Physical Exam to Consider

- Vital signs, including weight: note changes
- Palpate thyroid
- Complete GYN exam with particular regard to:
- Cervix for presence of:
  - Erosion or other symptoms of cervical cancer
  - Discharge
  - Presence of polyps
- Uterus for size, consistency, pain, palpation of masses
- Adnexal region for presence of masses or pain

Clinical Impression:

Differential Diagnoses to Consider

- Functional DUB (primary ovarian dysfunction)
- Uterine disorders
  - Fibroids
  - Endometrial hyperplasia or cancer
  - Endometriosis
  - Endometritis
- Cervical disorders
  - Cervicitis
  - Malignant lesions
  - Polyps
- Vaginal disorders
  - Congenital anomalies
  - Foreign body

  - Malignancy
- Pregnancy
  - Ectopic
  - Placenta previa
  - Septic abortions
  - Threatened abortion
- Systemic disease
  - Coagulation disorders
  - Aplastic anemia
  - Coagulation factor deficiencies
  - Blood dyscrasias
  - Leukemia
  - Thrombocytopenia
  - Von Willebrand's disease
- Endocrine disorder
  - Thyroid dysfunction
  - Diabetes
  - Adrenal disorders
  - Premature ovarian failure

Diagnostic Testing:

Diagnostic Tests and Procedures to Consider

- Pregnancy testing
- Pap smear
- Chlamydia and/or gonorrhea testing
- Thyroid testing: TSH, T3, T4
- Hormonal evaluation
  - FSH, LH,
  - Prolactin
  - Estradiol
  - Testosterone
- CBC with diff
- H & H
- Bleeding time, PT, PTT
- Pelvic ultrasound to evaluate for
  - Placenta previa
  - Uterine fibroids
  - Thickness of endometrial stripe
  - Intrauterine polyps
  - Ovarian or adnexal masses
- CT scan: abdomen & pelvis
- Endometrial biopsy

Providing Treatment:

Therapeutic Measures to Consider

- Consider differential diagnoses
- Functional DUB (primary ovarian dysfunction)
  - Trial of treatment with:
  - Oral contraceptives
  - Cyclical progestins
  - Begin 14 days before next anticipated menses
  - Provera 10 mg x 10 days
  - Prometrium 400 mg x 10-12 days

Providing Treatment:

Alternative Measures to Consider

- Improve nutritional status
- Regular planned exercise or activity patterns
- Counseling to treat emotional or social stress
- Herbal remedies:
  - Red raspberry
  - Black cohosh
  - Dong-quai
  - Vitex
- Iron foods to prevent/treat anemia
  - Sea vegetables
  - Egg yolk
  - Deep green leafy vegetables

- o   Liver

Providing Support:

Education and Support Measures to Consider

- Provide information about
  - o   Normal menstrual functioning
  - o   Work-up related to differential diagnosis
- Diagnosis
  - o   Informed choice regarding treatment options
  - o   Follow-up plan
  - o   Consultation &/or referral criteria
  - o   When to call for problems
  - o   Maintain menstrual calendar
  - o   Medication instructions

Follow-up Care:

Follow-up Measures to Consider

- Document
  - o   Presenting symptoms
  - o   Physical findings

- o   Diagnostic test results
- o   Working diagnosis
- o   Preliminary treatment plan
- o   Discussions with client
- o   Plan for continued care
- Return for continued care
  - o   As indicated by diagnosis
  - o   For persistent or worsening symptoms
  - o   For support during evaluation and/or treatment
  - o   For regular well-woman or gyn care following treatment

Collaborative Practice:

Criteria to Consider for Consultation or Referral

- Any diagnosis of cancer or pre-cancerous condition
- DUB caused by fibroids that is persistent and progressive
- DUB unresponsive to basic herbal or hormone therapy
- Medical or unknown cause of DUB
- For treatment outside the scope of the midwife's practice

Dysmenorrhea

Key Clinical Information

Painful periods may be functional or may be caused by endometriosis, infection or growing fibroids. When dysmenorrhea does not respond to treatment, evaluation for endometriosis should be considered. The pain of endometriosis frequently begins prior to the onset of menses unlike physiologic pain which is caused by uterine contractions expelling the menstrual flow. Pain with menstruation is often accompanied by heavy flow, headache, diarrhea or other symptoms, and may cause women lost days from work, or limit their ability to care for themselves or their family. Careful investigation into this common problem may provide options for relief or a decrease in symptoms.

Client History:

Components of the History to Consider

- Age
- Menstrual history
  - o   Age of menarche
  - o   Usual menstrual patterns
  - o   Age of onset of dysmenorrhea
- Characteristics of discomfort
  - o   Location
  - o   Duration
  - o   Severity
  - o   Timing in cycle at onset
  - o   Association with other body functions
- Bowel and bladder changes with pain
- Other associated symptoms
- Previous significant OB/GYN history
  - o   Current method of birth control
    - ▪   Hormonal contraceptive use
    - ▪   IUD use, type
  - o   PID/STIs
  - o   Endometriosis
  - o   Previous pelvic surgery
  - o   Any congenital pelvic anomaly

Physical Examination:

Components of the Physical Exam to Consider

- Vital signs

- Complete pelvic exam
  - o   Speculum exam
    - ▪   Appearance of cervix
    - ▪   Appearance of vagina
  - o   Bi-manual exam
    - ▪   Uterine size & contour
    - ▪   Uterine or cervical motion tenderness
    - ▪   Uterine and adnexal mobility
  - o   Evaluation for cystocele or rectocele
  - o   Rectal exam
- Abdominal palpation
  - o   Lower abdominal tenderness
- CVA tenderness

Clinical Impression:

Differential Diagnoses to Consider

- Functional dysmenorrhea
- Endometriosis
- PID
- Pelvic anomaly
- Pelvic tumor, i.e., fibroids
- Pelvic prolapse
- PMS
- Urinary tract dysfunction or infection
- Bowel disease

Diagnostic Testing:

Diagnostic Tests and Procedures to Consider

- Pap
- Chlamydia/Gonorrhea testing
- Urinalysis
- Stool for occult blood following rectal exam
- Pelvic ultrasound based on pelvic exam findings

Providing Treatment:

Therapeutic Measures to Consider

- Functional dysmenorrhea
  - Ibuprofen 300-600mg tid
  - Naproxen 275-500 mg bid
  - Begin 24 hours before menses expected
  - Hormonal control
    - Low-dose birth control pills
    - Mirena IUD
  - Suspected endometriosis
    - Low-dose birth control pills to regulate menses and diminish symptoms
    - Consider definitive diagnosis & treatment
    - Laparoscopy is used for evaluation & treatment
  - Other diagnoses, treat as appropriate

Providing Treatment:

Alternative Measures to Consider

- Heat to abdomen
- Balanced diet, plenty of fiber
- Increase exercise with episodes for endorphin release
- Herbal remedies
  - Evening primrose oil, 3-6 capsules/day
  - Dong-quai tea (not to be used while pregnant or nursing, or if menses are excessive)

- Crampbark tea or tincture, may combine with valerian root

Providing Support:

Education and Support Measures to Consider

- Explain normal reproductive anatomy and physiology
- Provide information about testing and treatment plan
- Provide information about self-help measures as requested
- Validate woman's concerns
- Identify
  - When to return for care
  - Indications for consult or referral

Follow-up Care:

Follow-up Measures to Consider

- Document
  - Presenting symptoms
  - Previous self-help measures used
  - Physical findings
  - Diagnostic test & results
  - Discussions with client
  - Plan for continued care
- Return to office or clinic
  - After treatment to evaluate effectiveness
  - As indicated by test results
  - For worsening symptoms

Collaborative Practice:

Criteria to Consider for Consultation or Referral

- For Rx treatment if not within the midwife's scope of practice
- For evaluation and treatment of suspected endometriosis
- For symptoms that do not improve with treatment
- For abnormal ultrasound, prolapse or occult bleeding

Endometrial Biopsy

Key Clinical Information

Endometrial biopsy is performed for a wide variety of indications. The most common indication is peri- or post-menopausal bleeding. Persistent dysfunctional uterine bleeding can also be further evaluated with endometrial biopsy. Evaluation of atypical glandular cells (AG-US) on pap smear is another indication for endometrial biopsy, however, in this instance endometrial biopsy is best performed in conjunction with colposcopy performed by an expert colposcopist due to the chance of highly aggressive disease associated with AG-US. Gentle technique will minimize discomfort during the procedure and aid in avoiding complications.

Client History:

Components of the History to Consider

- GYN history
  - Interval history related to indication for endometrial biopsy
    - Dysfunctional uterine bleeding (DUB)
    - Post-menopausal bleeding
    - Thickened endometrium on ultrasound
    - Infertility investigation
    - AG-US
  - LMP
    - Luteal phase for infertility investigation
    - Potential for pregnancy
  - Method of birth control if applicable
  - Last pap smear & results
- Medications
  - Use of analgesics prior to procedure
  - HRT
  - Hormonal contraception
- Medical conditions
  - Bleeding disorders
  - Heart valve replacement
  - Current undiagnosed fever
- Contraindications for endometrial biopsy
  - Presence of reproductive tract infection

- o   Pregnancy/positive HCG
- o   Untreated cervical cancer

Physical Examination:

Components of the Physical Exam to Consider

- Vital signs pre- and post-procedure
- Evaluate for presence of reproductive tract infection
- Bimanual exam to determine size and position of uterus

Clinical Impression:

Differential Diagnoses to Consider

- Endometrial biopsy for evaluation of
  - o   Post-menopausal bleeding
  - o   Post-menopausal HRT
  - o   Persistent DUB
  - o   AG-US

Diagnostic Testing:

Diagnostic Tests and Procedures to Consider

- Urine or serum HCG
- Pelvic ultrasound
- Endometrial biopsy procedure:
  - o   With speculum in place, examine cervix & vagina for signs of infection., if present do not proceed.
  - o   Cleanse cervix with povodine prep solution
  - o   Apply tenaculum to straighten uterus
    - ▪ Slow application decreases cramping
    - ▪ To upper lip of cervix for anteverted/anteflexed uterus
    - ▪ To posterior lip of cervix for retroverted/retroflexed uterus
    - ▪ Avoid 3 & 9 o'clock positions
  - o   Apply gentle steady traction to tenaculum
  - o   Sound uterus (this helps to dilate cervix and determine depth of endometrial biopsy collection device insertion)
    - ▪ Gently insert sound in direction of uterine curvature
    - ▪ Apply gentle pressure at os to relax os
    - ▪ When resistance lets go gently advance sound to fundus
    - ▪ DO NOT FORCE SOUND. If uterus is perforated remove sound and do not proceed
    - ▪ Remove sound
    - ▪ Note cm marking on sound
  - o   Insert endometrial biopsy collection device to fundus
    - ▪ Determine depth by sound measurement
    - ▪ Apply suction according per manufacturer's instructions
    - ▪ Rotate 360° while gently moving along length of uterus several times
    - ▪ Suction lost when tip removed from uterus
  - o   Deposit specimen into formalin
    - ▪ Cut end of collection device (into formalin)
    - ▪ Label formalin container
  - o   Obtain vital signs
    - ▪ Allow client to rest supine

- ▪ Vaso-vagal response may be delayed

Providing Treatment:

Therapeutic Measures to Consider

- Pre-procedure medication
  - o   Ibuprofen 600-800 mg
- Vasovagal syncope
  - o   Atropine sulfate indicated for heart rate under 40
    - ▪ Preferred route is IV, but may be given IM
    - ▪ Dose: 0.4 mg
  - o   Be prepared for CPR

Providing Treatment:

Alternative Measures to Consider

- Varies based on diagnosis or condition

Providing Support:

Education and Support Measures to Consider

- Provide information for informed consent
- Clients should anticipate potential side effects
  - o   Cramping
  - o   Light bleeding
- Clients should be aware of potential complications
  - o   Cervical stenosis preventing adequate biopsy
  - o   Uterine perforation
  - o   Post-procedure infection
- Initiate teaching regarding
  - o   Potential results
  - o   Tentative plan for continued care
  - o   Indications

Follow-up Care:

Follow-up Measures to Consider

- Document
  - o   Indication for procedure
  - o   Verification of non-pregnant status
  - o   Findings
  - o   Technique used
  - o   Client education
  - o   Client response
- Schedule contact for results
- Return for continued care
  - o   As indicated by biopsy results
  - o   With bleeding, pain, fever

Collaborative Practice:

Criteria to Consider for Consultation or Referral

- For endometrial biopsy if this procedure is not within the midwife's scope of practice
- Cervical stenosis
- Vagal response
- Pathology result diagnostic of
  - o   Endometrial cancer
  - o   Endometrial atypia
  - o   Endometrial hyperplasia

Endometrial Cancer

Key Clinical Information

Endometrial cancer involves the lining of the uterus. It may go undetected until abnormal bleeding occurs. Post-menopausal bleeding requires evaluation for endometrial cancer. Use of combination hormone replacement therapy decreases risk of endometrial cancer when compared to both non-hormone users, and those women with a uterus who take only estrogen. Women who use natural estrogen-containing products for the treatment of menopause should be advised to report any unexpected or unusual bleeding, and may consider the cyclic use of a progestin to diminish the growth of the endometrium.

Client History:
Components of the History to Consider
- Age
- Presenting symptoms
  - Bleeding
- OB/GYN history
  - Early menarche
  - Late menopause
  - Nulliparous
  - Infertility
  - Polycystic ovary syndrome
  - Estrogen producing tumors
  - Estrogen from natural sources
  - Previous or current breast cancer
- Family history
  - Northern European or North American
- Medical history
  - Diabetes
  - Hypertension
  - Biliary disease
- Medication use
  - Tamoxifen therapy
  - Estrogen replacement therapy
  -

Physical Examination:
Components of the Physical Exam to Consider
- Vital signs
- Speculum exam
  - Blood in vaginal vault
  - Appearance of cervix
  - Presence of lesions or masses
- Bimanual exam
  - Uterine size & contour
  - Cervical contour
  - Adnexal masses
  - Firmness & mobility of reproductive organs
- Inguinal lymph nodes
- Rectal exam
  - Confirm pelvic exam
  - Evlauate posterior pelvic
    - Masses
    - Mobility of tissues
    - Rectal involvement

Clinical Impression:
Differential Diagnoses to Consider
- Abnormal bleeding,
  - Pre- or post-menopausal
  - Consistent with endometrial abnormality

Diagnostic Testing:
Diagnostic Tests and Procedures to Consider
- Pelvic ultrasound
  - Abdominal
  - Transvaginal
  - Evaluation of endometrial stripe
    - 4-6 mm is WNL
- Endometrial curettage (D&C)
- Endometrial biopsy
- Hysteroscopy
- Sonohysterography

Providing Treatment:
Therapeutic Measures to Consider
- Referral for treatment is appropriate
- Surgical treatment is commonly indicated
- Radiation & chemotherapy may be indicated based on staging of disease

Providing Treatment:
Alternative Measures to Consider
- Alternative therapies should be aimed at supporting healing
- Some alternative therapies may interfere with medical therapies and need to be delayed or altered during treatment

Providing Support:
Education and Support Measures to Consider
- Discussion regarding need for work-up
- Results of physical exam & diagnostic testing
- Plan for referral and ongoing care
- Options for support services

Follow-up Care:
Follow-up Measures to Consider
- Document care provided
- Offer continued support, as appropriate

Collaborative Practice:
Criteria to Consider for Consultation or Referral
- For evaluation of abnormal bleeding
- Diagnosis of

- o Endometrial atypia
- o Endometrial hyperplasia
- o Endometrial cancer

- Referral to support services

Endometriosis

Key Clinical Information

Endometriosis is found in 5-5% of women or reproductive age during pelvic laparoscopy. As many as one third of these women have endometriosis related fertility issues. Pain is the primary presenting complaint in women who are diagnosed with endometriosis. Pelvic laparoscopy may be used to both diagnose and treat endometriosis. Endometriosis implants may affect the reproductive organs, the bowel, the bladder and the pelvic sidewalls.

Client History:
Components of the History to Consider

- Age
- G, P, LMP
- Menstrual history
  - o Age at menarche
  - o Usual menstrual patterns
  - o Age at onset of symptoms
- Presence of symptoms related to endometriosis
  - o Cyclic pre-and peri-menstrual pain
  - o Dysparunia
  - o Infertility
  - o Dysfunctional uterine bleeding
  - o Urinary urgency or frequency
  - o Onset, duration, and frequency of symptoms
  - o Affect on bowel and bladder function
- GYN history
  - o Use of hormonal contraceptives
  - o STIs
  - o GYN surgery
- Medical/surgical history
  - o Diverticular disease
  - o Appendicitis

Physical Examination:
Components of the Physical Exam to Consider

- Vital signs
- Bimanual exam, suggestive findings:
- Fixed, retroverted uterus
- Adnexal thickening, nodularity, or irregularity
- Uterus and/or adnexa immobile

Clinical Impression:
Differential Diagnoses to Consider

- Pelvic pain consistent with
  - o Endometriosis
  - o Fibroid uterus
  - o Chronic salpingitis
  - o Adhesions secondary to
    - ▪ PID
    - ▪ Peritonitis
    - ▪ Diverticular disease

Diagnostic Testing:
Diagnostic Tests and Procedures to Consider

- STI testing
- CBC

- Pelvic ultrasound:
  - o May be suggestive of endometriosis
  - o Used to rule out other differential diagnoses
- Laparoscopy with tissue sample to confirm diagnosis

Providing Treatment:
Therapeutic Measures to Consider

- Symptomatic treatment while awaiting diagnosis
  - o Anti-inflammatory medication
    - ▪ Naproxen sodium
    - ▪ Ponstel
  - o Initiation of hormonal birth control
- Laparocopy for diagnosis and preliminary treatment
- Medications initiated by physician after diagnosis for treatment of continued symptoms
  - o Danazol
  - o Progestins
  - o Oral/hormonal contraceptives
  - o GnRH agonist
- Surgical intervention
  - o Retreat with ablative therapy
  - o Hysterectomy with oopherectomy

Providing Treatment:
Alternative Measures to Consider

- Symptomatic treatment
  - o Local heat
  - o Castor oil packs
  - o See "The Roots of Healing" for additional suggestions
- Yoga
- Massage
- Acupuncture
- Meditation
- Pregnancy

Providing Support:
Education and Support Measures to Consider

- Provide information about
  - o Working diagnosis
  - o Evaluation process
  - o Potential modes of treatment
- Local support groups
- Endometriosis Association – (800) 992-3636

Follow-up Care:
Follow-up Measures to Consider

- Document
  - o Pertinent history

- o   Physical findings
- o   Diagnostic tests w/ results
- o   Discussions with client about options for continued care
- o   Referrals and anticipated evaluation & treatment
- Return for care
  - o   For support during diagnosis &/or treatment
  - o   For regular GYN/well-woman exams
  - o   With pregnancy

Consider Consultation or Referral:

- For Rx when not within the scope of the midwife's practice
- For clients with
  - o   Suspected endometriosis for diagnosis
  - o   Persistent pelvic pain
  - o   Pain accompanied by bowel or bladder involvement
  - o   Pain accompanied by fever or ↑WBC

Care of the Woman with Fibroid Uterus

Key Clinical Information

Fibroids are a common benign tumor of the uterus. Fibroids may enlarge continuously in the pre-menopausal woman, but generally regress during menopause. While fibroids are most often benign, there is a small chance of malignancy developing or being masked by the fibroids. In addition, blood supply to the fibroids may become occluded resulting in degeneration of the fibroids. Most fibroids are simply an over development of muscle cells of the uterus. They may occur any where in the uterus; the fundus, the wall of the uterus, inside the uterus, the cervix. Treatment is based primarily on relieving symptoms; pain, bleeding, and abdominal enlargement.

Client History:
Components of the History to Consider
- Age, G, P
- Interval history since last visit
  o Uterine size & contour
  o Previous pelvic ultrasounds
  o Previous GYN problems
- Menstrual history
  o Duration, frequency & length
  o Amount of flow
  o Dysmenorrhea
  o Intermenstrual bleeding
- Symptoms of uterine fibroids
  o Pelvic pressure
  o Abdominal enlargement
  o Changes in bowel or bladder function
  o Menstrual changes

Physical Examination:
Components of the Physical Exam to Consider
- Vital signs, including BP and weight
- General well-being
- Abdominal exam
  o Fundal height
  o Uterine contour
- Pelvic exam
  o Uterine size & position
  o Uterine contour
  o Uterine consistency
  o Presence of adnexal masses
  o Tenderness
  o Signs of other processes
    ▪ Discharge
    ▪ Pain on cervical motion
- Rectal exam

Clinical Impression:
Differential Diagnoses to Consider
- Enlarged uterus secondary to
  o Uterine fibroids
  o Pregnancy
    - Malignancy
    ▪ Uterine
    ▪ Cervical
    ▪ Ovarian
- Anemia secondary to
  o Menorrhagia

  o Occult GI bleeding

Diagnostic Testing:
Diagnostic Tests and Procedures to Consider
- Pelvic ultrasound
- Endometrial biopsy
- Hemoglobin & hematocrit
- Stool for occult bleeding

Providing Treatment:
Therapeutic Measures to Consider
- Hormonal regulation of menses
- Iron supplementation as indicated
  o Ferro-sequels 1-2 PO daily
  o Niferex 150 1-2 PO daily
  o Ferrous gluconate 1-2 PO daily
- Lupron-Depot prior to hysterectomy
  o Indicated to decrease uterine size prior to surgery
  o Dosing
    ▪ 3.75 mg IM monthly x 3 mo., *or*
    ▪ 11.25 mg IM x 1 (lasts 3 months)
  o Do not use for undiagnosed uterine bleeding
  o Exclude pregnancy prior to use
  o May cause vaso-motor symptoms
- Hysterectomy
  o Grossly enlarged uterus
  o Degenerative fibroids
  o Potential malignancy
  o Severe menorrhagia
  o Client preference
- Myomectomy
  o Excision of fibroid(s)
  o Retains fertility
  o Uterine scarring may require cesarean birth

Providing Treatment:
Alternative Measures to Consider
- Dietary sources of iron replacement
  o Organ meats & meats
  o Eggs
  o Blackstrap molasses
  o Dried fruits (raisins, apricots, prunes)
  o Deep green leafy vegetables
  o Sea vegetables
- Avoid phytoestrogens
- Calcium to prevent osteoporosis
- Homeopathic remedies (see standard indications)
  o Aurum mur.

o   Belladonna
o   Calc. Iod.
o   Tarentula hisp.

Providing Support:

Education and Support Measures to Consider

- Discussion regarding
  o   Anticipated testing
  o   Medications recommended
    - Indications
    - Side effects
    - Anticipated results
  o   Planned follow-up
  o   Warning signs
    - Excessive bleeding
    - Pain
- Provide information & support if surgery indicated
  o   Pre-operative testing
  o   Anticipated hospital stay
  o   Self-care following discharge
- Determine
  o   Concerns
  o   Family/personal support
  o   Coping mechanisms
- Allow grieving
  o   Loss of fertility/body part
  o   Body image changes with surgery
  o   Potential perceived loss of femininity

Follow-up Care:

Follow-up Measures to Consider

- Document
  o   Relevant history & record review
  o   Results of physical exam & testing
  o   Working diagnosis
  o   Client education & discussions
  o   Anticipated plan for care
  o   Consultations &/or referrals
- Return for care
  o   Re-evaluation of uterine size
    - Annual or semi-annual
    - Serial ultrasound sizing
  o   With significant change in bleeding pattern
  o   Progression of symptoms
  o   Pre-op history & physical if hysterectomy planned
  o   Informed consent as indicated for
    - Lupron-Depot
    - Hysterectomy

Collaborative Practice:

Criteria to Consider for Consultation or Referral

- Grossly enlarged uterus
- Client preference
- Progression of symptoms
- Evidence or suspicion of pathologic process
- Surgical and/or anesthesia consultation
- Social service support prn

Gonorrhea

Key Clinical Information

GC is often accompanied by chlamydia or trichomonas, and may infect eyes, mouth and joints as well as the reproductive tract. Significant effects of gonococcal infections include infertility, premature rupture of membranes, preterm labor, and infection of the newborn's eyes resulting in blindness if left untreated. Gonorrhea, like other STIs may increase the transmission risk of those exposed to HIV infection. Additional information may be obtained from the CDC at www.cdc.gov, the treatment guidelines may be downloaded to a Palm devise from the website.[35]

---

[35] CDC (2002) Sexually Transmitted Diseases Treatment Guidelines. Retrieved on-line at www.cdc.gov/std/treatement/TOC2002TG.htm

Client History:

Components of the History to Consider

- Allergies
- Medications
- GYN history
  - Most recent exam
    - Pap
    - STI testing
    - STI treatments
- Sexual history
  - Condom use
    - Male condom
    - Female condom
  - Birth control method
  - Monogamous or multiple partners for self or partner(s)
  - Greater or less than 5 partners
- Onset, duration and severity of symptoms
  - Urinary frequency and dysuria
  - Urethritis
  - Vaginal discharge
  - Pain with intercourse
  - Genital pain and discharge
  - Fever
  - Lower abdominal pain
- Medical/surgical history
- Social history
  - ETOH/Drug use
  - Social support
  - Living situation

Physical Examination:

Components of the Physical Exam to Consider

- Vital signs including temperature
- Pelvic exam
  - Bartholin's, urethra and Skene's for evidence of
    - Discharge
    - Inflammation
  - Vaginal or cervical discharge
    - Yellow or mucopurulent
  - Presence of PID
    - Pain on cervical motion
    - Adnexal or uterine tenderness
    - Lower abdominal pain
    - Plus one or more of the following
      - Temp > 38°C
      - Presence of inflammatory mass on pelvic exam or ultrasound
      - Sed. rate >15mm/hr
      - Mucopurulent cervicitis
      - Positive Gram stain

Clinical Impression:

Differential Diagnoses to Consider

- Chlamydia
- Gonorrhea
- PID
- Cervicitis
- Cervical cancer
- Ectopic pregnancy
- Ovarian cyst
- Ovarian tortion

Diagnostic Testing:

Diagnostic Tests and Procedures to Consider

- Gonorrhea testing with culture or gen-probe
- Chlamydia testing

- Wet mount
- Pelvic ultrasound
- WBC with sedimentation. rate
- HIV counseling and testing
- Gram stain
  - Gram negative intracellular diplococci
  - >10 wbc/hpf

Providing Treatment:

Therapeutic Measures to Consider

- Begin treatment based on symptoms
- One time dosing may be provided on site and administration ensured by direct observation
- Common treatment options for uncomplicated gonorcoccal
  - **Cefixime** 400 mg po (pregnancy category B) as one time dose, **OR**
  - **Ceftriaxone** 125mg IM (pregnancy category B) 1% lidocaine may be used as diluent to reduce pain of injection, **OR**
  - **Ciprofloxin** 500 mg po (pregnancy category C) as one time dose, **OR**
  - **Ofloxacin** 400 mg po (pregnancy category C), *plus* Azithromycin 1 gm po (pregnancy category B), one time dose, **OR**
  - **Levofloxin** 250 mg po one time dose
- **Plus**, if chlamydia has not been ruled out
  - **Azithromycin** 1 g po one time dose
  - **Doxycycline** 100 mg po (pregnancy category D) bid x 7 days
- **Alternate medication**
  - **Spectinomycin** 2 GM IM (pregnancy category B) Used for pregnant women, or those who cannot tolerate cephalosporins or quinolones.
  - **Ceftizoxime** 500 mg IM
  - **Cefoxitin** 2 g IM with probenecid 1 g po
  - **Cefotaxime** 500 mg IM
- **Pharyngeal infection**
  - **Ceftriaxone** 125mg IM (pregnancy category B) 1% lidocaine may be used as diluent to reduce pain of injection, **OR**
  - **Ciprofloxin** 500 mg po (pregnancy category C) as one time dose, **OR**
- **Plus**, if chlamydia has not been ruled out
  - **Azithromycin** 1 g po one time dose
  - **Doxycycline** 100 mg po (pregnancy category D) bid x 7 days

Providing Treatment:

Alternative Measures to Consider

- General supportive measures to promote healing
  - Rest
  - Sitz baths with comfrey leaf tea or Epsom salts
- Herbal support formulas
  - Adjunct to medical therapy
  - Use 2-3 times daily
- Prepare as tea or tincture
  - Red clover – 2 parts
  - Calendula – 2 parts
  - Yarrow – 1 part
  - Dandelion root – 1 part
- Homeopathic remedies
  - Adjunct to medical therapy
  - Use 30x grains three times daily
  - Arnica montana (promotes soft tissue healing)
  - Merc. sol (to offset side effects of antibiotic treatment)

Providing Support:

Education and Support Measures to Consider

- Client notification of results
    - o   Provide education regarding treatment regimen
    - o   Partner notification
    - o   Advise regarding State reporting requirements
    - o   Symptoms of acute PID, when and how to access care
- Client should refer recent partner(s) for evaluation and treatment
- Avoid sexual relations until treatment is completed, and symptoms have resolved
- Educate regarding STD transmission and prevention

Follow-up Care:

Follow-up Measures to Consider

- Document
    - o   Pertinent history
    - o   Physical findings
    - o   Test results
    - o   Treatment plan
    - o   Client education & response
    - o   Indications to return for care
- Return for care with symptoms of acute PID
- Return for test of cure if symptoms persist following treatment
- Offer HIV & other STI counseling & testing
- Return for testing with new partner for self or partner

Collaborative Practice:

Criteria to Consider for Consultation or Referral

- For Rx if not within the scope of the midwife's practice
- For suspected PID
- Any client requiring hospitalization
- For gonococcal infection of the throat, symptoms of meningitis, or disseminated infection
- For support services as indicated

Human Immuno-Deficiency Virus

Key Clinical Information

HIV infection is diagnosed by HIV-1 antibody testing in a two-step procedure. A screening test (EIA) is done, if it is reactive then a confirmatory test is done (either WB or IFA). 15-25% of infants born to untreated HIV infected mothers are infected with HIV, and breastfeeding is not recommended for those infants born to HIV positive mothers. HIV transmission to infants may be reduced to   2% by use of antiretroviral treatment during pregnancy and prophylactic Cesarean birth at 38 weeks gestation.[36] When referring to   a client's "partner" this means any sexual *or* needle-sharing partner.

HIV prevention vaccines (for use in HIV negative clients) and therapeutic HIV vaccines (to improve the immune system of HIV+ individuals) are currently undergoing clinical trials. No vaccines are available at this time.

---

[36] CDC (2002). Sexually Transmitted Diseases Treatment Guidelines. Retrieved on-line at www.cdc.gov/std/treatement/TOC2002TG.htm

Client History:

Components of the History to Consider

- Allergies
- Sexual history
  - Condom use
  - Sexual orientation for self and partner(s)
  - Previous HIV/STI testing
  - Previous diagnosis of STIs or abnormal pap
  - Treatement of previous STI or abnormal pap
- Risk factors for HIV-1 infection:
  - Greater than 5 sexual partners for self or partner(s)
  - Diagnosis or symptoms of any STI
  - IV drug use, self or partner
  - Exposure to blood or body fluids
- Risk factors for HIV-2 infection:
  - People from:
    - West Africa
    - Angola
    - France
    - Mozambique
    - Portugal
    - Clinical evidence of HIV infection with negative HIV-1 test
- Medical/surgical history
  - Chronic diseases or disorders
  - Signs & symptoms of acute retroviral infection
    - Fever
    - Malaise
    - Lymphadenopathy
    - Skin rash
  - Signs & symptoms of HIV infection
    - Fever
    - Weight loss
    - Diarrhea
    - Cough
    - Shortness of breath
    - Oral candidiasis
- Social history
  - Drug/ETOH use
  - Living situation
  - Access to services
  - Support systems

Physical Examination:

Components of the Physical Exam to Consider

- Vital signs, including temp
- Weight
- Evaluation for acute retroviral syndrome
  - Occurs in first weeks after infection prior to + antibody test
  - Immediate initiation of antiretroviral therapy amy delay onset of HIV-related complications
- Lymphadenopathy
- Skin rash
- Gyn exam as indicated by history

Clinical Impression:

Differential Diagnoses to Consider

- HIV infection&/or related illness
- AIDS
- Malignancy
- IV drug abuse/addiction
- TB
- Cervical cancer
- STIs
- Hepatitis

Diagnostic Testing:

Diagnostic Tests and Procedures to Consider

- HIV-1 antibody testing
  - Antibody screen will be positive >2-14 weeks post-infection
  - Perform pre-test counseling to obtain informed consent
    - Routes of transmission
    - Prevention measures
    - Information regarding testing
      - Venipuncture
      - Confidentiality
      - Test interpretation
      - Timing and return visit for results
      - Availability of anonymous testing
  - Collection: venous sample in tiger-top tube
  - Client must return for results and post-test counseling
- Other testing to consider
  - GC & chlamydia
  - Pap smear
  - Wet mount
  - Hepatitis A, B & C serology
  - Syphilis serology
  - Toxoplasma antibody test
  - TB testing
  - CD4+ T-Lymphocyte analysis & determination of viral load
  - Urinalysis
  - Chest X-ray

Providing Treatment:

Therapeutic Measures to Consider

- Antiretroviral therapy following initial evaluation
  - Nucleoside Reverse Transcriptase Inhibitors
  - Nonnucleotide Reverse Transcriptase Inhibitors
  - Protease Inhibitors
- Problem specific treatments as indicated

Providing Treatment:

Alternative Measures to Consider

- General measures to facilitate immune response
- Echinacea and other immuno-stimulants are not recommended for the HIV + individual
- For HIV immune support herbal formulas see The Roots of Healing pp. 254-255
- Creative support measures that encourage personal healing & living with HIV disease should be encouraged
  - Meditation or spiritual practices
  - Art therapy
  - Dance
  - Support groups
  - Religious involvement
  - Community involvement
  - Participation in HIV prevention programs

Providing Support:

Education and Support Measures to Consider

- Provide pre-and post-test counseling
- Obtain informed consent prior to testing
- HIV transmission and prevention teaching
- Partner notification
- Clients with positive HIV testing must receive or be referred for the following services:
  - Behavioral services
    - Risk reduction
    - Prevention management
    - Substance abuse services
    - Reproductive health counseling

o   Psychosocial services
- Mental health
- Crisis counseling
- Housing & financial support services

o   Medical evaluation and treatment
- Detailed medical history
- Physical exam including pelvic
- Comprehensive lab work
- TB testing
- Chest x-ray
- Psychosocial evaluation
- Monitoring of medical status

Client Resources
- CDC Division of HIV/AIDS Prevention: www.cdc.gov/hiv/dhap.htm
- AMA HIV/AIDS Patient Info: www.ama-assn.org
- HIV/AIDS Treatment Information Center www.aidsinfo.nih.gov
- National AIDS Hotline:
  o   English 1-800-342-AIDS
  o   Spanish 1-800-344-7432

Follow-up Care:

Follow-up Measures to Consider
- Document
  o   Pertinent history & behaviors
  o   Findings on physical exam
  o   Tests performed & results

o   Discussion with client
o   Client response
o   Referrals for services
o   Plan for continued care
- For post-test counseling and results
- HIV test negative
  o   Test result interpretation
  o   Assessment of risk behaviors & factors
  o   Review of behaviors to prevent infection
  o   Scheduling of repeat testing if indicated
  o   For treatment of STIs, abnormal pap etc.
- HIV test positive
  o   Test result interpretation
  o   Resources for emotional support
  o   Referral for case management and medical care
  o   Behavior changes to reduce risk of transmission or re-infection (increases viral load)
  o   Measures to decrease incidence of opportunistic infections

Collaborative Practice:

Criteria to Consider for Consultation or Referral
- HIV positive patients to HIV specialist for medical evaluation, treatment plan and coordination of case management
- HIV negative women with positive HIV risk factors offer/refer for psychosocial services

Hepatitis

Key Clinical Information

Hepatitis includes a number of liver diseases that may be broken down based on viral characteristics to Hepatitis A, Hepatitis B, Hepatitis C, Hepatitis D, and Hepatitis E. Hepatitis B & C are the forms of hepatitis that are most frequently seen by the midwife. Hepatitis B is 100 times more infectious that HIV. Risk of developing chronic infection is age related. Up to 90% of infected infants and only 10% of infected adults develop chronic HBV infections[37]. Chronic Hepatitis B infection can result in liver cancer. Find more information at the Hepatitis B Foundation (www.hepb.org).

Client History:

Components of the History to Consider

- Age
- Sexual history
- Risk factors for Hepatitis B
  - o Exposure to blood or body fluids
    - Healthcare workers
    - Household contacts
    - Blood recipients
    - Kidney dialysis
  - o Unprotected sex
    - Correctional facilities
    - Multiple sexual partners
    - STIs
    - Drug users
  - o Shared needles
    - IV drug users
    - Tatoo parlors
  - o Perinatal transmission
  - o Emigration , travel or adoption from endemic areas
- Medical/surgical history
- Social history

Physical Examination:

Components of the Physical Exam to Consider

- Vital signs
- Weight
- Skin color
  - o Evidence of jaundice
- Liver
  - o Margins
  - o Tenderness

Clinical Impression:

Differential Diagnoses to Consider

- Jaundice secondary to
  - o Hepatitis
  - o Biliary disease
- Asymptomatic HBV infection found via
  - o STI testing
  - o Blood donation

Diagnostic Testing:

Diagnostic Tests and Procedures to Consider

- Incubation lasts 1-4 months
- It may take up to 6 months to determine if a client has recovered or remains chronically infected
- HBsAg (hepatitis B surface antigen)
  - o Detected 1-12 weeks post-infection
  - o Positive result indicates infection with HBV
  - o Negative result indicates susceptibility to HBV
- HBsAb or anti-HBs (hepatitis B surface antibody)
  - o Positive result indicates immunity
  - o Negative result indicates infection
- HBcAb or anti-HBc (hepatitis core antibody)
  - o Indicates past or present infection
  - o May be present in those chronically infected
  - o False positive is possible

- With HBsAb indicates recovery
- With HbsAg indicates chronic infection

Providing Treatment:

Therapeutic Measures to Consider

- Hepatitis B vaccines
  - o Recombinant vaccines
  - o Age related doses by manufacturer
  - o Series of immunizations (3 doses)
  - o Given with HBIG immediately post-exposure
- HB immune globulin
  - o Given ASAP post-exposure (up to 7 days)
  - o 1 or 2 doses

Providing Treatment:

Alternative Measures to Consider

- Whole foods diet with minimum of toxins
- Milk thistle tea
- Silymarin 420 mg tid x 6 weeks
- Adequate rest

Providing Support:

Education and Support Measures to Consider

- Provide information about hepatitis
  - o Type
    - Route(s) of transmission
    - Prevention measures
  - o Medications for infant after birth
  - o Breastfeeding
    - Not contraindicated for immunized infant
    - Not recommended for non-immunized infant
- Discussion regarding
  - o Options for treatment & supportive care
  - o Potential effects of illness
  - o Medications
  - o Location of birth
  - o Parameters for referral

Follow-up Care:

Follow-up Measures to Consider

- Document
  - o Relevant history & symptoms
  - o Physical findings
  - o Laboratory results
  - o Discussions with client/family
  - o Client preferences
  - o Midwifery plan of care
- Return for care
  - o Routine prenatal care for carrier
  - o Weekly during acute phase of infection
  - o Periodic LFTs

Collaborative Practice:

Criteria to Consider for Consultation or Referral

- For Hepatitis B vaccine if not within the midwife's scope of practice
- For Rx of medications not within the midwife's scope of practice
- For HBV positive individuals for evaluation & treatment

Human Papilloma Virus

Key Clinical Information

There are more than 20 types of HPV that can affect the genital tract, but only a few that are considered high-risk types. Types 16, 18, 31, 33, and 35 are associated with cervical dysplasia, and may contribute to the development of anal and rectal cancer as well as cervical cancer. Women may be infected with more than one type of HPV. Current screening tests indicate the presence of one or more high-risk types of HPV, and do not indicate they specific types, nor the presence of low-risk types of HPV.

Client History:

Components of the History to Consider

- Age
- Allergies
- Medications
- Reproductive history
  - o LMP, chance of pregnancy
  - o Current method of birth control
  - o Sexual practices
    - ▪ Anal sex
    - ▪ Condom use
    - ▪ Number of sexual partners
  - o Previous
    - ▪ HPV testing
    - ▪ Pap smear results
- Review of systems
  - o Onset, duration and severity of current symptoms
  - o Location of lesions
  - o Other associated symptoms
- Risk factors for HPV infection
  - o Previous or current STIs
  - o Diminished immune response
  - o Unprotected sexual activity
  - o Multiple sexual partners for self or partner(s)
  - o Previous abnormal pap smear
- Social history
  - o Tobacco use (increases risk of progression)
  - o Drug &/or ETOH use

Physical Examination:

Components of the Physical Exam to Consider

- Pelvic exam
  - o Careful evaluation of internal & external genitalia for genital warts or lesions
  - o Consider application of 5% acetic acid (white vinegar) to highlight lesions
  - o Consider colposcopy of cervix and external genitalia
  - o Bimanual exam for presence of palpable abnormality of cervix or vagina

Clinical Impression:

Differential Diagnoses to Consider

- Genital warts
- Microscopic HPV
  - o Cervical
  - o Anal
  - o Vaginal
  - o Vulvar

- Musculosum contagiosum
- Syphylitic condyloma
- Other genital lesions

Diagnostic Testing:

Diagnostic Tests and Procedures to Consider

- Pap smear
  - o Slide (most cost effective for screening)
  - o Liquid-based cytology (allows for reflex testing for presence of HPV with ASC-US result)
- Other STI testing as indicated
  - o HPV testing
  - o HIV counseling and testing
  - o GC/CT
  - o RPR
- HCG as indicated, before treatment
- Stool for occult blood for women having anal intercourse

Providing Treatment:

Therapeutic Measures to Consider

- For Client applied therapy
  - o Imiquimod Cream 5% applied q hs 3-x week until clear.
    - ▪ Wash off after 6-10 hours
    - ▪ More info: 1-800-428-6397 or www.3M.com/ALDARA
  - o Podofilox 0.5% sol. or gel applied bid x 3 days, rest x 4 days, repeat up to 4 cycles
- Provider applied therapy
  - o Podophyllin resin apply weekly to lesions, wash off in 6-8 hours
  - o Trichloacetic acid apply weekly to lesions
  - o Bichloracetic acid apply weekly to lesions

Providing Treatment:

Alternative Measures to Consider

- Echinacea tea or tincture daily to boost immune response
- Rub broken end of fresh green bean over wart
- See The Roots of Healing for additional herbal formulas
- Visualization of area healed & whole
- Attention to nutrition; whole foods diet

Providing Support:

Education and Support Measures to Consider

- Male and female condoms provide limited protection
  - o Uncovered areas not protected
- Wart virus in not curable, but may become dormant
  - o Regression most likely in adolescents
- May spread virus with no visible warts

- Oral, pharyngeal, or anal warts may occur with exposure to these areas
- Review treatment plan and necessary instructions
  o Medication/remedy use
  o Anticipated response to treatment
  o Signs or symptoms indicating need to return for care
- Stress need for annual pap smears
  o Increased risk of abnormal pap
  o Smoking increases risk of progression
  o Immune response affects regression or progression
- Suggest partner be evaluated and treated if visible lesions present
- For more info contact the American Social Health Association : www.ashastd.org

Follow-up Care:

Follow-up Measures to Consider

- Document
  o Relevant history
  o Appearance, number & location of lesions
  o Pap smear & HPV results
  o Treatment plan

  o Referrals
- Return for care
  o As necessary for treatment chosen
  o Annually for pap smear
- Encourage smoking cessation

Collaborative Practice:

Criteria to Consider for Consultation or Referral

- When treatment option is outside the midwife's scope of practice
  o Prescription medication
  o Cryotherapy
  o Laser
  o Interferon injection of lesions
- For client with
  o Extensive lesions
  o Vulvar lesions
  o Anal lesions
  o Vaginal lesions
- For smoking cessation
- Social services

Herpes Simplex Virus

Key Clinical Information

Herpes virus is a common virus that may be sexually transmitted, and may cause significant discomfort to those with active lesions. The goal of therapy is to encourage the virus to become dormant, and to support the immune system so that it stays dormant and the client remains asymptomatic. Unfortunately, it is possible to spread the infection without a noticeable lesion. Infants who are exposed to HSV may acquire systemic infection resulting in serious illness or death. For this reason, Cesarean birth may be offered to pregnant womem with a history of recurrent HSV outbreaks during pregnancy.

Client History:

Components of the History to Consider

- Allergies
- Medications
- Duration and quality of present symptoms
  o Presence of vesicular lesions
  o Pain, tingling, dysuria
- Partner with oral or genital HSV
- Reproductive history
  o LMP, chance of pregnancy
  o Current method of birth control
  o Sexual practices
    ▪ Anal/oral sex
    ▪ Consistency of condom use
    ▪ Number of sexual partners
  o Previous
    ▪ HSV testing
    ▪ Pap smear results
  o History of genital or oral herpes
- Review of systems
  o Primary infection associated with
    ▪ Fever
    ▪ Headache
    ▪ Malaise

    ▪ Local lesions at site of infection
    ▪ Meningitis

Physical Examination:

Components of the Physical Exam to Consider

- Pelvic exam
  o Palpate inguinal lymph nodes
  o Examine external genitalia, buttocks and pelvic region for characteristic lesions
    ▪ Vesicles
    ▪ Shallow ulcers
- Examine for presence of other STI symptoms
  o Cervical discharge
  o Cervical or uterine motion tenderness

Clinical Impression:

Differential Diagnoses to Consider

- Primary herpes infection
  o Local
  o Systemic
- Recurrent herpes outbreak
- Non HSV lesions
  o Trauma
  o Chancre
- Bacterial meningitis

Diagnostic Testing:

Diagnostic Tests and Procedures to Consider

- Culture lesions for
    - o HSV
- Consider serum testing for HSV antibody titer
    - o Documents primary infection
    - o Important in early pregnancy
    - o Repeat 7-10 days
    - o Four-fold increase documents primary infection
- Additional STI testing as indicated

Providing Treatment:

Therapeutic Measures to Consider

- Valtrex (valacyclovir hydrochloride)
    - o Pregnancy category B
    - o Pregnancy registry 1-800-722-9292 ext. 39437
    - o Dose: 500 mg bid x 5 d begin medication within 24 hours of first symptom
- Famvir (famciclovir)
    - o Pregnancy category B
    - o Dose: 125 mg bid x 5 d begin medication within 6 hours of first symptom
- Zovirax (Acyclovir)
    - o Pregnancy category C
    - o Pregnancy registry 1- 800-722-9292 ext. 58465
    - o Dosages
        - ▪ Topical ointment 5% apply 3 x day x 7d
        - ▪ Initial outbreak: 200 mg po 5 x day x 10 days
        - ▪ Recurrent outbreak: 200 mg po 5 x day x 7 days
        - ▪ Suppression, severe recurrent outbreaks 400 mg po bid x 12 mo.
- Acetominophen or ibuprofen for pain relief

Providing Treatment:

Alternative Measures to Consider

- Lysine 1000 mg po bid x 3 months or with first sign of an outbreak
- Echinacea po tea, tincture, tablets or capsules tid x 2 weeks
- Sitz bath or salve made with:

- o Lemon balm
- o Calendula
- o Comfrey

Providing Support:

Education and Support Measures to Consider

- Avoid foods high in arginine: chocolate, cola, peanuts, cashews, pecans, almonds, sunflower and sesame seeds, peas, corn, coconut and gelatin.
- Include foods high in lysine: brewer's yeast, potatoes, fish
- Rest and comfort measures especially with initial outbreak as client may feel quite ill
- Discuss and provide written information about herpes its management and effects on sexuality, childbearing, self-image
- Review symptoms of meningitis signs and symptoms indicating the need to return for care

Follow-up Care:

Follow-up Measures to Consider

- Document
    - o History of outbreak
    - o Appearance, number & location of lesions
    - o Recommendations for care
    - o Client instructions
        - ▪ Medication use
        - ▪ When to return for care
    - o Referrals, prn
- For re-evaluation if symptoms persist > 10 days
- For worsening symptoms i.e. stiff neck, unremitting fever, inability to urinate

Collaborative Practice:

Criteria to Consider for Consultation or Referral

- For Rx medications if not within the midwife scope of practice
- For symptoms of herpes meningitis or systemic infection
- For care during pregnancy, labor and/or birth for women with active herpes

Monilia

Key Clinical Information

Monilia is so common that many women assume that every form of vaginitis is a 'yeast infection'. Monilial vulvovaginitis has many different appearances, from a curdy white vaginal discharge to the excoriated skin creases of the diabetic woman. Careful attention to the wet mount is necessary to determine the presence of yeast, and the absence of additional causes of vaginitis.

Client History:

Components of the History to Consider

- Age
- Allergies
- Medications
    - o Antibiotic use
    - o Steroid use
- Reproductive health history
    - o G, P, LMP
    - o Current method of birth control

- o Douching
- o Sexual practices
    - ▪ Anal/vaginal intercourse
    - ▪ Sex toys
- Symptoms
    - o Onset, location, duration
    - o Description
        - ▪ Intense itching
        - ▪ Curdy discharge
        - ▪ Moist, raw skin
- Other associated symptoms

- o   Burning with urination
- o   Pain
- Medical history
  - o   Diabetes or gestational diabetes
  - o   HIV status
  - o   Cancer
  - o   Immunocompromised condition
- Social history
  - o   Use of tight or damp clothing
  - o   Change in sexual partners/habits

Physical Examination:

Components of the Physical Exam to Consider

- Pelvic exam
  - o   Presence of red, excoriated external genitalia
  - o   White, adherent, curdy discharge within vagina
  - o   Collect wet mount specimen
- May also be present
  - o   On skin folds
  - o   As cutaneous infection
  - o   As oral infection
- Observe for signs or symptoms of STIs

Clinical Impression:

Differential Diagnoses to Consider

- Monilial vulvovaginitis
- Bacterial vaginitis
- Chlamydia
- Gonorrhea
- Chronic cervicitis
- Foreign body
- Medical conditions
  - o   Diabetes mellitus
  - o   HIV
  - o   Secondary to antibiotic use

Diagnostic Testing:

Diagnostic Tests and Procedures to Consider

- Wet mount for
  - o   Budding yeast
  - o   Mycelia
  - o   Branching hyphae
- Vaginal Ph testing
- Severe or recurrent infection
  - o   Fasting blood sugar
  - o   HIV testing
- Other STI testing if indicated by history

Providing Treatment:

Therapeutic Measures to Consider

- Diflucan 150 mg po x 1 or 2 doses

- Terazol (Terconazole) 3 or 7 day therapy
- Monistat Derm for cutaneous symptoms
- Over the counter antifungals:
  - o   Mystatin (Mycostatin)
  - o   Miconazole (Monistat)
  - o   Clotrimazole (Gyne-Lotrimin, Mycelex)
  - o   Butoconozole (Femstat)

Providing Treatment:

Alternative Measures to Consider

- Acidophilus capsules 1 per vagina qhs x 5-7 days
- Boric acid capsules 1 per vagina qhs x 5-7 days (CAUTION: *Poisonous if taken orally*!)
- Herbal douche 2 x week (use acidophilus capsules other nights)
  - o   1 Tbs ti tree oil
  - o   2 Tbs. cider vinegar
  - o   2 cups warm water

Providing Support:

Education and Support Measures to Consider

- Dry genital region thoroughly before dressing (use blow-drier on 'warm' setting)
- Wear cotton panties, loose clothing (boxer shorts are good)
- Wear no panties to allow maximum ventilation
- Avoid excessive sugar or alcohol in diet
- Tub bath with 1 cup vinegar in water
- Avoid intercourse while using medication

Follow-up Care:

Follow-up Measures to Consider

- Document
  - o   Relevant history
  - o   Physical & wet mount findings
  - o   Recommended treatment plan
  - o   Client education
- Return for care
  - o   If symptoms not improved within 5 days
    - ▪   For additional testing
    - ▪   Consider vaginal culture
  - o   As indicated by other test results

Collaborative Practice:

Criteria to Consider for Consultation or Referral

- For Rx of medication if not within the midwife's scope of practice
- For yeast infection that is recurrent or unresponsive to therapy
- For fasting glucose over 126 gm/dl (diagnostic of diabetes)
- For positive HIV titer

Nipple Discharge

Key Clinical Information

Nipple discharge in the absence of lactation must be evaluated. It may represent a physiologic variation from normal or the presenting symptom of a pathologic process. In evaluating galactorrhea of > 6-12 months duration the possibility of a pituitary tumor must be considered. Fortunately, many tumors are exceedingly slow-growing, and not malignant.

Client History:
Components of the History to Consider
- G, P, LMP
- Current method of birth control
- Medication intake, esp. phenothiazine derivatives
- Onset & duration of symptoms
  - Nature of discharge, bloody, greenish or milky
  - Associated symptoms, pain, tenderness, masses, etc.
  - Recent breast changes
  - Presence of menstrual dysfunction
- Breast history
  - Lactation, duration & most recent dates
  - Mastitis
  - Fibrocystic breast disorder
  - Breast abscess
  - Breast cancer
  - Breast surgery
- Review medical/surgical history
- Family history of
  - Breast disease
  - Endocrine disorder

Physical Examination:
Components of the Physical Exam to Consider
- Full breast examination looking for:
  - Breast asymmetry or retraction
  - Masses
  - Presence of spontaneous nipple discharge
  - Crusting of discharge on nipple
  - Skin changes; thickening, coarseness, edema, scaling, redness
- Palpate axillary lymph nodes
- Observe for hirsutism
- Thyroid palpation

Clinical Impression:
Differential Diagnoses to Consider
- Galactorrhea post breastfeeding
- Galactorrhea secondary to pregnancy
- Mastitis or breast infection
- Breast malignancy
- Pituitary adenoma

Diagnostic Testing:
Diagnostic Tests and Procedures to Consider
- Consider differential diagnoses
- Purulent discharge: infection
  - History of current or recent lactation
  - Presence of fever, pain, redness of breast
  - Culture of discharge
  - Ultrasound for fluctuant mass

- Bloody discharge: breast cancer
  - Mammogram
  - Referral for biopsy
- Milky discharge: pregnancy or galactorrhea of unknown etiology
  - Pregnancy testing
  - Endocrine evaluation
    - Thyroid testing, TSH
    - Prolactin (normal < 100ng/ml)
    - Coned-down view of sella turcica
    - MRI for abnormalities of prolactin or sella turcica

Providing Treatment:
Therapeutic Measures to Consider
- Treatment is based on final diagnosis
  - Breast infection: see Mastitis
  - Breast cancer: refer for evaluation and treatment
  - Endocrine disorders, per dx

Providing Treatment:
Alternative Measures to Consider
- Provide emotional support
- Comfort measures
  - Castor oil packs to breast
  - Bach flower remedies to balance emotional state
- Alternative treatments based on diagnosis

Providing Support:
Education and Support Measures to Consider
- Provide information related to
  - Diagnosis; evaluation, treatment, prognosis
  - Community support groups or organizations
  - Need for follow-up and with whom

Follow-up Care:
Follow-up Measures to Consider
- Document
  - Relevant history & review of systems
  - Findings on physical exam
  - Results of diagnostic testing
  - Discussions with client
  - Consultation regarding client care
  - Plan for ongoing care related to problem
- Return for care
  - By diagnosis: for follow-up &/or care of problem
  - Pregnancy: options counseling as indicated
  - Galactorrhea, simple: follow with periodic prolactin levels to confirm stability
  - Galactorrhea, pathologic: following referral for further evaluation, and medical or surgical treatment
  - For routine well woman/gyn care

Collaborative Practice:

Criteria to Consider for Consultation or Referral

- For diagnostic testing if not within the scope of the midwife's practice

- For abnormal breast findings that are not physiologic or simple infection
- For endocrine evaluation

Pediculosis & Scabies

Key Clinical Information

Lice and scabies can be a particularly challenging problem in midwifery practice. An infestation of lice can be hard to eradicate, and since they are mobile, may affect the office environment & housekeeping practices after a client has been diagnosed.

Client History:

Components of the History to Consider

- Allergies
- Medications
- LMP
- Current method of birth control
- Symptoms
  - Onset, duration, location
  - Itching
  - Presence of nits
  - Presence of skin tracks
- Exposure to lice, nits, or scabies
  - Household contacts
  - Intimate contacts
  - Public contacts
  - International travel

Physical Examination:

Components of the Physical Exam to Consider

- Presence of
  - Lice (1 mm crab-like organism)
  - Nits (small white orb attached to hair shaft)
  - Skin tracks from scabies burrows
  - Secondary signs due to itching
- Physical signs of STIs
- Lymph nodes for enlargement

Clinical Impression:

Differential Diagnoses to Consider

- Pediculosis
- Scabies
- Impetigo
- Other parasitic infestation

Diagnostic Testing:

Diagnostic Tests and Procedures to Consider

- As indicated by history and/or physical findings
  - Microscopic examination of parasites
  - Wet mount
  - STI testing
  - Culture of skin lesions
  - Evaluation of type of parasite

Providing Treatment:

Therapeutic Measures to Consider

- Pyrethrins

  - Pregnancy risk factor C
  - Preferred over lindane as it is not systemically absorbed
- Lindane 1% lotion, cream or shampoo
  - Pregnancy risk factor B
  - Use no more than twice during pregnancy due to toxic characteristics

Providing Treatment:

Alternative Measures to Consider

- Lice
  - Shave affected area
  - Vinegar rinse of affected areas bid, blot dry
- Prepare wash of Painted Daisy
  - Source of pyrethrins
  - Use wash to affected area tid

Providing Support:

Education and Support Measures to Consider

- Provide written medication instructions
- Recommend treatment for all contacts
- Avoid sexual contact until treatment complete
- Review transmission mechanisms
- Cleanse bedding and clothing
  - Hot water wash with bleach
  - Hot dryer
- Vacuum living quarters
- Wash throw rugs

Follow-up Care:

Follow-up Measures to Consider

- Document
  - Presenting symptoms
  - Physical findings & confirmatory testing
  - Recommended treatment
  - Client education
  - Anticipated return for care
- Return for care
  - 1 week if symptoms not eliminated
  - PRN for reinfestation

Collaborative Practice:

Criteria to Consider for Consultation or Referral

- For Rx medication if not within the scope of the midwife's practice
- For identification of unusual parasites

Pelvic Pain, Acute

Key Clinical Information

Pelvic pain may have many potential causes, both GYN and non-GYN related. Acute pelvic pain requires prompt diagnosis in order to institute corrective action. The ability to differential between acute & non-acute pain is one that the midwife must acquire so that appropriate emergency care can be obtained in a timely manner.

Client History:
Components of the History to Consider
- Age
- Medications
- Allergies
- Location, onset, duration, severity of symptoms
- Associated symptoms
  - Fever & chills
  - Nausea and vomiting
  - Diarrhea
  - Constipation or obstipation
  - Vaginal discharge
    - Bleeding
    - Mucopurulent
- Reproductive history
  - LMP, G, P
  - Last exam, pap & STI testing
  - Previous diagnosis of
    - STIs
    - Endometriosis
    - Ectopic pregnancy
  - Change in sexual partner for self or partner
  - Current method of birth control, i.e. IUD
- Review of systems, focus on
  - Genitourinary
  - Gastro-intestinal
- Medical/surgical history
- Social history
  - Physical or sexual violence
  - Drug/ETOH use
  - Living situation
  - Mental health status

Physical Examination:
Components of the Physical Exam to Consider
- Vital signs
- Abdominal palpation with focus on
  - Distention
  - Rebound tenderness
  - Guarding
  - Presence or absence of bowel sounds
- Pelvic exam with focus on
  - Presence of cervical discharge
  - Cervical motion tenderness
  - Uterine enlargement or tenderness
  - Palpation of adnexal mass

Clinical Impression:
Differential Diagnoses to Consider
- Lower abdominal trauma
- Reproductive system
  - Muco-purulent cervicitis

  - Ectopic pregnancy
  - PID
  - Spontaneous abortion or miscarriage
  - Ovarian cyst
  - Torsion of ovary
  - Endometriosis
  - Degenerating fibroids
  - Septic abortion
- Urinary system
  - Renal calculi
  - Acute cystitis
- Gastro intestinal system
  - Acute appendicitis
  - Diverticulitis
  - Ulcerative colitis
  - Incarcerated inguinal hernia
  - Bowel obstruction

Diagnostic Testing:
Diagnostic Tests and Procedures to Consider
- Urinalysis
- Serum or urine HCG
- STI testing
- Gram stain of cervical discharge
  - Presence of gram negative intracellular diplococci
  - >10 WBC/hpf
- Pelvic ultrasound
- CBC with differential
- ESR

Providing Treatment:
Therapeutic Measures to Consider
- Treatment varies with diagnosis (see PID)
- Medical care is indicated for acute abdominal or pelvic pain
- Acetaminophen or ibuprofen for fever or pain
  - Take medication with sips of water
  - Avoid eating or drinking until definitive diagnosis

Providing Treatment:
Alternative Measures to Consider
- Rest
- Reassurance & support
- Symptomatic treatment as applicable while test results pending
  - Local heat
  - Positioning

Providing Support:
Education and Support Measures to Consider
- Provide information regarding
  - Working diagnosis
  - Evaluation plan
  - Consultation and/or referral

Follow-up Care:

Follow-up Measures to Consider

- Document
  - o Relevant history & ROS
  - o Physical findings
  - o Diagnostic testing ordered
  - o Initial assessment & working diagnosis
  - o Immediate plan while awaiting results
  - o Discussions with client
    - ▪ Working diagnosis
    - ▪ Tentative plan
    - ▪ Alternate plans
    - ▪ How to access care if condition worsens
  - o Potential follow-up plans
    - ▪ After results
    - ▪ If client worsens
    - ▪ If client improves
- Return for care
  - o 24-48 hours if non-acute status is determined

  - o ASAP for worsening symptoms

Collaborative Practice:

Criteria to Consider for Consultation or Referral

- For discussion regarding
  - o Differential diagnosis
  - o Evaluation plan
  - o Treatment options
  - o Clients requiring hospitalization
- Refer for medical evaluation for
  - o Temp 102° F with rebound tenderness or guarding
  - o Suspected
    - ▪ Pelvic abscess
    - ▪ Ectopic pregnancy
    - ▪ Other surgical emergency
  - o Uncertain diagnosis
  - o Clients with no improvement in 24-48 hours with treatment

Pelvic Pain, Chronic

Key Clinical Information

Chronic pelvic pain is a common finding in women's health and may be related to reproductive functioning, the bladder or bowels, or residual effects from a previous infection of the genital tract. Low-grade pelvic pain is not uncommon in women who have been subject to sexual assault or molestation. Client support during investigation of this problem is essential. Validation of the client's discomfort and concerns are needed as much as a skilled history, review of systems, and thorough physical examination.

Client History:

Components of the History to Consider

- Age
- Medications
- Allergies
- Location, onset, duration, severity of symptoms
- Character of symptoms
  - o Precipitating factors
  - o Relation to menses
  - o Affect on bowel & bladder function
  - o Affect on sexual functioning
- Relief measures used and client response
- Associated symptoms
  - o Fever & chills
  - o Nausea and vomiting
  - o Vaginal discharge
- Reproductive history
  - o LMP, G, P
  - o Last exam, pap & STI testing
  - o Previous diagnosis of
    - ▪ STIs
    - ▪ Endometriosis
    - ▪ Ectopic pregnancy
  - o Change in sexual partner for self or partner
  - o Current method of birth control, i.e. IUD
- Review of systems, focus on
  - o Genitourinary
  - o Gastro-intestinal

- Medical/surgical history
- Social history
  - o Physical or sexual violence
  - o Drug/ETOH use
  - o Living situation
  - o Mental health status

Physical Examination:

- Components of the Physical Exam to Consider
- Vital signs
- Complete physical with focus on
  - o Abdominal exam
    - ▪ Palpate for masses and/or pain
    - ▪ Note guarding or rebound tenderness
    - ▪ Ascultate bowel sounds
- Pelvic exam
  - o Vaginal discharge
  - o Bleeding
  - o Cervical discharge or lesions
  - o Pain on cervical motion, uterine or adnexal palpation
  - o Uterine contour & position
  - o Adnexal massess
- Rectal exam

Clinical Impression:

Differential Diagnoses to Consider

- Physiologic
  - o Mid-cycle pain
  - o Pelvic relaxation
- Infection

- o   Chlamydia
- o   Gonorrhea
- o   Low-grade PID
- o   Urinary tract infection
- GYN pathology
  - o   Endometriosis
  - o   Uterine fibroids
  - o   Chronic pelvic pain post-PID
  - o   Ovarian mass or cancer
- Pelvic pathology
  - o   Peritoneal adhesions
  - o   Hernia
  - o   Gastro-intestinal cause
- Psychogenic cause

Diagnostic Testing:

Diagnostic Tests and Procedures to Consider

- Urinalysis
- Stool for occult blood
- Pregnancy testing
- Pap smear
- STI testing
- CBC, with differential
- Pelvic ultrasound

Providing Treatment:

- Therapeutic Measures to Consider
- Treatment is based on diagnosis
- Anti-inflammatory medications
  - o   Ibuprofen 600 mg tid x 5-7 days
  - o   Naproxen sodium 500 mg bid x 7-10 days

Providing Treatment:

Alternative Measures to Consider

- Encourage client participation in evaluation process
- Provide reassurance, comfort, active listening
- Provide coping skills for living with chronic pain
- Dietary support
  - o   Eat a well balanced diet
  - o   Encourage whole foods diet

- o   Decrease fatty foods, caffeine & alcohol
- o   Drink plenty of fluids
- Provide information about community resources
  - o   Acupuncture
  - o   Expressive therapy
  - o   Support groups
- Local symptomatic relief measures
  - o   Heat
  - o   Positioning
  - o   Physical activity

Providing Support:

Education and Support Measures to Consider

- Discuss differential diagnosis, evaluation and treatment plan
- Encourage client to keep symptom and menstrual record
- Review danger signs, i.e. fever, acute pain, syncope

Follow-up Care:

Follow-up Measures to Consider

- Document
  - o   Primary complaint with relevant history
  - o   Findings on exam & testing
  - o   Discussions with client
  - o   Working diagnosis
  - o   Initial plan for continued care/treatment
  - o   Alternate plans
  - o   Consultations & referrals
- Return for continued care
  - o   At frequent intervals until pathology ruled in/out
  - o   Consider laparoscopic evaluation for diagnosis, prn
  - o   Periodically for support if no pathology found

Collaborative Practice:

Criteria to Consider for Consultation or Referral

- For testing not within the scope of the midwife's practice
- For evaluation of suspected endometriosis
- For pain of suspected or documented pathologic origin
- For persistent low-grade pelvic pain unresponsive to therapy
- For pain with apparent psychogenic basis for mental health therapy

Pelvic Inflammatory Disease

Key Clinical Information

Pelvic inflammatory disease (PID) may have many causes and my mimic many other disorders. It is commonly associated with both chlamydia & gonorrhea, however, it may occur in women who are not sexually active simply by ascension of bacteria through the genital tract. It is essential that the sexual partner(s) of women with suspected PID are treated before resumption of sexual activity. PID may cause significant scarring in the fallopian tubes as well as in the pelvis. This may contribute to chronic pelvic pain and other related disorders.

Client History:

Components of the History to Consider

- Allergies
- Medications
- Location, onset, duration, severity of symptoms
- Associated symptoms

- o   Vaginal discharge, or odor
- o   Fever
- o   Nausea and vomiting
- o   Diarrhea
- o   Malaise
- Reproductive history
  - o   LMP, G, P

- o   Last pap & STI testing
- o   Sexual activity
- o   Previous diagnosis of STIs
- o   Change in sexual partner for self or partner
- o   Current method of birth control, i.e. IUD
- o   Recent surgery, delivery or termination of pregnancy
- Medical/surgical history

Physical Examination:

Components of the Physical Exam to Consider

- Vital signs
- Abdominal palpation with focus on
  - o   Distention
  - o   Rebound tenderness
  - o   Guarding
  - o   Presence or absence of bowel sounds
- Pelvic exam with focus on
  - o   Presence of muco-purulent cervical discharge
  - o   Collection of cervical cultures
  - o   Cervical motion tenderness
  - o   Uterine enlargement or tenderness
  - o   Palpation of adnexal mass

Clinical Impression:

Differential Diagnoses to Consider

- PID
- Ectopic pregnancy
- Ovarian cyst
- Septic abortion
- Endometriosis
- Degenerating fibroids
- Acute cystitis
- Acute appendicitis
- Diverticulitis
- Ulcerative colitis

Diagnostic Testing:

Diagnostic Tests and Procedures to Consider

- Urinalysis
- Serum or urine HCG
- STI testing
- Gram stain & culture of cervical discharge
  - o   Presence of gram negative intracellular diplococci
  - o   >10 WBC/hpf
- Pelvic ultrasound
- CBC with differential
- ESR

Providing Treatment:

Therapeutic Measures to Consider

- Choice and location of treatment varies with
  - o   Severity of illness
  - o   Anticipated client compliance
- Home-based treatment
  - o   Cefoxitin 2 gm IM, *plus* probenicid 1G po, *or*
  - o   Ceftriaxone 250mg IM, *plus* doxycycline 100 mg po bid x 14 days

- o   Ofloxacin 400 mg po bid x 14 days, *plus either*
- o   Clindamycin 450 mg po qid x 14 days, *or*
- o   Metronidazole 500 mg po bid x 14 days
- Hospital-based treatment
  - o   Cefoxitin 2 gm IV q 6 hr, *or*
  - o   Cefotetan 2 gm IV q 12 hours *plus* doxycycline 100 mg po or IV q 12 hr
  - o   Clindamycin 900 mg IV q 8 hr, *plus* gentamycin loading dose(2mg/kg) IV or IM, followed by 1.5 mg/kg IV or IM q 8 hours

Providing Treatment:

Alternative Measures to Consider

- Alternative therapies are not a substitute for prompt medical care
- Herbal and homeopathic remedies for healing, stress and treatment of symptoms
  - o   Echinacea
  - o   Rescue Remedy
- Visualization

Providing Support:

Education and Support Measures to Consider

- Provide information related to
  - o   Diagnosis
  - o   Treatment plan
  - o   Transmission of infection
  - o   Mandatory STI reporting
  - o   Prevention of recurrence
  - o   Need to evaluate and/or treat partner(s)
- Provide written information about
  - o   Medication instructions
  - o   Warning signs
  - o   When to return for care

Follow-up Care:

Follow-up Measures to Consider

- Document
  - o   Presenting problem & relevant history
  - o   Findings on physical exam & testing
  - o   Working diagnosis
  - o   Initial plan for continued care
  - o   Discussions with client about care
  - o   Consultations or referrals
- Return for continued care
  - o   Within 24-48 hours for home-based therapy
  - o   With test results
  - o   For test of cure following treatment
- Consider HIV testing if not done with initial work-up

Collaborative Practice:

Criteria to Consider for Consultation or Referral

- For Rx medications when not within the midwife's scope of practice
- Acutely ill women requiring hospitalization
- Pregnant women with PID
- Clients who do not improve within 24-48 hours of treatment

Premenstrual Syndrome

Key Clinical Information

Premenstrual syndrome or PMS is a common cyclical hormonal disorder that may manifest with physical ir emotional signs & symptoms. Women who suffer from PMS frequently feel that they are not in control of their moods or actions. Treatment is aimed at finding relief measures that are acceptable to the individual woman, and support her in the context of her life. Attention to lifestyle, diet, home life and other life choices is an integral part of the assessment & treatment for PMS.

Client History:

Components of the History to Consider

- Age
- Reproductive history
  - LMP, G, P
  - Age at menarche, years of menstruation
  - Age with onset of symptoms
  - Methods of birth control use
  - Current stage of reproductive life
  - Review of last exam, pap etc.
- Symptom profile
  - Onset duration and severity of symptoms
  - Potential for harm to self or others
  - Symptoms of depression or other mental health conditions
  - Relief measures used and rate of success
- Medications
- Medical/Surgical history
  - Allergies
  - Endocrine disorders
  - Heart disease, hypertension
  - Other medical conditions
- Social history
  - Drug/ETOH, tobacco use
  - Usual physical activity
  - Diet review
  - Social & family support
  - Stressors
- Review of systems

Physical Examination:

Components of the Physical Exam to Consider

- Age appropriate physical exam
  - If none within previous 6-12 months
  - With new onset of symptoms
  - To update pertinent systems
- Thyroid palpation
- Pelvic exam
  - Visualization of
    - External genitalia
    - Vagina
    - Cervix
  - Palpation of
    - Uterus
    - Adnexa
  - Rectal exam

Clinical Impression:

Differential Diagnoses to Consider

- Premenstrual syndrome
- Peri-menopausal changes
- Mood disorder
- Endocrine disorder

Diagnostic Testing:

Diagnostic Tests and Procedures to Consider

- Testing is based on age & findings on H&P
- Thyroid panel
- TSH
- LH/FSH
- Renal function testing
- Hepatic function testing

Providing Treatment:

Therapeutic Measures to Consider

- Combination hormone replacement therapy
  - Hormonal contraceptives
  - Estrogen/progesterone replacement
- Anti-depressants
  - SSRIs
    - Prozac
      - 20 mg daily
      - Pregnancy category C
    - Zoloft
      - 50 mg daily
      - Pregnancy category C
    - Wellbutrin
      - 100 mg bid
      - Increase to 100 mg tid
      - Pregnancy category B
- Calcium supplementation
  - 400 mg qid

Providing Treatment:

Alternative Measures to Consider

- Herbal balancing formula: (for additional formulas see *The Roots of Healing* pp. 124-134)
  - Mix equal parts
    - Chamomile
    - Red raspberry leaf
    - Chasteberries (Vitex)
    - Prepare as tea or tincture
    - Use daily
- Diuretic formula for premenstrual phase of cycle:
  - Dandelion leaf or root – 2 parts
  - Stinging nettle – 2 parts
  - Peppermint – 1 part
  - Black cohosh – 1 part
  - Mix and prepare as tincture (preferable) or tea.
  - Use 10 gtts tincture tid, or tea morning and night
- Premenstrual depression
  - St. John's wort
  - Use with caution if using hormonal birth control, may alter effectiveness
- Homeopathic remedies
  - Use 30x tabs. qid for acute symptoms, or 100x pellets daily as constitutional remedy

- o   Calcarea phos. – general sense of weakness and fatigue accompanied by breast tenderness, genital sweating and itching.
- o   Pulsatilla – for tears and anxiety, nausea, tension. Menses are unpredictable
- o   Sepia – symptoms of exhaustion, irritability, low back pain, deceased sex drive, anger and intolerance

Providing Support:

Education and Support Measures to Consider

- Reinforce need for:
  - o   Excellent and balanced nutrition
  - o   Regular exercise
  - o   Personal time
- Discuss potential lifestyle changes
  - o   Reduce stress
  - o   Foster self-image and autonomy
  - o   Encourage family & friends to help a
    - ▪   Allow for personal time
    - ▪   Shared responsibility
- Review menstrual cycle & function
- Explore fertility/sexuality issues
- Provide information of support groups/community resources
  - o   Music or art therapy

- o   Dance
- o   Women's groups

Follow-up Care:

Follow-up Measures to Consider

- Document
  - o   Symptoms & relevant history
  - o   Physical findings
  - o   Testing & results
  - o   Discussions with client
  - o   Initial plan for continued care
  - o   Alternate plans
  - o   Indications for referral
  - o   Consultations or referrals
- Return for continued care
  - o   For persistent or worsening symptoms
  - o   For medication follow-up
  - o   For routine well-woman care

Collaborative Practice:

Criteria to Consider for Consultation or Referral

- For underlying medical or gynecological problem
- For mental health issues greater than PMS
- To support groups

Syphilis

Key Clinical Information

Syphilis is a complex disorder with the following possible stages: *primary infection* (ulcer or chancre at infection site); *secondary infection* (rash, mucocutaneous lesions, and lymphadenopathy); *latent stage*, and *tertiary infection* (cardiac, neurologic, ophthalmic, auditory, or gummatous lesions). Early latent syphilis is when the illness has been acquired within one year, while late latent syphilis is when the disease was acquired more than one year previously, yet still is in the latent stage. Treatment is most successful when the disease is caught early. Perinatal transmission commonly results in development of congenital syphilis in the newborn.

Client History:

Components of the History to Consider

- Age
- Reproductive history
- LMP. G, P
- Perinatal losses
- Last exam, pap & STI screen
- Previous diagnosis or treatment of STIs
- Sexual activity
- Current method of birth control if not pregnant
- Duration, onset and severity of symptoms
- Medical/Surgical history
  - o   Allergies
  - o   Medications
  - o   Chronic or acute health conditions
  - o   HIV status, if known
- Latent phase
  - o   No clinical manifestation
  - o   Testing is essential

- Review of systems for S/S of infection
  - o   Symptoms of systemic illness
  - o   Generalized malaise
  - o   Fever
  - o   Skin & soft tissue
    - ▪   Symmetric, macular, papular rash
    - ▪   Alopecia
    - ▪   Condyloma lata
    - ▪   Mucous membrane lesions
    - ▪   Chancre
    - ▪   Granuloma development
  - o   HEENT
    - ▪   Pharyngitis
    - ▪   Hoarseness
  - o   Gastrointestinal
    - ▪   Anorexia
  - o   Neurologic
    - ▪   Headache
    - ▪   Symptoms of CNS involvement
    - ▪   Auditory or visual symptoms
  - o   Cardiopulmonary

- Shortness of breath
- Hypertension

Physical Examination:

Components of the Physical Exam to Consider

- Vital signs, including BP & temperature
- General physical exam
- Observe skin & soft tissue for signs of primary infection
  - Alopecia
  - Generalized adenopathy
  - Rash
- Cardiopulmonary assessment
  - Presence of murmur
  - Lung sounds
- Neurologic assessment
  - Cranial nerve abnormalities
  - Diminished reflexes
  - Change in personality
- Pelvic exam
  - Primary chancre (develops 2-12 weeks post-exposure)
    - Characteristic painless, firm ulcer
  - Other mucous membrane ulcers
  - Codylomata lata
  - Evaluation for signs of other STIs
  - Collection of specimens for testing

Clinical Impression:

Differential Diagnoses to Consider

- Syphilis
  - Primary
  - Secondary
  - Latent, (early or late)
  - Tertiary
- Acute bacterial infection
- Viral infections
  - Mononucleosis
  - Hansen's disease
- HPV related condyloma

Diagnostic Testing:

Diagnostic Tests and Procedures to Consider

- RPR or VDRL titers
  - Positive 1-4 weeks after chancre
  - Positive VDRL or RPR > FTA-ABS or MHA-TP to confirm
  - FTA -ABS = fluorescent treponemal antibody absorbed
  - MHA-TP = microhemagglutination assay for antibody to *T.pallidum*
- Chlamydia and gonorrhea testing
- HCG testing
- Hepatitis screen
- HIV counseling and testing
- High risk population during pregnancy: RPR or VDRL
  - Initial prenatal visit
  - 28 weeks gestation
  - On admission for delivery
- Test for syphilis with presence of any sexually transmitted infection

Providing Treatment:

Therapeutic Measures to Consider

- Parenteral penicillin G is treatment of choice
- Primary, secondary syphilis & early latent syphilis
  - Benzathine penicillin G
    - 2.4 million units IM as one time dose
    - In pregnancy may repeat dose in 7 days
  - PCN allergy:

- Doxycycline 100 mg po bid x 14 days
  - pregnancy category D
- Tetracycline 500 mg po qid x 14 days
  - pregnancy category D
- Late latent syphilis or syphilis of unknown duration
  - Benzathine penicillin G 7.2 million units total dose
    - IM as weekly doses of 2.4 million units
    - 3 week series
  - PCN allergy:
    - Doxycycline 100 mg po bid x 28 days
      - pregnancy category D
    - Tetracycline 500 mg po qid x 28 days
      - pregnancy category D

Providing Treatment:

Alternative Measures to Consider

- ✒ Alternative measures are not a substitute for prompt antibiotic treatment
- General measures to promote healing

Providing Support:

Education and Support Measures to Consider

- Reinforce need for sex partners to be tested
- Partner exposed within 90 days may be infected yet seronegative
- Partner exposed > 90 days should be treated presumptively while awaiting serology
- Time periods before treatment used for identifying at-risk partners
  - 3+ months duration of symptoms for primary syphilis
  - 6+ months duration of symptoms for secondary syphilis
  - 12 months for early latent syphilis
- Provide
  - Prevention education
  - Medication information
  - Information about STI reporting & contact follow-up
  - Written return visit information

Follow-up Care:

Follow-up Measures to Consider

- Document
  - Presenting symptoms & relevant history
  - Physical & test findings
  - Diagnosis
  - Discussion/education with client regarding disease
  - Report as required for STIs
  - Document treatment given
  - Anticipated or recommended return for care
  - Consultations or referrals
- Return for continued care
  - As indicated for pregnancy
  - Re-evaluate and retest at 6 and 12 months
  - Retreat for
    - Persistent symptoms
    - Failure to have 4-fold decline in nontreponemal test titers
  - HIV testing for treatment failures

Collaborative Practice:

Criteria to Consider for Consultation or Referral

- For Rx of medications not within the scope of midwife's practice
- For acute illness with infection
- As needed for contact follow-up
- For tertiary or neurosyphilis
- Pediatric referral for infants born to mothers with syphilis

References

22. ACOG (2002). <u>Compendium of Selected Publications</u>. Washington, DC: ACOG.

23. Barger, M. K. Ed. (1988). <u>Protocols for Gynecologic and Obstetric Health Care.</u> Philadelphia, PA: W. B. Saunders.

24. Barton, S. Ed. (2001). <u>Clinical Evidence</u>. London. BMJ Publishing Group.

25. CDC (2002).Sexually Transmitted Diseases Treatment Guidelines 2002. Retrieved on-line at: www.CDC.gov/std/treatment/ TOC2002TG.htm

26. Emmons, L., Callahan, P., Gorman, P., Snyder, M. (1997) Primary care management of common dermatologic disorders in women. <u>Journal of Nurse-Midwifery, 42,</u> 228-253.

27. Frye, Anne. (1998). <u>Holistic Midwifery</u>. Portland, OR. Labrys Press

28. Foster, S (1996). <u>Herbs for Your Health</u>. Loveland, CO: Interweave Press.

29. Gordon, J. D., Rydfors, J. T., et al. (1995) <u>Obstetrics, Gynecology & Infertility</u> (4th Ed.) Glen Cove, N.Y., Scrub Hill Press.

30. MacLaren, A., Imberg, W., (1998) Current issues in the midwifery management of women living with HIV/AIDS. <u>Journal of Nurse-Midwifery, 43.</u> 502-521.

31. Nyirjesy, I., Billingsley, F. S., Forman, M.R. (1998) Evaluation of Atypical and Low-Grade Cervical Cytology in Private Practice. <u>Obstetrics & Gynecology, 92,</u> 601-607.

32. Scott, J. R., Diasaia, P.J., et al. (1996). <u>Danforth's Handbook of Obstetrics and Gynecology</u>. Philadelphia, PA, Lippincott - Raven.

33. Soule, D. (1996). <u>The Roots of Healing.</u> Secaucus, NJ: Citadel Press.

34. Speroff, L., Glass, R. H., Kase, N. G. (1999) <u>Clinical Gynecologic Endocrinology and Infertility</u> Philadelphia, PA, Williams & Wilkins.

35. Varney, H., (2004). <u>Varney's Midwifery</u> (4th ed.). Boston, MA: Jones and Bartlett.

36. Winegardner, M.F. (1998, February 25). The atypical pap smear: new concerns. <u>The Clinical Advisor.</u> 26-31.

37. Wright, V. C., Lickrish, G.M., Eds. (1989) <u>Basic and Advance Colposcopy:</u> A practical handbook for diagnosis and treatment. Houston, TX: Biomedical Communications, Inc

Chapter

9

Care of Women with Primary Health Care Needs

Many midwives include primary care within the scope of midwifery practice. For those who don't this chapter can help you decide when consultation or referral may be appropriate.

Women utilize health care services more often, in general, than men do. One goal of including primary care within the scope of midwifery practice is to increase the opportunities for midwives to provide education & support for women to make healthy choices. Many women only see their GYN healthcare provider during their reproductive years, and do not have ready access to a primary care physician or nurse-practitioner.

The practice guidelines in this section provide a brief overview of possible primary care health conditions. The midwife is responsible for caring only for those conditions that are within her or his scope of practice, and may opt to expand that scope with education and experience. An experienced colleague with which to consult provides a safe basis for learning and optimal care for the midwifery client.

Care of the Woman with Cardiovascular Problems

Key Clinical Information

Heart disease account for nearly ½ of all deaths in women. Most research about the prevention & treatment of heart disease has been performed using male subjects. Midwives, who are often used to caring for essentially healthy women, must keep in mind the risk factors, signs and symptoms of heart disease, hypertension and stroke.[38] Many women may be unaware that they have a problem until significant symptoms develop. Women with diabetes may additionally develop peripheral vascular problems. Clients should participate in personal review of fixed risk factors and modifiable risk factors, and encouraged to identify lifestyle changes to decrease their risk of coronary artery disease.

---

[38] Madankumar R (2003). An overview of hypertensive disorders in women. *Primary Care Update for OB/GYNs* 10;14-18.

Client History:

Components of the History to Consider

- Age
- Medical/surgical history
  - o Allergies
  - o Medications
  - o Conditions
    - ▪ Diabetes
    - ▪ Hypertension
    - ▪ Dyslipidemia
    - ▪ Depression
- Family history
  - o Coronary artery disease (males <55, females<65)
  - o Stroke
  - o Hypertension
  - o Diabetes
- Social history
  - o Alcohol use
  - o Tobacco use (cigarettes, snuff, chewing tobacco)
  - o Support systems
  - o Stressors
  - o Usual coping methods
  - o Daily physical activity
  - o Usual diet
- Risk factors for heart disease
  - o Tobacco use
  - o Sedentary lifestyle
  - o Poor nutrition
  - o Obesity
  - o Hypertension
  - o High cholesterol/triglycerides
  - o Diabetes
  - o Heredity
  - o Increasing age
- Review of systems
  - o Headache
  - o Chest pain
  - o Palpitations
  - o Shortness of breath with exertion
  - o Syncope
  - o Numbness or weakness
  - o Peripheral and/or dependent edema

Physical Examination:

Components of the Physical Exam to Consider

- BP
  - o Measure supine & standing
  - o Diagnosis of hypertension
    - ▪ 6-9 BP readings over 2-3 visits
    - ▪ Persistent BP of 140/90 on more than one occasion
    - ▪ BP 160-170/105-110 on one occasion
    - ▪ Persistent systolic BP of 140 or above
    - ▪ Persistent diastolic BP of 90 or above
- Pulses
  - o Rate & rhythm
  - o Bruits
  - o Decreased pulsed in carotids or extremities
- Height, weight and body mass index
  - o weight lbs/height in^2 x 705
- Fundoscopic exam
- Chest
  - o Contour
  - o Respiratory rate and effort
  - o Auscultate breath sounds
  - o Use of accessory muscles
- Cardiac evaluation
  - o Auscultation of heart

- o Rate & rhythm
- o Presence or absence of
  - ▪ Murmur
  - ▪ Thrills
- o Palpation of heart
- o Percussion of chest
- Left border cardiac dullness
- General inspection of the client
  - o Obesity – esp. abdominal fat
  - o Signs of prior stroke/CVA
- Skin and soft tissue
  - o Color
    - ▪ Pallor
    - ▪ Cyanosis
    - ▪ Blanching
  - o Edema
- Extremities
  - o Capillary refill
  - o Evaluation for non-healing wounds/ulcers

Clinical Impression:

Differential Diagnoses to Consider

- Hypertension
- Dyslipidemia
- Coronary artery disease
- Valvular heart disease
- Diabetes mellitus
- Chronic obstructive pulmonary disease

Diagnostic Testing:

Diagnostic Tests and Procedures to Consider

- CBC
- Urinalysis for protein, glucose
- Lipid profile
  - o Cholesterol <200 mg/dL
  - o HDL >35 mg/dL, LDL <130 mg/dL
  - o Triglycerides <200 mg/dL
- Chemistry profile
  - o Potassium & sodium
  - o Creatinine (>1.3 mg/dL)
  - o Fasting glucose (<110 mg/dL)
  - o Serum uric acid
- Liver & renal function profiles
- ECG – 12 lead
- Cardiac stress test
- Echocardiogram
- Pulmonary function testing

Providing Treatment:

Therapeutic Measures to Consider

- Initiation of medical therapies by primary care provider or referral specialist as indicated by clients condition & midwife scope of practice/practice setting
- Uncomplicated hypertension
  - o Diuretics
  - o ß-blockers
  - o Avoid oral contraceptives if hypertension is not controlled
- Elevated cholesterol
  - o Statins
  - o Niacin
  - o Bile-acid binding resins
  - o Fibrates

Providing Treatment:

Alternative Measures to Consider

- Alternative measures are not a substitute for medical treatment in a client who does not have a favorable response with lifestyle changes
- General measures to promote healing/well-being
  - o Adequate rest
  - o Nutritional support
    - Well balanced diet
    - Vegetarian or whole foods diet
    - Fish oils
    - Garlic
    - Sea vegetables for minerals
- Herbs
  - o Atherosclerosis
    - Billberry promotes micro-circulation
  - o Hypertension
    - Garlic
    - Hawthorn
    - Reishi
  - o High Cholesterol
    - Garlic
    - Psyllium
- Exercise or physical activity
  - o At least 10 minutes daily
  - o Increase as tolerated to 40+ min/day
- Stress reduction activities
  - o Biofeedback
  - o Relaxation techniques
  - o Meditation or yoga
  - o Support groups
  - o Schedule personal time
- Review personal life goals

Providing Support:

Education and Support Measures to Consider

- Education related to lifestyle changes
  - o Work toward maintaining healthy weight
  - o Physical activity 30-45 min./day
  - o Tobacco cessation
- Dietary changes as needed
  - o Avoid or limit alcoholic beverages to 1/day
  - o Decrease salt intake
  - o Balanced diet
  - o Grains & grain products: 7-8 servings/day
  - o Vegetables: 4-5 servings/day
  - o Fruits: 4-5 servings/day
  - o Low-fat dairy or legume products: 2-3 servings/day
  - o Meat, poultry, fish: 1 serving/day
  - o Reduce salt intake to <2400 mg/day
  - o Decrease saturated fats & cholesterol
  - o Low fat, high fiber diet
  - o High protein, low carbohydrate diet
- Ambulatory BP monitoring
- Information regarding
  - o Personal cardiac risk
  - o Potential cardiac risks of HRT
- Medication information
  - o Correct dosing
  - o Side effects
  - o Anticipated benefits
  - o Need for long term treatment and follow-up
- Referral system
- Signs and symptoms that indicate a need for
  - o Emergency care
  - o Prompt care
  - o Referral
  - o Return to office

Follow-up Care:

Follow-up Measures to Consider

- Document
  - o Primary indication for visit
  - o Signs and symptoms of problem
  - o Current treatments
  - o Physical findings
  - o Test results
  - o Working diagnosis
  - o Referrals or consultations
  - o Treatment
  - o Plan for continued care
- Return for continued care
  - o As indicated by lab results
  - o For support during
    - Smoking cessation (see smoking cessation)
    - Dietary and lifestyle changes
  - o For reproductive health care
  - o Hypertension
    - For BP monitoring
    - Evaluation of lifestyle changes
    - Significant medication side effects
    - Determination of need for referral for care
  - o Dyslipidemias
    - Serial evaluation of lipid profile
    - Evaluation of lifestyle changes
    - Significant medication side effects
    - Determination of need for referral for care

Collaborative Practice:

Criteria to Consider for Consultation or Referral

- Immediate referral for
  - o BP systolic >200 or diastolic >120
  - o Signs or symptoms suspicious for stroke or MI
- For evaluation and/or treatment
  - o Suspected cardiovascular dysfunction
  - o Elevated lipid levels consistent with dyslipidemia
  - o Hypertension
  - o Diabetes
- For conditions not within the midwife's scope of practice
- For Rx if not within the midwife's scope of practice

Care of the Woman with Dermatologic Disorders

Key Clinical Information

Many illnesses and conditions may present with skin changes. Skin lesions may represent a local condition or be a manifestation of a viral infection such as rubella. A good dermatologic text with color photographs can be very handy for the midwife providing primary care.

Client History:
Components of the History to Consider
- Age
- Medical/surgical history
  - o Allergies and sensitivities
  - o Current medications (especially recent onset of use)
  - o Chronic & acute conditions
  - o Previous surgery
  - o Previous skin conditions
- Symptom profile
  - o Potential exposures
    - ▪ Infections
    - ▪ Infestations
    - ▪ Bites/stings
      - • Insects
      - • Snakes
      - • Spiders
      - • Jelly-fish, etc.
    - ▪ Sun exposure
    - ▪ Chemicals/toxins
  - o Onset, duration, severity of symptoms
  - o Distribution an characteristics of skin lesion(s)
  - o Associated factors/additional symptoms
    - ▪ Fever/chills
    - ▪ Nausea/vomiting
    - ▪ Pain
    - ▪ Swelling
    - ▪ Review of systems
  - o Remedies used and their effects
- Acne:
  - o Vulgaris &/or nodulocystic: presents with comedones, inflammatory papules and pustules, erythema and scarring, lesions primarily facial, may spread to back and shoulders
  - o Rosacea: chronic acneform conditions
    - ▪ Stage I: persistent erythema with scattered telangiectases
    - ▪ Stage II: symptoms of stage I with papules, pustules and prominent facial pores
    - ▪ Stage III: persistent deep erythema, dense telangiectases, papules, pustules, and plaque-like edema ⇒ peau d'orange texture.
  - o Ophthalmic rosacea: photophobia, conjunctivitis, iritis, & chronically inflamed eye margins
- Bacterial infections
  - o Cellulitis: acute spreading lesion presenting with red, hot tender skin and subcutaneous tissue, borders are irregular and raised due to edema
  - o Impetigo: acute purulent infection characterized by 1-3 cm denuded weeping area surrounded by honey-

colored crust, erythematous halo suggests strep infection, large confluent lesions may occur
- Dermatitis:
  - o Contact: erythema, may progress to scale and plaque formation or desquamation with moist epidermis and lacy border, associated symptoms include puritis, burning, stinging
  - o Eczema (Atopic dermatitis): intensely itching skin lesions characterized by erythema, papules, scaling, excoriations and crusting, most commonly seen in the crease of elbow & knees, behind the ears, hands and feet
- Infestations
  - o Lyme disease:
    - ▪ Stage I: hallmark symptom is a "bullseye" lesion of 3-15 cm at the site of tick bite, flu-like symptoms and lymphadenopathy may develop
    - ▪ Stage II: severe fatigue, malaise as well as dermatologic, cardiovascular, musculoskeletal and neurologic symptoms may develop
  - o Scabies: lesions appear as gray or skin-colored linear or wavy ridges ending in a minute vesicle or papule, associated with severe itching
  - o Pediculosis
    - ▪ Capitis: puritis of scalp is primary complaint
    - ▪ Pubis: puritis of pubic area is primary complaint
- Viral infections
  - o Rubella: reddish-pink rash beginning on face & spreads to trunk
  - o Herpes
  - o Varicella: vesicular lesions that become ulcerated then crust
  - o Zoster: grouped vesicles with erythematous base that are along nerve path, lesions become pustular then crust
  - o Simplex: blisters and ulcerated sores may occur anywhere on body
- HIV-related skin disorders
  - o Thrush
  - o Hairy leukoplakia
  - o Herpes simplex and zoster
  - o Kaposi sarcoma
- Nongenital warts
  - o Common wart: flat, flesh-colored papule on elbows, knees, finger & palms
  - o Flat wart: smooth, small, grouped lesions on hands, legs, face
  - o Plantar wart: small to large singular or grouped nodules on plantar surfaces of feet
- Mulluscum contagiosum: dome shaped papules with umbilicated centers and central waxy core
- Fungal infections

- o   <u>Tinea pedis:</u> scaling, fissures, and maceration between toes
- o   <u>Tinea manuum:</u> scaling, papules & clustered vesicles, usually on dominant hand
- o   <u>Tinea corporis:</u> sharply circumscribed annular lesions on trunk or extremities
- o   <u>Tinea unguium:</u> brown or yellowish discoloration of nail, spreads under the nail
- o   <u>Tinea versicolor:</u> scaly hypo- or hyper-pigmented areas on trunk, arms & neck
- Psoriasis:
  - o   Plaque type: characterized by deeply erythematous sharply defined oval plaques, may have overlying silvery scale, puritis
  - o   Guttate: 1-2 cm papules, primarily seen on the trunk, puritis
  - o   Erythrodermic: presents with generalized, intense erythema, puritis
  - o   Pustular: sterile pustules 2-3 mm that coalesce then desquamate, puritis
- Skin cancer symptoms
  - o   Sore that won't heal
  - o   Bleeding from lesion
  - o   Warning signs of melanoma
    - ▪   Asymmetry of shape
    - ▪   Border irregularity
    - ▪   Color variation
    - ▪   Diameter larger than 6 mm
- Related family history
  - o   Melanoma
  - o   Psoriasis

Physical Examination:

Components of the Physical Exam to Consider

- General physical exam, with focus on presenting complaint
- Vital signs, including temperature
- Thyroid
- Lymph nodes
- Systemic signs of disease
- Observation and palpation of the lesion(s) for
  - o   Location and distribution of lesion(s)
  - o   Size and number of lesion(s)
  - o   Symmetry of lesion(s)
  - o   Surface contour of lesions
    - ▪   Flat
    - ▪   Raised,
    - ▪   Macular
    - ▪   Papular
    - ▪   Bullous
  - o   Margin characteristics
    - ▪   Geographic, irregular
    - ▪   Clear, smooth, linear
    - ▪   Blended
    - ▪   Raised
    - ▪   Rolled
    - ▪   Varied
  - o   Coloration of lesion(s)
    - ▪   Pigment color(s)
    - ▪   Patchy
    - ▪   Confluent
  - o   Description of lesion(s)
    - ▪   Scaling
    - ▪   Crusting
    - ▪   Ulceration
    - ▪   Erosion
  - o   Presence of exudate

Clinical Impression:

Differential Diagnoses to Consider

- Bacterial or viral infections
- Acne
- Psoriasis
- Infestations
- Exposure to irritants or toxins
- Allergic reaction
- Medication reactions
- Skin cancers
- Skin reactions as a sign of systemic disease

Diagnostic Testing:

Diagnostic Tests and Procedures to Consider

- Wet prep of exudate
- Cultures of lesions
  - o   Fungal – dematophyte test medium
  - o   Bacterial – routine culture, consider Gram stain
  - o   Herpes – viral culture medium
- Skin biopsy
  - o   Punch biopsy
  - o   Excisional biopsy
- Skin scraping
  - o   Suspected scabies
- Serology & titers
  - o   Rubella
  - o   RPR
  - o   HIV
- Testing for systemic disorders
  - o   TSH
  - o   ANA (Lupus)
  - o   Lyme titer

Providing Treatment:

Therapeutic Measures to Consider

- General relief measures
  - o   Acetaminophen
  - o   Ibuprofen
  - o   Benadryl
  - o   Topical aloe vera w/lidocaine
- Acne
  - o   Topical agents
    - ▪   Tretinoin - 0.025 % cream or 0.01% gel, increase strength as tol. and indicated
    - ▪   Benzoyl peroxide - gel or wash 2.5-10%
    - ▪   Clindamycin phosphate - gel, lotion & solution
    - ▪   Erythromycin - gel, ointment or solution
    - ▪   Tetracycline (Topocycline®)
  - o   Oral agents
    - ▪   Tetracycline 250-500 mg bid
- Acne Rosacea
  - o   Erythromycin - ointment or solution, apply bid
  - o   Metronizazole - gel, apply bid
  - o   Ketaconazole 2% - apply 1-2 x daily
  - o   Clindamycin phosphate
    - ▪   Gel, lotion or solution
    - ▪   Apply bid
- Bacterial infections
  - o   Cellulitis: Requires prompt antibiotic therapy
    - ▪   Dicloxacillin 0.5-1 g po q 6 h
    - ▪   Erythromycin 500 mg po q 6 h
  - o   Impetigo: Topical *or* systemic antibiotics
    - ▪   Throrough washing with soap and water or Hibiclens®
    - ▪   Apply topical mupirocin (Bactroban)
    - ▪   Oral therapy
      - •   Dicloxacillin 500 mg po qid

- Ciprofloxin 500 mg po bid
- Sulfa-trimethoprim DS 1 po bid

- Dermatitis:
  o Topical corticosteroid preparations (many other products are available)
  o Highest potency: Betamethasone dipropionate 0.05 % cream, oint. or sol. (Diprolene AF)
  o High potency: Flucinonide 0.05% cream, gel, ointment or solution (Lidex)
  o Med-high potency: Amcinonide 0.1% cream (Cyclocort)
  o Medium potency: Hydrocortisone valerate 0.2% ointment (Wescort)
  o Low potency: Triamcinolone acetonide 0.1% cream or lotion (Aristocort, Kenolog)
  o Mild potency: Desonide 0.05% cream (Tridesilon)
  o Lowest potency: Dexamethasone 0.1% gel (Decadron)
- Infestations
  o Lyme disease
    ▪ Erythromycin 250 mg po qid x 10-21 days
    ▪ Amoxicillin 500 mg po tid x 10-21 days (full 21 days for pregnancy)
    ▪ Doxycycline 100 mg po bid x 10-21 days (not for use in pregnancy)
- Scabies
  o Permethrin 5% (pregnancy category B)
    ▪ Apply to entire body from neck down
    ▪ Wash off in 8-12 hours
    ▪ Reapply in 48 hours x 1 only
  o Launder all bedding and clothing
  o Treat all household and other contacts
- Pediculosis
  o Permethrin 1% rinse (NIX®)
    ▪ Apply x 10 minutes then rinse
    ▪ Remove nits with fine-tooth comb
  o Launder all bedding and clothing
  o Treat all contacts
- Viral infections
  o Herpes
    ▪ Varicella
    ▪ Zoster
    ▪ Simplex
- Nongenital warts – topical salicylic acid plaster, pad, solution
- Mulluscum contagiosum – treat topically with ablative therapy (TCA, BCA) if desired
- Fungal infections
  o Topical agents
    ▪ Allylamine – apply to affected areas 1-2 x daily. Pregnancy category B
    ▪ Ciclopirox olamine – apply to affected areas bid. Pregnancy category B
    ▪ Haloprogin - apply to affected areas bid. Pregnancy category B
    ▪ Imidazole – apply to affected areas 1-2 x daily. Pregnancy category B
    ▪ Tolnaftate – apply bid. No pregnancy studies
    ▪ Undecyclic acid – apply to affected areas after bathing. No pregnancy studies
  o Oral antifungals (not recommended for pregnancy)
    ▪ Griseofulvin – 250-500 mg bid x 2 weeks – 12 mo. based on indication
    ▪ Ketaconazole – 200-400 mg daily for 3-18 mo. based on indication
    ▪ Itraconazole - 200 mg daily for 3 mo., or 200 mg bid x 7 days monthly x 2-4 mo.

Providing Treatment:

Alternative Measures to Consider

- General measures to promote tissue healing and boost immune response
  o Well balanced diet
  o Avoid alcohol, spicy foods, hot drinks
  o Adequate rest
  o Exposure to light and air (unless contraindicated by medication use)
  o Limit occlusive skin coverings
- Symptomatic relief
- Itching
  o Cool colloidal oatmeal baths
  o Herbal wash
    ▪ Chamomile
    ▪ Calendula
    ▪ Aloe
    ▪ Lemon balm
- Fungal infections and pediculosis
  o Allow ventilation of affected area(s)
  o Use vinegar in bath water
  o Launder and air clothing and bedding
  o Tea tree oil applied topically (also for acne)

Providing Support:

Education and Support Measures to Consider

- Provide information regarding
  o Diagnosis
  o Testing
  o Anticipated course
  o Relief measures
  o Skin care
  o Care of contacts, as applicable
  o Prevention methods
  o Hygiene, laundering of bedding etc., as applicable
- Instructions to return for care as indicated by diagnosis, *or*
  o If condition worsens or recurs
  o Warning signs & symptoms
- Discuss treatment plan options
- Medication instructions

Follow-up Care:

Follow-up Measures to Consider

- Document
  o Relevant history and ROS
  o Physical findings
    ▪ Lesion distribution
    ▪ Related manifestations
  o Working diagnosis
  o Recommended treatment
  o Consultation or referral
  o Plan for continued care
- Return for continued care
  o For test of cure as applicable
  o For worsening of symptoms
  o Medication reaction(s)
  o Evaluation for need for consultation or referral

Collaborative Practice:

Criteria to Consider for Consultation or Referral

- Skin lesions accompanied by fever, malaise or other constitutional symptoms
- Suspected or biopsy-proven skin cancer
- Initial diagnosis of HIV infection, or evidence of progressive disease
- Documented or suspected systemic illness, i.e., Lyme disease, Lupus, etc.

- Dermatologist referral for treatment of resistant acne with isotretinoin
- Inexperience with dermatologic conditions
- Fro conditions not within the midwife's scope of practice

- For Rx of medications id not within the midwife's scope of practice

Care of the Woman with Endocrine Disorders

Key Clinical Information

The endocrine system regulates and affects most body systems, and its' disruption may cause a multitude of symptoms that initially may appear unrelated. In any evaluation of health problems consideration should be given to the potential impact of the endocrine system on symptoms development. Women are more likely than men to be affected by endorine disorders. Menstrual dysfunction may be only presenting complaint or there may be dramatic evidence of an endocrine disorder, such as hair loss, development of a noticeably enlarged thyroid, or the pigment changes associated with adrenal insufficiency.

Client History:

Components of the History to Consider

- Age
- Review history
  - Weight changes
  - Previous complaints or problems
  - Nutrition & activity patterns
- Reproductive history
  - LMP, G, P
  - Method of birth control
  - Potential for pregnancy
  - Menstrual history
- Medical/surgical history
  - Allergies
  - Current medications
    - Many drug classes affect thyroid function
  - Chronic conditions
  - Surgeries
- Family history
  - Chronic & acute conditions
  - Endocrine disorders
- Recent symptoms: onset, duration, description
- Review of systems for symptoms of endocrine disorders
  - **Hypothyroid**
    - Lethargy, malaise
    - Cold intolerance
    - Weight gain
    - Menorrhagia, amenorrhea
    - Depression, irritability, apathy
  - **Hyperthyroid**
    - Nervousness
    - Anxiety
    - Heat intolerance
    - Diplopia
    - Shortness of breath
    - Weakness
    - Oligomenorrhea
  - **Hyperparathyroid**
    - Asymptomatic, or
    - General vague symptoms
    - Fatigue
    - Anorexia

- Weakness
- Arthralgia
- Poyuria
- Constipation
- Nausea and vomiting
- Mental disturbance
  - **Hypoparathyroid**
    - Parasthesias of hands, feet and circumoral area
    - Mental & emotional status derangement
    - Lethargy
  - **Hypopituitary**
    - Failure to lactate
    - Symptoms associated with
      - LH & FSH deficiency
      - TSH deficiency
      - ATCH deficiency
  - **Hyperpituitary**
    - Amenorrhea
    - Galactorrhea
    - Infertility, ⇓ libido, vaginal dryness
    - Hirsutism
    - Headache, visual field changes due to tumor impingement
  - **Diabetes mellitus**
    - Polydipsia
    - Polyuria
    - Polyphagia
    - Weight loss
    - Blurred vision
    - Parasthesias
    - Fatigue
  - **Hypofunction of adrenal cortex**
    - Fatigue & weakness
    - Anorexia, nausea & vomiting
    - Cutaneous and mucosal hyperpigmentation
    - Weight loss
    - Hypotension
    - Abdominal pain, constipation & diarrhea
    - Salt craving
    - Syncope
    - Personality changes and irritability
  - **Hyperfunction of adrenal cortex**
    - Thick body, thin extremities, round face

- Cervicodorsal & supraclavicular fat pads
- Thin fragile skin, easy bruising, poor wound healing
- Acne, hirsutism
- Hypertension
- Hyperglycemia

Physical Examination:

Components of the Physical Exam to Consider

- Complete physical exam including vital signs
- Focus on signs of endocrine disorders
  - Hypothyroid
    - Cool, pale, tough, dry skin
    - Hoarse, husky voice
    - Myxedema
    - Bradycardia, cardiomyopathy, pericardial effusion
    - Anemia
    - Cerebellar ataxia
    - Goiter
    - Thinning, brittle hair
  - Hyperthyroid
    - Tremors
    - Weight loss
    - Exophthalmos
    - Sweating
    - Palpitations, tachycardia, atrial fibrillation
    - Warm, moist skin
    - Lid lag
    - Goiter, diffuse or nodular
    - Brisk reflexes
    - Thyroid bruit
  - Hyperparathyroid
    - Weakness
    - Arthralgia
    - Poyuria
    - Renal calculi
  - Hypoparathyroid
    - Increased neuromuscular excitability, muscle cramps, tetany
    - Cataract development
    - Abnormalities of skin hair, teeth and nails
  - Hypopituitary
    - Evaluation of visual fields
    - Neurologic exam
  - Hyperpituitary
    - Observe for symptoms of hypogonadism
  - Diabetes mellitus
    - Obesity, or recent weight loss
    - Signs of fungal vulvovaginitis
    - Fruity odor to breath
  - Hypofunction of adrenal cortex
    - Cutaneous and mucosal hyperpigmentation
    - Weight loss
    - Hypotension
    - Syncope
    - Personality changes and irritability
  - Hyperfunction of adrenal cortex
    - Thick body, thin extremities, round face
    - Cervicodorsal & supraclavicular fat pads
    - Thin fragile skin, easy bruising, poor wound healing
    - Acne, hirsutism
    - Hypertension
    - Hyperglycemia

Clinical Impression:

Differential Diagnoses to Consider

- Menstrual dysfunction

- Unusual body habitus
- Hyperthyroid
- Hypothyroid
- Thyroid tumor
- Pituitary dysfunction
- Hyperfunction of adrenal cortex
- Hypofunction of adrenal cortex
- Pancreatic dysfunction
- Diabetes mellitus
- Polycystic ovary syndrome

Diagnostic Testing:

Diagnostic Tests and Procedures to Consider

- **General evaluation**
  - Urinalysis
  - Chemistry profile
- **Thyroid testing**
  - Hypothyroidism TSH ⇑
  - Hyperthyroid TSH ⇓, T4 ⇑, or T3 ⇑ with normal T4
  - Thyroid antibodies + in patients with autoimmune disorders of thyroid
- **Parathyroid Disorders**
  - Abnormal serum calcium, usually found incidentally on chemistry screening
  - **Hyperparathyroid**
    - Serum calcium ⇑ (> 10.5 mg/dl)
    - Serum phosphate ⇓ (< 2.5 mg/dl)
    - ⇑ Serum parathyroid hormone (PTH) levels confirm diagnosis
  - **Hypoparathyroid**
    - Serum calcium ⇓ (<8.8 mg/dl)
    - Serum phosphate ⇑ (>4.5 mg/dl)
    - Low or absent parathyroid hormone (PTH) levels confirm diagnosis
- **Pituitary**
  - **Hypopituitary**
    - ACTH
    - TSH
    - T4
    - FSH & LH
    - Estradiol
    - Prolactin
    - Electrolytes
    - BUN & creatinine
    - CAT scan or MRI of sella turcica
  - **Hyperpituitary**
    - HCG
    - Serum prolactin levels (>300μg/ml = prolactinoma [non-pregnancy woman])
- **Disorders of glucose metabolism**
  - **Diabetes mellitus**
    - Fasting blood sugar
    - >126 gm/dl diagnostic for DM
    - >110 gm/dl < 126 gm/dl = abnormal glucose metabolism
    - 70-110 gm/dl = normal glucose metabolism
- **Evaluation of adrenal cortex**
  - Consider referral for testing & evaluation

Providing Treatment:

Therapeutic Measures to Consider

- Initiation of medical therapies by diagnosis
- Maintenance by CNM in consultation with PCP

Providing Treatment:

Alternative Measures to Consider

- General measures to promote well-being

- o   Emotional support
- o   Adequate nutrition
  - ▪   Sea vegetables
  - ▪   Trace minerals
  - ▪   Iodine
  - ▪   Blue green algae
- o   Bilberry
  - ▪   Improves microcirculation in diabetes
- o   Adequate rest
- o   Regular physical activity

Providing Support:
Education and Support Measures to Consider
- Provide information regarding diagnosis
- Potential effects on client, family, reproductive capacity
- Testing recommendations
- Medication
  - o   Instructions for use
  - o   Side effects
- Signs & symptoms indicating a need to return for care
- Necessary follow-up
- Provide information on local resources prn
- Listening to & addressing client concerns

Follow-up Care:
Follow-up Measures to Consider
- Document
  - o   Relevant client history & ROS

- o   Physical findings to support diagnosis
- o   Working diagnosis
- o   Testing recommendations
- o   Consultation or referral
- o   Plan for continued care
  - ▪   Individualized plan documented in record
  - ▪   Diagnosis
  - ▪   Recommended frequency of return visits
  - ▪   Follow-up testing - type and frequency
  - ▪   Medications – type, dose, titration parameters
  - ▪   PCP or physician notification parameters
- Return for continued care
  - o   As indicated for support and continuing reproductive health care
  - o   Provide follow-up care of selected problems in medically stable patient
  - o   Work with client's primary care provider to develop management plan & delegate care prn

Collaborative Practice:
Criteria to Consider for Consultation or Referral
- For testing or Rx if not within the scope of midwife's practice
- Clients with confusing presentation
- Clients with endocrine dysfunction for relevant work-up and initiation of treatment
- Ongoing care of endocrine disorders

Care of the Woman with Gastrointestinal Disorders

Key Clinical Information

Problems of the gastrointestinal tract may range from simple nausea to the presence of obstructing colon cancer. Inquiry into usual bowel function is an essential component of the client history. GI symptoms may present as signal of a GI disorder, or as a sign or symptom of an endocrine, reproductive or nervous system disorder. Many women manifest their stress with GI symptoms; nausea, diarrhea, "butterflies in the stomach". Social history may reveal a psychosocial component to the disorder.

Client History:
Components of the History to Consider
- Age
- Reproductive history
  - o   LMP
  - o   Method of birth control
  - o   Last exam, pap & STI testing
- Medical/surgical history
  - o   Allergies
  - o   Current medications
    - ▪   Aspirin use
    - ▪   NSAID use
  - o   Chronic & acute conditions
    - ▪   Diverticulitis
    - ▪   Gall bladder disease
    - ▪   Peptic ulcer disease
  - o   Past surgical history
    - ▪   Cholecystectomy
    - ▪   Oopherectomy
    - ▪   Appendectomy

- Current symptoms
  - o   Description of discomfort
    - ▪   Location
    - ▪   Onset
    - ▪   Duration
    - ▪   Severity
  - o   Associated symptoms
  - o   Exacerbating or alleviating factors
- Review of systems
  - o   GI history
    - ▪   Usual diet
    - ▪   Unusual substances
    - ▪   Eating patterns
    - ▪   Elimination patterns
- Family history
  - o   Ulcers
  - o   Diverticular disease
  - o   Gastro-esophogeal reflux disorder
  - o   Colon cancer
- Social history

- o   Living situation
- o   Stresses
- o   Drug, ETOH, & tobacco use
- o   Nervous habits
- o   Support systems

Physical Examination:

Components of the Physical Exam to Consider

- Vital signs including weight
- General physical exam with focus directed by history
- Observe for evidence of endocrine dysfunction
- Examination of mouth & throat
  - o   Presence & condition of teeth
  - o   Presence & size of tonsils
  - o   Ability to swallow
- Auscultation of heart and lungs
- Abdominal exam
  - o   Inspection for shape, symmetry, pulsations
  - o   Auscultation for bowel sounds, bruits
  - o   Percussion
  - o   Palpation, light & deep
    - ▪   Pain
    - ▪   Rigidity
    - ▪   Guarding
    - ▪   Rebound tenderness
    - ▪   Masses
- Bimanual abdomino-pelvic exam
  - o   Pain
  - o   Masses
- Rectal exam

Clinical Impression:

Differential Diagnoses to Consider

- Lactose intolerance
- Dyspepsia
- Hiatal hernia
- H-Pylori infection
- Gastro-esophogeal reflux disorder
- Gastroenteritis
- Peptic ulcer disease
- Irritable bowel syndrome
- Diverticulitis
- Constipation
- Diarrhea
- Pica
- Hemorrhoids
- Gallbladder disease
- Cholelithiasis
- Pancreatitis
- Hepatitis
- Malignancies
- Abdominal pain, unknown etiology

Diagnostic Testing:

Diagnostic Tests and Procedures to Consider

- CBC with peripheral smear
- ESR (erythrocyte sedimentation rate)
- H-pylori testing
- Urinalysis or urine culture
- Chlamydia &/or gonorrhea cultures
- Wet prep
- HCG
- Stool testing
  - o   Occult blood
  - o   Ova and parasites
  - o   Culture

- Liver function testing
- Hepatitis screen
- Amylase and lipase levels
- CA-125
- Endoscopy
  - o   Upper endoscopy
  - o   Sigmoisoscopy
  - o   Colonoscopy
- Ultrasound
  - o   Pelvic
  - o   Gallbladder & pancreas
- CT of abdomen
- X-ray
  - o   Upper GI series
  - o   Lower GI
  - o   Barium swallow
  - o   Barium enema

Providing Treatment:

Therapeutic Measures to Consider

- Treatment based on differential diagnosis
- Antacids
  - o   5-10 ml/1-4 tablets po 1-3 h ac & hs
- H2 Receptor antagonists
  - o   Cimetadine (Tagamet) – 400 mg bid or 800 mg qhs
  - o   Ranitidine (Zantac) – 150 mg bid or 300 mg qhs
  - o   Famotidine (Pepcid) – 20 mg bid or 40 mg qhs
  - o   Nizatidine (Axid) – 150 mg bid
  - o   Omeprazol (Prilosec) – 20 mg daily
- Antimicrobial treatment for *H. pylori* infection
  - o   *Regimen 1*
    - ▪   Bismuth 2 tabs qid x 2 weeks
    - ▪   Metronidazole 250 mg tid
    - ▪   Tetracycline 500 mg tid
  - o   *Regimen 2*
    - ▪   Bismuth 15 ml qid x 2 weeks
    - ▪   Metronidazole 500 mg tid
    - ▪   Tetracycline 500 mg tid
  - o   *Regimen 3*
    - ▪   Metronidazole 500 mg tid x12 days
    - ▪   Amoxicillin 750 mg tid
  - o   *Regimen 4*
    - ▪   Omeprazole 20 mg bid x 2 weeks
    - ▪   Amoxicillin 500 mg qid
- Healing agents
  - o   Sucralfate (Carafate)
    - ▪   1 g tab ac & hs
    - ▪   1-2 g bid to prevent recurrence
  - o   Misoprostol – 100-200 mcg qid w/ meals & hs (not for use in pregnancy)
- Laxatives
  - o   Bulk forming agents: Metamucil, Fiberall, Perdiem
  - o   Emolients: docusate products
  - o   Saline derivitives: magnesium, sodium, or potassium salts
  - o   Lubricants: mineral and olive oil products
  - o   Hyperosmotics: glycerin suppositories
  - o   Stimulants: aloe, cascara sagrada, danthron, senna
- Antidiarrheal medications
  - o   Opiates: paregoric, codeine
  - o   Absorbents: polycarbophil
  - o   Antiperistaltics: loperamide, diphenoxylate
- Antiemetics
  - o   Antihistamines: promethizine, cyclizine, meclizine
  - o   Phenothiazines: Compazine, sparine, Tigan

Providing Treatment:

Alternative Measures to Consider

- ☛Alternative therapies are not a substitute for prompt medical evaluation with acute symptoms
- Diarrhea
  o Increase fiber to regulate fluid balance in stool
  o Bearberry or uva-ursi (not recommended in pregnancy)
  o Bilberry
- Constipation
  o Increase fiber and fluids
  o Cascara sagrada – 10 gtts fluid extract, stimulates bowel function
  o Psyllium seed – increases bulk to stool
  o Senna – use sparingly, very effective, but may cause cramping
- Reflux
  o Chamomile tea
  o Papaya enzyme tablets - with meals and hs
  o Hazelnuts - with meals and hs
  o Goldenseal - pinch of powdered root or tincture 10 gtts tid
  o Licorice - tincture or standardized products; use for 4-6 weeks max.

Providing Support:

Education and Support Measures to Consider

- Hydration
  o Drink ample fluids
  o Limit caffeine & alcohol intake
- Lactose intolerance
  o Limit all dairy products
  o Check labels for dairy in packaged products
- Fiber intake; high fiber foods
  o Dried beans
  o Whole kernel corn
  o Peas
  o Apples (with peel)
  o Berries
  o Whole grain breads and cereals

- Physical activity
  o 20 minutes daily stimulates bowels
- Provide information related to
  o Testing
  o Working diagnosis
  o Medications & treatments
    ▪ Anticipated results
    ▪ Side effects
  o Plan for follow-up care
  o Signs & symptoms indicating need to return for care
  o Referral criteria and mechanism

Follow-up Care:

Follow-up Measures to Consider

- Document
  o Relevant history & ROS
  o Clinical findings
  o Preliminary diagnosis
  o Treatment recommendations
  o Consultations or referrals
  o Plan for continued care
- Return for continued care
  o 7-14 days
  o As indicated by test results
  o For follow-up of chronic problems
  o For worsening signs or symptoms

Collaborative Practice:

Criteria to Consider for Consultation or Referral

- For evaluation or Rx not within the scope of the midwife's practice
- For confirmed or suspected
  o Acute abdomen
  o Intestinal obstruction
  o Gall bladder disease
  o Ovarian cancer
  o Colorectal malignancy
  o GI bleeding
- For GI problem unresponsive to therapy within 7-21 days

Care of the Woman with Mental Health Disorders

Key Clinical Information

While midwifery assessment of mental health conditions may include diagnosis and treatment of mild self-limiting disorders, it is assumed that all women with ongoing psychiatric problems will be referred to a mental health professional for further evaluation and treatment Active listening is a crucial part of the assessment process, places the midwife in a prime position of evaluate the mental well-being of the women who come to her for care. A strong network of referral options is beneficial in directing women to the type of care that will best meet their needs.

Client History:

Components of the History to Consider

- Chief complaint, in client's own words
  o History of current problem
    ▪ Symptoms
    ▪ Onset

    ▪ Duration
    ▪ Precipitating factors
    ▪ Previous treatment
  o Client's feelings of danger to self or others
  o Suicide attempts or ideation
- Reproductive history
  o LMP, current menstrual status

- o   G, P, children at home
- o   Losses as applicable
- Medical & surgical history
  - o   Allergies
  - o   Current medications
  - o   Medical conditions, i.e.,
    - ▪ Endocrine problems
    - ▪ Arthritis
    - ▪ Chronic fatigue
    - ▪ Multiple sclerosis
    - ▪ Cancer
- Social history
  - o   ⊕Cultural background
    - ▪ Effect on primary complaint
    - ▪ Social stigma related to seeking help
    - ▪ Cultural variations in symptoms presentation
  - o   Family & community support systems
  - o   Alcohol, drug or tobacco abuse
  - o   Emotional or physical abuse
  - o   Employment/financial status
  - o   Life stresses
- Related family history
  - o   Mental illness
  - o   ETOH or drug abuse/addiction
  - o   Medical conditions that may affect emotional well-being
- Review of systems
  - o   Evaluate for physiologic basis of symptoms

Physical Examination:

Components of the Physical Exam to Consider

- Mental status exam, with focus on
  - o   Cooperation, participation, eye contact
  - o   Affect
  - o   Physical manifestations of anxiety; tics, agitation
  - o   Speech patterns
  - o   Thought processes; i.e., organization & content
    - ▪ Description and theme of mood
    - ▪ Effect on daily life
    - ▪ Delusions
    - ▪ Paranoia
  - o   Suicidal ideation; thoughts, plans, intent, means
  - o   General cognitive status; orientation, memory, attention, abstract thinking
- Complete general physical exam, with focus on
  - o   Thyroid
  - o   Cardio-pulmonary status
  - o   Neurologic functioning
  - o   Reproductive (hormonal) systems

Clinical Impression:

Differential Diagnoses to Consider

- Affective disorders
- Eating disorders
- Personality disorders
- Psychosis
- Endocrine dysfunction; i.e. thyroid, diabetes, adrenal
- Hormonal dysfunction; i.e. PMS, peri-menopause, postpartum depression
- Excessive caffeine or stimulant use
- Substance abuse
- Hypoxia due to cardiac, respiratory, or other pathology
- Neurologic disorder; i.e. encephalopathy or seizure disorder

Diagnostic Testing:

Diagnostic Tests and Procedures to Consider

- Evaluate for physical disorder as cause of mental status change based on physical exam

- o   TSH
- o   FSH, LH
- Evaluate for symptoms of mental/emotional disorders based on symptoms & presentation
- **Affective (mood) disorders**
  - o   *Depression*
    - ▪ Depressed mood
    - ▪ Diminished interest in all activities
    - ▪ Weight loss/gain
    - ▪ Insomnia/hypersomnia
    - ▪ Psychomotor agitation/retardation
    - ▪ Fatigue or loss of energy
    - ▪ Feelings of worthlessness or guilt
    - ▪ Inability to concentrate
    - ▪ Recurrent thoughts of death: suicidal ideation, plan or intent
  - o   *Mania*
    - ▪ Decreased need for sleep
    - ▪ Rapid or "pressured" speech
    - ▪ Distractibility
    - ▪ Flight of ideas
    - ▪ Increased goal-directed activity
    - ▪ Inflated self0esteem or grandiosity
    - ▪ Engagement in risk taking behaviors
  - o   *Bipolar disorders*
    - ▪ Symptoms of depression and mania
      - • Symptoms alternate
- **Anxiety disorders**
  - o   *Generalized anxiety disorder*
    - ▪ General anxiety about "everything"
  - o   *Panic disorder*
    - ▪ Subjective symptoms of panic attack
      - • Tightness in the chest or throat
      - • Difficulty breathing without evidence of obstruction
      - • Dry mouth
      - • Trembling
      - • Palpitations
    - ▪ Physical symptoms of panic attack
      - • ⇑ BP, tachycardia, tachypnea
      - • Restlessness, trembling, exaggerated startle response
      - • Pallor, sweating, erythema, cold & clammy hands
      - • Vomiting, loss of bowel or bladder control
  - o   *Phobias*
    - ▪ Irrational fear out of proportion to stimulus
  - o   *Obsessive-compulsive disorder*
    - ▪ Persistent recurrence of
      - • Intrusive thoughts (obsessions)
      - • Ritualized behaviors (compulsions)
  - o   *Post-traumatic stress disorder*
    - ▪ Development of symptoms following a significant traumatic event
    - ▪ Symptoms include
      - • Flashbacks to the event
      - • Emotional numbing to external stimuli
      - • Autonomic, cognitive and dysphoric symptoms
- Eating disorders
  - o   *Bulimia*
    - ▪ Preoccupation with weight and food intake
    - ▪ Feelings of being out-of-control related to food intake

- Binge eating
- Purging
- Fasting
- Over-exercising
- Laxative or diuretic abuse
  o *Anorexia nervosa*
    - Preoccupation with weight and food intake
    - Focus on control of food intake
    - Loss of 15% of body weight
    - Amenorrhea for at least 3 consecutive cycles
    - Denial
    - Self-repulsion
    - Distortion of body image
- **Personality disorders**
  o Person with a set of inflexible & maladaptive character traits
  o Ingrained patterns of perceiving and relating to others & environment
  o Classifications
    - Cluster A: paranoid, schizoid, schizo-typical
    - Cluster B: histrionic, narcissic, antisocial, & borderline
    - Cluster C: avoidant, dependent, obsessive-compulsive, & passive aggressive
- **Psychoses (thought disorders)**
  o Presence of 2 or more of the following within a 1 month period
    - Delusions
    - Auditory hallucinations
    - Disorganized speech
    - Grossly disorganized or catatonic behavior
    - Negative sx, i.e. flat affect or psychomotor retardation

Providing Treatment:
Therapeutic Measures to Consider

- Consider HRT for new onset mild mental health dysfunction in peri-menopausal or menopausal women with no precipitating events (see HRT)
- Commonly prescribed medications by class
- *All have potentially serious side effects, check profile before prescribing and against client symptoms/presentation*
- **Antidepressants**
  o Selective serotonin reuptake inhibitors (SSRI) – may cause ⇓ libido
    - Prozac 10-60 mg/d
    - Paxil 10-30 mg/d
    - Zoloft 25-150 mg/d
  o Tricyclic – long history of use
    - Elavil 50-200 mg/d
    - Tofranil 50-150 mg /d
    - Pamelor 50-150 mg/d
  o Monoamine oxidase inhibitors (MAOI) *not recommended for CNM Rx*
    - Nardil 15-90 mg/d
    - Parnate 10-30 mg/d
  o Other antidepressants
    - Wellbutrin 150-450 mg/day
    - Desyrel 200-400 mg/day
    - Serzone 50-500 mg/d
- **Anxiolytics & Hypnotics**
  o Benzodiazepines
    - Xanax 0.5-6 mg/d, half life 6-20 h
    - Klonapin 0.5-8 mg/d, half life18-50 h
    - Valium 2-60 mg/d, half life 30-100 h
  o Other
    - Buspar 10-40 mg/d
    - Atarax 200-400 mg/d

- Ambien 5-10 mg/d
- **Mood stabilizers**
  o Lithium carbonate 600-1800 mg/d
  o Lithium carbonate slow-release 450-1350 mg/d
  o Lithium citrate 10-30 mL/d
- **Anti-convulsants (used as mood stabilizers)**
  o Tegretol 400-1200 mg/d
  o Depakene/Depakote 500-1250mg/d
- **Neuroleptics (antipsychotics)**
  o Medication use by diagnosis
- *Affective (mood) disorders*
  o Depression
    - Antidepressants for ⇓ mood, sleep dysfunction, obsessive self-flagellation
    - Anxiolytics if anxiety also present
  o Bipolar disorders & mania
    - Mood stabilizers (lithium & anticonvulsants)
- *Anxiety disorders*
  o Anxiolytics for acute and chronic anxiety or panic
  o Antidepressants for panic attacks, phobias, or OCD
- *Post Traumatic Stress Disorder*
  o Antidepressants for depression or obsessive thoughts or behaviors
  o Anxiolytics for panic, general anxiety or mild paranoia
  o Antipsychotics for
    - Agitation
    - Anxiety if anxiolytics have poor response or contraindicated
    - For persistent paranoid thinking
- *Eating disorders*
  o Antidepressants for mood disorder and obsessive thinking
  o Anxiolytics if anxiety present
  o Antipsychotics if thinking is delusional
- *Psychoses (thought disorders)*
  o Neuroleptics (antipsychotics) referral for Rx

Providing Treatment:
Alternative Measures to Consider

- Warm, loving, safe, environment
- Interactive psychotherapy, i.e.
  o Individual or group counseling
  o Art therapy
  o Music therapy
  o Expressive therapy
- Herbal or homeopathic support for *minor* mood disorders
  o Anxiety
    - Hops
    - Kava-kava
    - Passionflower
    - Reishi
    - Valarian
  o Depression
    - Chamomile
    - Lemon balm
    - St. John's Wort
  o Hormonal effects
    - Dong-quai
    - Black cohosh
    - Evening primrose
- Support groups, i.e.,
  o Religious
  o Women's groups
  o Bereavement support
  o Related to other medical diagnosis (i.e., breast cancer support)

Providing Support:

Education and Support Measures to Consider

- Provide information related to community resources
  - o   Health education services
  - o   Support groups
  - o   Crisis hotline number(s)
- Women with abusive partners
  - o   Safety planning
  - o   How to access safe-housing
  - o   Effects of medications on ability to be vigilant
- Women with medical treatment and/or referral
  - o   Medication
    - ▪   Name
    - ▪   Dosing instructions
    - ▪   Indication
    - ▪   Desired effects
    - ▪   Potential side effects
    - ▪   Pregnancy category (prn)
  - o   Referral information and goal of referral
- Midwifery plan for continued care
- Signs and/or symptoms indicating need for
  - o   Return for care
  - o   Immediate care
  - o   Emergency care

Follow-up Care:

Follow-up Measures to Consider

- Document
  - o   Primary reason for visit
  - o   Relevant history & ROS

- o   Clinical findings
- o   Clinical impression
- o   Therapeutic measures
- o   Consultation and/or referral
- o   Midwifery plan for continued care
- Return for care
  - o   Verify client compliance with referral(s)
  - o   Provide support and education related to diagnoses
  - o   Provide treatment
    - ▪   Counseling
    - ▪   Continuing medication use
    - ▪   Need for referral
  - o   Routine women's health care & contraception prn

Collaborative Practice:

Criteria to Consider for Consultation or Referral

- For diagnosis not within the midwife's scope of practice
- For Rx not within the midwife's scope of practice
- Psychiatric emergency
- Suicidal or homicidal ideation
- Psychosis
- Potential life-threatening drug reaction
- Need for hospitalization
- Symptoms that suggest a complex psychiatric disorder
- Concomitant substance abuse
- Persistent psychosocial problems
- Failure to respond to medication or prescribed treatment
- Formal psychotherapy indicated or requested

Caring for the Woman with Musculoskeletal Problems

Key Clinical Information

The midwife may assess for musculoskeletal conditions during a college, sports or school physical, prior to a client beginning a vigorous exercise program, or as the result of new-onset symptoms. The two most frequently diagnosed musculoskeletal problems diagnosed in women are osteoarthirits and back strain.

Client History:

Components of the History to Consider

- Primary indication for visit
- Evaluation of symptoms
  - o   Location
    - ▪   Unilateral vs bilateral
    - ▪   Symmetric
    - ▪   Joint vs muscle
  - o   Onset
    - ▪   Precipitating factors
    - ▪   Mechanism of injury
    - ▪   Gradual vs sudden
    - ▪   Effect of time of day/weather
  - o   Duration
    - ▪   Chronic vs acute
    - ▪   Constant vs intermittent
  - o   Severity of symptoms
    - ▪   Mild ω severe
  - o   Measures used for relief of symptoms and their effects
    - ▪   OTC or Rx meds
    - ▪   Heat/Ice

- ▪   Rest
- ▪   Compression
- Symptoms of possible tumor or infection
  - o   Atypical pain
  - o   Fever
  - o   Chills
  - o   Weight loss
- Medical/surgical history
- Age (consider patient's lifespan stage)
- Allergies
- Current medications
- Last Td immunization
- History of GI upset, or bleeding with prior NSAID use
- Osteoporosis risk ⇑ with
  - o   Early menopause (natural or surgical)
  - o   Hx of anorexia nervosa
  - o   Amenorrhea due to athletic activity
- Family history
  - o   Osteoarthritis
  - o   Osteoporosis
- Social history

- o   Physical activity patterns
- o   Nutritional status
- o   Physical abuse/neglect
- o   Physical exertion/strain related to
  - ▪   Job
  - ▪   Hobby
  - ▪   School
  - ▪   Sports
- o   Drug or ETOH use
- Review of systems

Physical Examination:

Components of the Physical Exam to Consider

- Vital signs, including temperature
- Evaluate for neurovascular status of tissues distal to site of injury
- Evaluate affected area for
  - o   Heat, redness, or swelling
  - o   Range of motion, crepitus, clicks
  - o   Muscle tension or limitation
- Palpation
  - o   Tenderness
  - o   Point tenderness
  - o   Soft tissue spasm
  - o   Mass
- Neurological assessment
  - o   Strength/weakness
  - o   Muscle wasting
  - o   Sensation
- Vascular assessment
  - o   Color
  - o   Pulses
  - o   Capillary refill
- Presence or absence of
  - o   Echymosis
  - o   Hematoma
  - o   Limb or joint deformity

Clinical Impression:

Differential Diagnoses to Consider

- Osteoarthirits
- Back strain
- Physical abuse
- Joint strain or sprain
- Malignancy or tumor
- Infection
- Systemic disorders (i.e., multiple sclerosis)
- Vascular disease
- Peripheral neuropathy and/or radiculopathy
- Fractures

Diagnostic Testing:

Diagnostic Tests and Procedures to Consider

- Bone mineral density testing
- Bony tenderness, with night pain
  - o   X-ray
  - o   MRI
  - o   Bone scan
  - o   Referral for diagnostic evaluation
- Anticipated NSAID administration > 3 months
  - o   Baseline testing
    - ▪   Liver function
    - ▪   Platelets
- Concern re: infection
  - o   CBC w/ diff
  - o   ESR
- Evaluation of mass
  - o   Ultrasound
  - o   X-ray

- o   CT

Providing Treatment:

Therapeutic Measures to Consider

- NSAIDs are frequently the first line of therapy
  - o   Naproxen sodium
  - o   Ibuprofen
- Muscle relaxants
  - o   Equagesic – musculoskeletal pain with anxiety
    - ▪   Dose: 1-2 tablets tid or qid
    - ▪   Short term use only
  - o   Flexeril – muscle spasm
    - ▪   Dose: 10 mg tid; max 60 mg daily
    - ▪   Limit use to 21 days or less
  - o   Robaxin – painful musculoskeletal conditions
    - ▪   Dose: 1.5 mg qid x 2-3 days m
    - ▪   Maintenance: 4 gm daily in divided doses
- Sprain or strain
  - o   Air cast (ankle)
  - o   Compression bandage
  - o   Splinting
- Consider physical therapy
- Consider trial of antidepressants for suspected fibromyalgia (see Care of the Woman with Mental Health Disorders)

Providing Treatment:

Alternative Measures to Consider

- Rest of affected area
- Ice to affected area for first 24 hours followed by heat
- Elevation of affected area when possible
- For soft tissue injury
  - o   Comfrey leaf compresses
  - o   Homeopathic arnica montana
  - o   Massage therapy
  - o   Hydrotherapy
- Arthritis
  - o   Extremely low fat diet (5 gm day) shown to ⇓ pain, swelling, and progression of disease
  - o   Non-weight bearing exercise maintains muscle strength and range of motion
  - o   Condroitin and/or glycosamine

Providing Support:

Education and Support Measures to Consider

- Review mechanism of injury, as indicated
- Teach proper body mechanics
  - o   Wide base of support
  - o   Avoid reaching, twisting, hands over head
- Active and passive range of motion exercises
  - o   Stretching
  - o   Provide exercise information related to diagnosis
  - o   Back stretching/abdominal strengthening
  - o   Non-weight bearing exercise for arthritis, i.e. swimming
- Provide information about medication
  - o   Drug name, dose, frequency of use
  - o   Side effects
- Provide information about additional recommendations
- Stress importance of well balanced diet, limited ETOH
- Chronic pain may result in depression
- Signs & symptoms indicating need to return for care

Follow-up Care:

Follow-up Measures to Consider

- Document
  - o   Primary complaint
  - o   Relevant signs & symptoms
  - o   Physical findings
  - o   Testing, if ordered
  - o   Clinical impression

- o   Treatments
  - ▪   Medications
  - ▪   Recommendations
  - ▪   Referrals
  - o   Plan for continued care
- Return for continued care
  - o   Within 7-14 days
  - o   If problem worsens or persists
  - o   If depression occurs related to chronic pain syndrome(s)
  - o   Prn for medication management

Collaborative Practice:

Criteria to Consider for Consultation or Referral

- For evaluation of problems outside the scope of the midwife's practice
- For Rx of medications not within the scope of the midwife's practice
- For persistent back pain, without evidence of pathology consider referral to:
  - o   Osteopath
  - o   Chiropractor
  - o   Acupuncturist
  - o   Neurologist

- Orthopedic referral, if limited results from treatment, for:
  - o   Bursitis
  - o   Tendonitis
  - o   Carpal tunnel
  - o   Sprain or strain
  - o   Knee effusion
  - o   Epicondylitis
  - o   Herniated disc (consider neurology consult depending on your area)
  - o   Osteoporotic & other fractures
- Podiatric or orthopedic referral
  - o   Bunion
  - o   Plantar Fascitis
  - o   Morton's neuroma
- Rheumatology consult for
  - o   Suspected or diagnosed arthritis
  - o   Suspected fibromyalgia
- Mental health referral for chronic pain syndromes
- Evaluation & treatment of significant problems
  - o   Neurologic origin
  - o   Fracture
  - o   Muscular sclerosis, etc.

Care of the Woman with Respiratory Disorders

Key Clinical Information

Most common primary care presentation of respiratory disorders includes sinusitis, bronchitis, asthma, and chronic cough. Less commonly seen problems such as TB, pneumonia, and respiratory malignancies should be kept in mind. Often the primary presenting complaint in the woman with metastatic cancer to the lungs is cough. Women with HIV/AIDS may present with *pneumocystic carinii*, or drug resistant tuberculosis.

Client History:

Components of the History to Consider

- Primary complaint
- Symptom review
  - o   Onset, duration, severity of symptoms
  - o   Cough
  - o   Sputum production
  - o   Color of sputum/nasal discharge
  - o   Shortness of breath
  - o   Difficulty with respiration; wheezing
  - o   Frontal headache
  - o   Fever &/or chills
  - o   Other symptoms
    - ▪   Weight loss
    - ▪   Night sweats
    - ▪   Malaise
- Relief measures used and their effects
- Medical & surgical history
  - o   Allergies
  - o   Medications
  - o   Medical conditions
    - ▪   Heart disease
    - ▪   Respiratory disease
      - •   Asthma
      - •   COPD
      - •   Emphysema
      - •   Sinus infection(s)
      - •   Pneumonia
    - ▪   Cancer
  - o   Exposure to asthma triggers
    - ▪   Allergens
    - ▪   Irritants
    - ▪   Drugs
  - o   Exercise or cold air
- HIV status, if known
- Social history
  - o   History of IV drug use, alcohol abuse, tobacco use
  - o   Living conditions
  - o   Nutritional status
  - o   Job related exposure to respiratory irritants
- Review of systems

Physical Examination:

Components of the Physical Exam to Consider

- Vital signs including
  - o   Weight
  - o   Temperature
  - o   Pulse & respiratory rate
- Color
  - o   Pallor
  - o   Rubor
  - o   Cyanosis
- Respiratory evaluation

- o Rate and pattern of breathing
- o Depth and symmetry of lung expansion
- o Auscultation
  - Quality and intensity of breath sounds
  - Adventitious breath sounds
- o Pneumonia
  - Crackles
- o Asthma
  - Diffuse wheezes or rhonchi
  - Prolonged expiratory phase
- o Percussion
  - Dull – Consolidation or pleural effusion
  - Resonant – Normal, asthma or interstitial lung disease
  - Hyperresonant – Emphysema or pneumothorax
  - Intercostal or supraclavicular retractions
- Evidence of respiratory distress
  - o Peripheral cyanosis
  - o Elevated pulse & respiratory rate

Clinical Impression:

Differential Diagnoses to Consider

- Asthma
- Bronchitis
- Chronic cough, due to
  - o Smoking
  - o Post nasal drip
  - o Work related exposure to inhaled irritants
- Sinusitis
- HIV/AIDS
- Community acquired pneumonia or bronchitis
- Respiratory malignancies

Diagnostic Testing:

Diagnostic Tests and Procedures to Consider

- Suspected pneumonia
  - o Chest x-ray (order for fever + abnormal breath sounds, and/or + PPD)
  - o Gram stain and culture of purulent sputum
- Asthma
  - o Peak flow or spirometry
- Bronchitis
  - o Testing if pneumonia or asthma suspected at follow-up visit
  - o Afebrile, normal breath sounds, cough > 2 weeks duration ⇒ pertussis serology
- Chronic cough
  - o Sinus x-rays
  - o TB testing
  - o Chest x-ray
- Consider HIV counseling and testing
- Tuberculosis
  - o TB Mantoux
    - 0.1 ml injected intradermally
    - 2 step procedure indicated for select groups
  - o Chest x-ray
  - o PPD Interpretation - *MM of Induration Considered Positive*
    - 5 mm
      - HIV infected patients
      - Close contact of newly diagnosed patient with active TB
      - Scars on x-ray suggest prior healed active TB
    - 10 mm
      - Immigrants from areas with endemic TB prevalence

- Low-income &/or medically underserved
- IV drug users
- Chronic illness or exposure that may increase risk of contracting TB
- Infants and young children
  - 15 mm
    - No known risk factors for TB

Providing Treatment:

Therapeutic Measures to Consider

- Community acquired pneumonia or bronchitis:
  - o Erythromycin 250-500mg qid x 10 days (pregnancy category B)
  - o Azithromycin 500mg on day 1, then 250 mg q day x 4 additional days (pregnancy category B)
  - o Sulfa-trimethoprim 1 DS tablet BID x 10 days (third trimester of pregnancy only)
  - o Amoxicillin – clavulanic acid 250-500 tid x 10 days
  - o Cefuroxime 250-500 mg bid x 10 days
- Asthma
- Use a combination of
  - o Bronchodilators (fast acting for acute attacks)
  - o Anti-inflammatory medications (to decrease airway edema and secretions)
- Bronchodilators
  - o Albuterol
    - Inhaled β-agonist
    - 2 puffs q 4-6 h prn
  - o Ipratropium
    - Anti-cholinergic
    - 3-6 puffs q 6 h
  - o Metaproterenol
    - Inhaled β-agonist
    - 2 puffs q 4-6 h prn
  - o Salmeterol
    - Inhaled long-acting β-agonist
    - 2 puffs q 12 h
  - o Theophylline
    - Methylanthine
    - 600-900 mg/d in 2-3 doses
    - Titrate by serum levels
- Anti-inflammatory medications:
  - o Beclomethosone
    - Inhaled steroid
    - 2-5 puffs qid
  - o Cromolyn sodium
  - o Mast-cell stabilizer
    - 2-4 puffs qid
  - o Flunisolide
    - Inhaled steroid
    - 2-4 puffs bid
- Bronchitis
  - o Cough suppressants
  - o Antibiotics generally not indicated, unless pneumonia is suspected
  - o Albuterol inhaler (afebrile but diffuse abnormal breath sounds)
  - o 2 puffs q 4 h prn
- Pertussis - suspected or confirmed
  - o Erythromycin 1 gm/day in divided doses x 14 days
  - o Sulfa-trimethoprim DS 1 po bid x 14 days
- Chronic cough
  - o Treatment based on definitive diagnosis
- Tuberculosis
  - o See CDC guidelines for treatment of tuberculosis
  - o www.cdc.gov

Providing Treatment:

Alternative Measures to Consider

- General measures to promote healing
- Rest, adequate nutrition
- Increase fluid intake, especially hot liquids
- High-protein, high-calorie diet
- Use positioning to aid drainage of secretions
- Herbal remedies
  - o Marshmallow
  - o Echinacea (not for use in immunocompromised clients)
  - o Licorice (do not use with pregnancy, or in those with hypertension, heart or liver disease)
  - o Astragalus (safe for those with immune disorders)[39]

Providing Support:

Education and Support Measures to Consider

- Provide detailed instruction for medication regimen(s)
  - o Dosage, frequency
  - o Potential side effects
  - o Indications for cough suppressants
- Signs of improvement
  - o Symptoms diminish within 1-3 days
  - o Afebrile within 2-5 days (pneumonia)
- Provide information re: environmental controls
- When/where to return for care
  - o Signs & symptoms indicating need to return for care
  - o Need to go to ED for severe symptoms
  - o Anticipated course & follow-up plan
- Additional recommendations
  - o Rest
  - o Isolation from family, prn

Follow-up Care:

Follow-up Measures to Consider

- Document
  - o Presenting complaint
  - o Relevant history & review of systems
  - o Clinical findings
  - o Working diagnosis
  - o Testing results
  - o Recommendations for care
    - ▪ Medications
    - ▪ Treatments
    - ▪ Referrals
  - o Plan for continued care
- Return for continued care
  - o 7-10 days
  - o Sooner if symptoms persist or worsen in spite of therapy
- Persistent sx at revisit re-evaluate for asthma

Collaborative Practice:

Criteria to Consider for Consultation or Referral

- For evaluation of problems not within the midwife's scope of practice
- Rx for medications not within the midwife's scope of practice
- For clients potentially requiring hospitalization
  - o Respiratory rate ∞30
  - o Superclavicular or intercostal retractions
  - o O2 saturation of < 95%
  - o Cyanosis
  - o WBC > 25,000/mm
  - o Symptoms of respiratory distress
  - o Supportive care indicated
- Suspected
  - o TB: + PPD or Mantoux test
  - o Pertussis
  - o Pneumocystis carinii
  - o Pneumonia
- HIV/AIDS

---

[39] Foster, pp 6-7.

Care of the Woman with Urinary Tract Problems

Key Clinical Information

Urinary tract problems include common urinary tract infections, pylonephritis, incontinence issues, and structural problems such as cystocele. All urinary tract problems create discomfort for the woman, whether it be physical, emotional or social. Many women restrict their activities due to urinary frequency or fear of wetting. Many women do not address the issue of incontinence with their midwife or health care provider out of embarrassment, or a belief that it is a natural consequence of aging that they must live with. Thoughtfully worded questions during the history may encourage discussion of this problem, and exploration of potential solutions.

MEDICATIONS FOR URINARY TRACT INFECTIONS:

Medication	Dose	Side Effects
Amoxicillin/Clavulanate	250/125 mg q 8 hours	Rash, GI upset
Cefaclor	250-500 mg q 8 hours	Caution if PCN allergy
Cephalexin	250 q 6 hours or 500 q 8	Caution if PCN allergy
Ciprofloxin	250-500 mg b.i.d	Dizziness, headache, GI upset
Fosfomycin	Single-dose packet	Diarrhea, headache
Lomeofloxacin	400 mg once daily	Dizziness, headache, GI upset
Nitrofurantoin	50-100 q 6 hours	Nausea, pulmonitis, neuropathy
Ofloxacin	400 mg b.i.d.	Dizziness, headache, GI upset
Sulfa/trimethoprim	800/160 mg b.i.d.	Rash, Stevens-Johnson Syndrome
Trimethoprim	100 mg q 12 hours	GI upset, delayed rash

Client History:

Components of the History to Consider

- Urinary symptom history
  - History of previous urinary tract infections
  - Frequency, volume, and timing of voids
  - Presence of
    - Urgency
    - Pain, flank & or dysuria
    - Fever & chills
  - Changes in lifestyle related to urinary tract
  - Relief measures used and results
  - Genital hygiene habits
  - Onset, duration, type and severity of symptoms
- Common UTI symptoms include
  - Dysuria
  - Frequency and urgency
  - Lower abdominal pain
  - Flank pain
  - Malaise
- Urge incontinence
  - Characterized by involuntary bladder contractions
  - May be neurologic or caused by irritant
- Stress incontinence
  - Occurs when intra-abdominal pressure is greater than urethra's closing pressure
  - May be worsened by
    - Childbearing
    - High impact activities
    - Heredity
    - Atrophy
- Mixed incontinence
  - Stress & urge incontinence
- Overflow incontinence
  - Obstruction
  - Detruser incoordination
  - Urethral tortion
- Iatrogenic incontinence
  - Surgical scarring or trauma
  - Medications
- Reproductive history
  - G, P, LMP
  - Vaginal births
  - STIs
  - Sexual activity
    - Anal/vaginal intercourse
    - Lubrication
    - Sex toys
  - Vasomotor symptoms

- Medical/Surgical history
  - o Allergies
  - o Current medications
  - o Neurologic disorders
  - o Medical conditions i.e. diabetes
  - o Genital or pelvic surgery
- Social history
  - o Caffeine intake
  - o Fluid intake
  - o Bowel status/hygiene habits
- Review of systems

Physical Examination:

Components of the Physical Exam to Consider

- Vital signs, including temperature
- Pelvic exam with focus on
  - o Urethra
  - o Presence of cystocele or rectocele
  - o Signs or symptoms of GYN infections
  - o Signs or symptoms of menopausal genital atrophy
  - o Signs or symptoms of genital trauma
  - o Evaluation of pelvic floor strength & function
- CVA tenderness and other signs of pylonephritis

Clinical Impression:

Differential Diagnoses to Consider

- Urinary tract infection
  - o Cystits
  - o Urethritis
  - o Pylonephritis
- Urinary incontinence
  - o Urge
  - o Stress
  - o Mixed
  - o Overflow
  - o Iatrogenic
- Interstitial cystitis
- STI affecting the urinary tract
  - o Chlamydia/gonorrhea
  - o Herpes

Diagnostic Testing:

Diagnostic Tests and Procedures to Consider

- Urinary tract infections
  - o Urinalysis (dip or microscopic)
  - o Most common pathogens E. Coli, Staph saprophyticus, proteus, enterococcus
  - o Diagnosis considered + if > 100,000 colony count in clean catch specimenUrinalysis (dip or microscopic)
  - o Culture for recurrent or persistent symptoms, and in pregnancy
- Pregnancy testing as indicated
- Urinary calculi
  - o Ultrasound
  - o Strain urine
- Incontinence
  - o Urodynamics
  - o Post void catheterization to determine residual

Providing Treatment:

Therapeutic Measures to Consider

- Urinary tract infection
  - o Pyridium for pain relief 200 mg tid x 2 D
  - o Appropriate antibiotic therapy
- Pylonephritis
  - o IV fluids
  - o Pain relief
  - o Appropriate antibiotic therapy
- Urge incontinence

- o Detrol 2 mg BID
- o Ditropan XL 5 or 10 mg 1 po daily
- Stress Incontinence
  - o Biofeedback: www.neocontrl.com
  - o Hormonal treatment for urogenital atrophy
    - ▪ Estring
    - ▪ Vaginal estrogen cream
    - ▪ See HRT
  - o Medications
    - ▪ Pseudoephedrine HCL
    - ▪ Phenylpropanolamide
  - o Pessary fitting
    - ▪ Ring
    - ▪ Ring with support
    - ▪ Gelhorn
    - ▪ Use vaginal cream with pessary
      - • Trimo-san
      - • Acigel

Providing Treatment:

Alternative Measures to Consider

- Urinary Tract Infection:
  - o Cranberry Tablets
  - o Flush urinary system; drink large amounts of water
  - o Homeopathic remedies:
    - ▪ Aconitum – for early recent infection, with or without flank pain
    - ▪ Cantharis – Searing lancing pain accompanied by urgency and frequency
  - o Herbal tea/tincture made of:
    - ▪ Echinacea root – 3 parts
    - ▪ Corn silk – 1 part
    - ▪ Pippsissewa – 1 part
    - ▪ Cleavers – 2 parts
    - ▪ Usnea lichen tincture – 2 parts
    - ▪ Bearberry (uva ursi) 2 parts (not for use in pregnancy)
    - ▪ Drink ½ cup every hour (20-40 drops of tincture) until symptoms subside, then continue 3-5 x daily for 10 days.

Providing Support:

Education and Support Measures to Consider

- Information regarding treatment options
- UTI
  - o Medication instructions
  - o Avoid caffeine
  - o Drink plenty of water
  - o Void frequently
  - o Void after intercourse
  - o Blot from front to back after voiding
- Urge incontinence
  - o Void
    - ▪ Frequently
    - ▪ With initial urge
  - o Do not limit fluids
  - o Kegel exercises
  - o Medication instructions
- Stress incontinence
  - o Kegel exercises
  - o Biofeedback plan
  - o Pessary use and fitting
- Signs and symptoms requiring return for continued care
  - o Signs of infection/stones
  - o Worsening symptoms
- Option for referral for surgical consultation

Follow-up Care:

Follow-up Measures to Consider

- Document
  - o Reason for visit
  - o Pertinent history & ROS
  - o Clinical findings & tests ordered
  - o Working diagnosis
  - o Treatment recommendations
  - o Consultation or referral
  - o Plan for continued care
- UTI
  - o Re-culture following treatment for
    - ▪ Acute pylonephritis
    - ▪ Recurrent symptoms
    - ▪ Pregnancy
- Urge/stress incontinence
  - o Keep 2-5 day urinary diary
  - o Follow-up for
    - ▪ Biofeedback
    - ▪ Re-evaluation of
      - Pelvic floor strength
      - Response to medications
      - Need for pessary
      - Need for surgical consult
- Pessary use
  - o Check q 3 months
  - o Clean
  - o Evaluate for tissue breakdown

Collaborative Practice:

Criteria to Consider for Consultation or Referral

- For evaluation of problems not within the midwife's scope of practice
- For Rx of medications not within the midwife's scope of practice
- Acute pylonephritis
- UTI during pregnancy
- Urology referral
  - o Unresolved, recurrent or persistent infection
  - o Persistent renal calculi
  - o Suspected obstruction
- OB/GYN referral
  - o Evaluation of persistent urinary incontinence
  - o Pelvic prolapse
  - o Pessary fitting
  - o Surgical repair

References

1. Alliance for Aging Research. (1997). <u>Controlling High Blood Pressure in Older Women:</u> Clinical Reference Manual. National Heart, Lung and Blood Institute. Alliance for Aging Research.

2. American Heart Association. (1998) Cardiovascular disease in women: A scientific statement from the AHA. <u>Clinician Reviews.</u> Vol. 8 No. 4, 145-160.

3. Benetti, M. C., Marchese, T. (1996). Primary care for women; Management of common musculoskeletal disorders. <u>Journal of Nurse-Midwifery, 41,</u> 173-187.

4. Bromberg, W. D., (1998, August 25). Urinary tract infections: The basics. <u>The Clinical Advisor.</u> 60-64.

5. Brucker, M. C., Faucher, M. A. (1997) Pharmacologic management of common gastrointestinal health problems in women. . <u>Journal of Nurse-Midwifery, 43,</u> 145-162.

6. Clark, C., Paine, L.L. (1996). Psychopharmacologic management of women with common mental health problems. <u>Journal of Nurse-Midwifery 42,</u> 254-274.

7. Czarapata, B. J. (1999). Managing urinary incontinence. <u>Patient Care for the Nurse Practitioner.</u> April 1999. 37-48.

8. Davis, L., Stecy, P., (1997). Pharmacologic management of cardiovascular problems in women. <u>Journal of Nurse-Midwifery, 42,</u> 176-185.

9. Drazen, J.M., Weinberger, S. E. (1998) Disorders of the respiratory system. In Fauci, A. S., Braunwald, E., et al (Eds.) <u>Harrison's Principles of internal medicine</u> (pp. 1407-1410). NY, NY: McGraw-Hill.

10. Emmons, L., Callahan, P., Gorman, P., Snyder, M. (1997) Primary care management of common dermatologic disorders in women. <u>Journal of Nurse-Midwifery, 42,</u> 228-253.

11. Fauci, A. S., Braunwald, E., et al. (Eds.) (1998) <u>Harrison's Principles of Internal Medicine</u> (14th Ed.) New York, NY: McGraw Hill.

12. Foster, S. (1996). <u>Herbs for Your Health.</u> Loveland, CO: Interweave Press.

13. Harris, G.D., (1999). Managing hypertension in female patients. <u>Women's Health in Primary Care.</u> 2 (5). 395-417.

14. Madankumar R (2003). An overview of hypertensive disorders in women. *Primary Care Update for OB/GYNs* 10;1:14-18.

15. MacLaren, A., Imberg, W., (1998) Current issues in the midwifery management of women living with HIV/AIDS. <u>Journal of Nurse-Midwifery, 43.</u> 502-521.

16. Mays, M., Leiner, S. (1997). Pharmacologic management of common lower respiratory tract disorders in women. The Journal of Nurse-Midwifery 42, 163-175.

17. Mays, M., Leiner, S. (1996). Primary care for women: Management of common respiratory problems. The Journal of Nurse-Midwifery 441, 139-154

18. Moser M., (1996). Clinical Management of Hypertension. Caddo, OK. Professional Communications, Inc.

19. National Cholesterol Education Program. (1993). Second report on the detection, evaluation and treatment of high blood cholesterol in adults. National Institutes of Health.

20. Payton, R.G., Gardner, R., Reynolds, D. (1997) Pharmacologic considerations and management of common endocrine disorders in women. Journal of Nurse-Midwifery 42, 186-206.

21. Rovner, E.S., Weine, A.J. (2000) Overactive bladder and urge incontinence: Establishing the diagnosis. Women's Health in Primary Care. 3 (2), 117-126.

22. Schmitt, M., (1999). Skills Workshop: Evaluating the shoulder. Patient Care for the Nurse-Practitioner, March 1999, 42-50.

23. Shaw, B. (1996). Primary Care for women; Management and treatment of gastrointestinal disorders. The Journal of Nurse-Midwifery, 41, 155-172.

24. Siris, E. S., Schussheim, D. H. (1998). Osteoporosis: Assessing your patient's risk. Women's Health in Primary Care. 1(1), 99-106

25. Smith, T., (1984). A Woman's Guide to Homeopathic Medicine. New York, NY, Thorsons Publishers Inc.

26. Soule, D. (1996). The Roots of Healing. Secaucus, NJ: Citadel Press.

27. Speroff, L., Glass, R. H., Kase, N. G. (1994) Clinical Gynecologic Endocrinology and Infertility (5th Ed.) Philadelphia, PA, Williams & Wilkins.

28. Swartz, M. H. (1994) Textbook of Physical Diagnosis: History and examination. (2nd Ed.) Philadelphia, PA, W. B. Saunders Co

29. Weintraub, T. A., Paine, L.L., Weintraub, D. H. (1996) Primary care for women: Comprehensive assessment and management of common mental health problems. The Journal of Nurse-Midwifery, 41, 125-138.

Index